# MANAGEMENT IN NURSING

## MARJORIE CUTHBERT
Division of Nursing
Lincoln School of Health Sciences
La Trobe University

## CHRISTINE DUFFIELD
Faculty of Nursing
University of Technology, Sydney

## JOANNE HOPE
Division of Nursing
Lincoln School of Health Sciences
La Trobe University

W. B. Saunders

Baillière Tindall

**Harcourt Brace Jovanovich, Publishers**
Sydney    Philadelphia    London    Toronto

W. B. Saunders/Baillière Tindall

An imprint of
Harcourt Brace Jovanovich Group (Australia) Pty Limited
30-52 Smidmore Street, Marrickville, NSW 2204

Harcourt Brace Jovanovich Limited
24/28 Oval Road, London NW1 7DX

Harcourt Brace Jovanovich, Inc.
Orlando, Florida 32887

*National Library of Australia Cataloguing-in-Publication Data*

Management in Nursing.

ISBN 0 7295 0380 8.

1. Nursing services – Australia – Administration – Case studies. 2.
Nurse administrators – Australia – Case studies. 1. Cuthbert, Marjorie.
I. (Marjorie Isobel). II. Duffield, Christine Margaret. III. Hope, Joanne.

362 173068

Printed in Australia

# CONTENTS

# PART 2: PROCESSES: THE FUNCTIONS OF MANAGEMENT

## 2.2 THE NURSE AS A RESOURCE MANAGER  171
*Mary Courtney and Kristina Malko*

## 2.3 OUTLINE OF EVALUATION SYSTEMS FOR NURSE MANAGERS  209
*Robert Martin and Marjorie Cuthbert*

# PREFACE

This book grew out of the dissatisfaction by the editors in their work as lecturers that there was no nursing management text written specifically for Australian health care services. The gestation period was lengthy because we are all involved in the changes in the education system as nurse training makes the change from hospitals to colleges and now to universities, and from diplomas to degrees in 1992.

We had a number of discussions about the content of the book and out of these discussions arose the format of structure, process and outcome based on the Donabedian model for evaluation first proposed in 1966. We decided that nurses and their unit managers need an understanding of the environmental factors and structures which affect the process of providing quality health care. We also decided to include as many strategies and tools as possible that could help make their very complex and often difficult job somewhat easier.

Because of the structure of the book it may seem at times that there is some repetition of subject matter in each of the sections. At first this caused us some concern. However we wanted each chapter to stand alone and as each author is writing from the different perspectives presented by each section we decided to accept this repetition.

We have written with concern for students and their lecturers and included objectives, summaries and case studies. Lecturers may choose to set an assignment based on the whole case study or to use only a part of one. It is up to you. A number of the case studies have been written in gender free language and reflect the multitude of cultures which make up our health care workforce. This was done for the express purpose of breaking down some of the stereotypes that currently exist — that the chief executive officer is necessarily male while the director of nursing is necessarily female; that doctors are males and nurses female; that professional staff are white Anglo-Saxons while cleaning and catering staff are of migrant stock.

This book necessarily reflects the biases of the authors and to a large extent their needs as teachers of nursing management. In the first unit we attempt to give the reader a thorough understanding of the principles underlying the practice of nursing management within the Australian health care system. This however should not preclude the book from being useful to students of nursing management in other countries. The concepts of nurse management, organisational structures and constraints, nurse staffing, patient assignment patterns, and legal obligations and limitations are all discussed in this unit.

In the second unit we look at the process of nurse management including communication patterns, resource management, management and research and evaluation systems. Finally we look at ways of assessing outcomes and include some tools developed in Australian hospitals which can be of assistance.

If you find this book useful we would like to hear about it and so would our publishers. We would also like to hear about it if you don't and would appreciate comments, and constructive suggestions for improvement because if there is a demand we will do it again with a bigger, brighter edition.

# PART ONE

# Structures: Foundations of Management

# The concept of management

CHRISTINE DUFFIELD AND JANICE LEWIS

On completion of this chapter the reader should be able to:

1. identify the change forces impinging on the role and functions of the first-line nurse manager;

2. differentiate between management, administration, supervision and leadership;

3. identify management tasks;

4. provide an overview of management and organisation theories;

5. describe the planning process;

6. describe a change model and its application to nursing management.

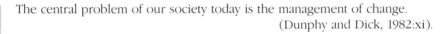

> The central problem of our society today is the management of change.
>
> (Dunphy and Dick, 1982:xi).

Perhaps nowhere is this statement more accurate than throughout the health care system in Australia. Change, mostly unplanned, is emerging as a central feature. The purpose of this chapter is to provide a context for the study of management and its associated principles. The major changes which surround and potentially impinge upon the role and functions of the first-line nurse manager will be outlined, followed by a brief overview of the Australian health care system. The discussion of these two aspects will provide a contextual background for the study of management throughout this book. The three sections which follow define management, the development of management and organisation theories, and the planning process for first-line managers. The last portion of the chapter covers change theory which will assist first-line managers to assess ways of effecting change in light of the challenges they face.

## 1. AN AUSTRALIAN CONTEXT

There are a variety of organisational and professional changes over which first-line nurse managers have little direct control. However, these may affect the interpretation of their role, the functions they perform or the ways in which they must manage. It is important that first-line nurse managers be aware of these change influences, if only to understand the boundaries within which they must function. Any change can modify established behaviour patterns, thereby altering the interpretation of roles.

Decentralisation has occurred throughout most health care agencies as well as within nursing services, thus devolving responsibility and authority to the level at which knowledge is held. This move has resulted in changes in the role and the concomitant skills required of first-line nurse managers. In the United States the skills required of this level of nurse manager now include hiring, firing and promoting staff; the determination of salary and staffing levels and staffing standards; and accountability for budget deficits and excesses (Hodges, 1987). Traditionally these skills have not been included in undergraduate courses overseas, and as a result most first-line nurse managers have been inadequately prepared in these areas (Hodges, 1987). This situation is no different in Australia and is exacerbated by the changes outlined below which increase the expectations of the first-line nurse manager's role. This role is essential for the smooth and efficient functioning of the entire organisation and vital for achieving a quality product, client care.

Probably one of the most substantial and enduring pressures on the health care system is the rapid escalation of health costs as a result of inflation, devaluation of the dollar and the high costs associated with an increase in the complexity and profusion of technology. Adding to the pressure on health costs are the increasing numbers of elderly, the increased throughput in care agencies with a resultant decrease in length of stay, and an increase in client acuity (Carroll and Dwyer, 1987; Davis and George, 1988; Grant and Lapsley, 1990). As a result, the costs of health care in Australia overall have risen from $7239 million in 1977/78 to $21 053 million in 1986/87. Despite this increase in dollar outlay, the amount of Gross Domestic Product spent on health has remained constant at 8 per cent (Davis and George, 1988; Grant and Lapsley, 1990).

Not surprisingly, health care managers generally have had to become more accountable for expenditure. Computerised information systems have proliferated to provide essential data on the use and distribution of human and consumable resources. Senior nursing personnel are now actively involved in budgeting and financial planning. This increased involvement by nurse managers in fiscal determination, coupled with decentralisation, has ensured that first-line nurse managers have also become increasingly responsible and accountable for their own budgets, particularly in the area of staff wages. These costs and the associated productivity of staff are variables over which first-line nurse managers have some control. Effective managers can predict and thus alter their leadership style in order to achieve the most effective staff response. The technique or style used by a supervisor can influence important performance-related outcomes (Burke, Weitzel and Weir, 1982).

In addition to staff costs, first-line nurse managers must also be aware of the costs associated with the introduction of new technologies, which can be substantial and are not entirely monetary in nature. For example, Brewer (1983) found that the introduction of technology into the health care system is a source of great stress for the nursing workforce. At a time when 'burnout' and increased stress levels are being blamed for nursing staff shortages, any factor which exacerbates this situation is intolerable. Technology can also affect the role played by care providers, requiring nurses to be better educated to deal not only with the technological device itself, but also with the more complex physical and psychosocial problems faced by patients. Nurses must also come to terms with the more intricate moral and ethical issues involved in the current use of technology. Consequently, traditional nursing skills may not adequately equip nurses to make decisions or care for patients in today's highly technological environment.

While technology proliferates in the health arena, the focus of basic nursing programmes in the higher education sector is on the psychosocial aspects of the caring role. Similarly, students entering these programmes perceive that the caring aspect is the most important function of nurses (Adams, Donoghue, Duffield and Pelletier, 1988). Unfortunately, the philosophy of nursing programmes, while compatible with entering students' perceptions, is in conflict with the nature of health care provision in the workplace.

Farmer (1978) believes that the introduction of technology alters and extends the role of the nurse and consequently the role of the nurse manager. For example, uncertainty in nursing technology adversely affects nursing performance and requires greater direction from first-line nurse managers (Alexander and Bauerschmidt, 1987). As a consequence, first-line managers at the very least should be involved in the selection and purchase of equipment and technology, and ideally should be able to weigh up the associated costs and benefits for nursing staff and their clients.

The nursing profession itself has also undergone rapid changes recently. Perhaps the most notable has been the demand that pre-registration education for nurses be undertaken in the higher education sector. The educational preparation of nurses at a beginning level is significant in determining the subsequent professionalisation of nurses as well as their preparation for future managerial roles. To advance, the nursing profession requires personnel who have been appropriately and adequately prepared to act as role models and career planners for those nurses working under their direction (Pembrey, 1984).

The challenge for first-line nurse managers of today is to successfully incorporate tertiary graduates into the workforce. This requires managers who are able to provide an appropriate organisational climate so that these graduates can contribute to the profession and provide quality care. Early evidence in New South Wales suggests that the first-line nurse manager is most influential in this regard (Lumby, 1989). Unsuccessful assimilation will aggravate the problem of nursing shortages experienced in recent years.

The issue of nursing shortages poses another challenge for nurse managers. The failure to recruit and maintain staff is an important management problem. Reasons cited for high staff turnover have included inadequate salary levels, unsociable working hours, stress associated with work and the rigidity of administrative systems (New South Wales Department of Health, 1985). This situation is aggravated as more nurses leave the health care sector. While all these factors cannot be changed by the first-line nurse manager, there are specific job and nursing attributes, described in later chapters, which are under the control of managers. These determine to a great extent the perceptions held by nursing staff of their autonomy and job satisfaction, thereby affecting the decision to leave (Weisman, Alexander and Chase, 1981). In other words, nurse managers can significantly affect wastage and turnover rates of staff. As the 'Magnet Hospital' study found, the retention of staff correlated with the effectiveness of the first-line nurse manager (McClure, Poulin, Sovie and Wandelt, 1983). Managers of today must focus on the quality of an individual nurse's contribution and reward this effort. This means a nurse manager must be able to plan for retention and manage more effectively than has been done previously. Large turnover rates for nursing staff are costly, not only financially, but also in terms of the loss of continuity, productivity and quality which also result (Vogt, Velthouse, Vox and Thames, 1983; Butler, 1987; Huston and Marquis, 1989).

Another factor likely to alter the role of the first-line nurse manager is the introduction of a clinical career structure in all states. This innovation was intended to provide an incentive to continue in the workforce for those nurses who wished to remain at the bedside. While many in the profession praised such a development, some nurse managers regarded the development of clinical positions as a threat to their role, particularly if they perceived they had clinical as well as managerial responsibilities. 'Trained incapacity' denotes a condition whereby workers are no longer able to perform roles for which they have been prepared because some of their functions have been reallocated to other workers (Brewer, 1982). This could equally apply to nurse managers who feel they have lost some of their clinical responsibilities to the clinical nurse specialist and are left wondering what their role is meant to entail.

The last issue to be raised relates to the consumers of health care, the clients. There is a clear demand for an increased involvement of members of the community in health care decisions. Many hospitals now have client care representatives, and consumers are also represented on committees. This trend is reflected in the higher education system, where the role of client advocate is an important component of nursing curricula and is reflected in the perceptions of the nursing role (Pelletier, Adams, Donoghue and Duffield, 1989). An increase in the number of complaints received by the Complaints Unit of the New South Wales Health Department (New South Wales Department of Health, 1988) may be a further indication that clients in this country are becoming more active consumers.

The involvement of consumers is significant, because as they become more aware of the increasing costs of a product, they demand evidence of the quality of the item provided, in this case client care. However, the views of consumers are not necessarily the same as those who provide that care. They are more often concerned with humane treatment, reasonable cost and the outcome of care (Hamilton, 1982). Most quality assurance programmes do not deal with the issue of outcome, focusing instead on the structure of the organisation or the processes of care within it. An increasing emphasis on the outcome of care for a client can be expected, and nurse managers must be actively involved in this. Once the outcome for clients becomes the focus, more attention will be directed towards the nursing care provided on the ward, an area which is very much under the jurisdiction of the first-line nurse manager.

With this in mind, managers will need to establish the most cost-effective methods of caring for clients while ensuring that quality is enhanced. The nexus between cost-effectiveness, quality of care and equity issues can be dealt with in an integrated way through the use of Diagnosis Related Groups (DRGs) (Hindle and Scuteri, 1988), in which costs are allocated to client care units. The costs of production such as nursing functions are currently being determined in this country (Hindle and Scuteri, 1988) and nurse managers must ensure that nursing services are appropriately and accurately costed in this model.

# 2. THE AUSTRALIAN HEALTH CARE SYSTEM

Nurse managers must function within the structural parameters of the Australian health care system. However, their power to effect change within the system is great since here, as in many countries, the nursing profession comprises a significant proportion of the workforce. In the most recent census for which complete results are available (1981), 1.7 per cent of the entire employed workforce in this country were registered nurses. Medical practitioners accounted for only 0.4 per cent. Overall, throughout Australia in 1986 there were 257 731 persons in health occupations of which 141 980 (55 per cent) were registered nurses (Palmer and Short, 1989). The health care delivery system and the nursing profession are inextricably linked. The health care system is one of the largest employer groups in the industrial arena and changes within this system can have profound effects on the nursing profession and its managers. Nurses, on the other hand, constitute the largest single employee category within this system and can similarly have a significant impact on the health care system, particularly the public hospital sector where most nurses are employed. The 1986 strike by nurses in Victoria over a range of issues, including the condition of the state's health care system (Bessant and D'Cruz, 1989), is solemn testimony to this nexus.

There have been significant changes to the funding arrangements of health care which are not entirely related to the ideological beliefs held by the national government of the day. In fact, the financial arrangements between the Commonwealth and State governments have largely been structured so as to allow the Commonwealth government to implement its own policies regarding health insurance (Palmer and Short, 1989). Since 1983 there has been a national tax-funded health scheme (Medicare). It is financed by a 1.25 per cent levy on taxable incomes. As part of the Medicare scheme, the Commonwealth Government pays each state a Medicare Compensation Grant in addition to the Identified Health Grants paid specifically for health provision. This is to ensure that no state is financially disadvantaged by the introduction of Medicare through a loss of income related to changes in inpatient and outpatient charges. In return, each state provides public inpatient and outpatient treatment at no cost to the consumer. Once funds have been allocated to states for health care purposes, they are free to dispose of the funds (except for those allocated for specific purposes such as AIDS research) as they deem necessary. So while funding for health is largely Commonwealth based, with states adding resources as need or ideology dictates, the organisation of health care and the provision of most services is under state control.

Within this national funding arrangement, states have chosen different organisational models, implementing changes from time to time as governments change. Decentralisation has increasingly been the impetus behind governmental change. Irrespective of the structure of the health care system, nursing conditions, rates of pay and industrial classifications are negotiated by the trade union representing the nursing profession in the particular state. This accounts for differences between states in the organisational structure and classification of employees. For example, in New South Wales a nursing unit manager is appointed to manage a particular ward or unit; clinical nurse specialist status is awarded to a registered nurse who fulfils the criteria of either 12 months' experience and an appropriate post-basic qualification, or four years' post-basic experience, three of which are in a specified clinical area (New South Wales Department of Health, 1986). The broad definition of the responsibilities of clinical nurse specialists includes one who acts as a resource person and who has expert nursing knowledge related to her unit or speciality (New South Wales Department of Health, 1986). As the title is awarded to an individual and relinquished on the resignation or, at times, transfer of that nurse, there is no designated number of positions per ward or unit.

While the broad definition of responsibilities allocated to clinical nurse specialists is similar, the selection criteria, with respect to years of relevant clinical practice and academic qualifications, vary from state to state, as do responsibilities within the organisation. In Western Australia, the clinical nurse specialist is on the third hierarchical level of that state's career structure as opposed to the second level in New South Wales. In addition, ward level clinical nurses are responsible for providing the leadership and direction necessary for effective clinical management and the area manager assumes nurse management responsibilities for an area, not just one ward or unit (RANF 1987).

# 3. MANAGEMENT

If the first-line nurse manager is to perform effectively and efficiently in this environment of change, it is essential that a clear idea of that role, its responsibilities, and how it relates to other roles in the organisation be acquired.

As Douglass (1988) points out, no single definition of management has been universally accepted. Management can be seen as involving the co-ordination of human and material resources towards objective accomplishment (Kast and Rosenzweig, 1981); or as the process of getting activities completed efficiently with and through other people (Robbins, 1989); or as the process of planning, organising, leading and controlling the efforts of organisation members and of using all other organisational resources to achieve stated organisational goals (Stoner, Collins and Yetton, 1985).

Despite the differing emphasis in the definitions, basic common elements can be identified. Management:

☐ is a goal oriented activity;

☐ is through other people;

☐ is a process involving the application of principles and techniques — a practice methodology;

☐ takes place in an organisation.

An organisation is a group of people who have joined together in a systematic structure for a specific purpose. Organisations are ubiquitous, including everything from local sporting clubs to giant multinational conglomerates. All nurses work in organisations, whether they be large city hospitals, small community nursing posts or anything in between.

Defining a practice methodology for managers has led to much debate. Is management an art or is it a science? Koontz, O'Donnell and Weihrich (1984) argue that management, like all arts (for instance nursing, musical composition, engineering), makes use of an organised body of knowledge — science — and applies it in the light of realities to gain a desired practical result. Science and art are not mutually exclusive but are complementary: the most productive art is always based on an understanding of the science underlying it. Thus, to be a good nurse manager, one must have a solid preparation in the underlying principles and techniques of management. This conclusion is of particular significance to nurses. In previous times it was not usual for nurses to have any formal preparation for the management role. The basic assumption seems to have been that any nurse who was a good clinical practitioner would also be a good manager. Many nurses were thrust into management and had to learn the job as they went, relying on tradition, experience and intuition. While these informal methods can be effective in a stable environment, where situations are predominantly recurrent and when there is time on the job to learn necessary management skills, intuition and experience alone are not sufficient in a rapidly changing environment.

Conceptualisation or discussion of precisely what the role of the nurse manager should be is impeded by what Meleis and Jennings (in Henry et al, 1989) describe as the paucity of use and development of nursing theory in nursing administration. The theoretical basis of nursing administration is derived largely from other academic disciplines such as sociology, management and psychology. Meleis and Jennings argue that just as the medical model has proved an unsatisfactory basis for clinical nursing practice, so management theories drawn from other disciplines are not a suitable basis for nursing administration. Nurse managers play a unique role in creating an environment in which professional nursing practice can occur and endure. As theory is central to the concept of science and the art of practice is based on a scientific foundation, the lack of well-developed theories of nursing management is a cause for professional concern. Nurse managers must synthesise two disciplines — nursing and management. Although the momentum for research in nursing administration is growing, there is still a long way to go. In the climate of change pervasive within the Australian health care system in general and within the nursing profession in particular, it has never been more necessary for nurses to be able to assume powerful management roles in order to capitalise on this change. The absence of well-developed theories in nursing administration should not preclude nurse managers from seeking guidance for managerial action in other disciplines and applying these principles to their nursing practice. The art has to be supported by a strong foundation in the science, and nurses must have adequate and appropriate preparation for the management role.

## 3.1 TERMINOLOGY

To many people, the terms management, administration and supervision can be used interchangeably. Despite some arguments to the contrary (for example, McFarland, Skipton-Leonard and Morris, 1984), management and administration are like terms. In Australia, management seems to be the term used in private enterprise, and administration the term favoured in public enterprise. This may explain why the latter is the terminology most commonly used in nursing. Supervision, on the other hand, is a component of management or, if preferred, administration. Ordinarily it is a term used to apply to those in the first line of management: Robbins (1989) uses supervisor and first-line manager as equivalent terms.

Management is often referred to in terms of line and staff positions. Line management positions are associated directly with the achievement of the organisation's goals. These managers are directly responsible for delivering the service that the organisation offers. Staff management positions, on the other hand, provide a service or specialist advice to those in line positions. Staff managers are usually those who work in such areas as accounting, financial control, personnel, office management, cleaning and other support services. Thus staff managers contribute to the achievement of the organisation's goals, albeit indirectly.

## 3.2 LEADERSHIP

Lundborg (1982) describes a leader as a person whom others will follow willingly and voluntarily. Altman, Valenzi and Hodgetts (1985) define leadership as the process of influencing others to direct their efforts towards the achievement of some particular goal or goals.

Leadership is often used as an all-encompassing term for what a manager does. As Austin (1981) points out, a considerable amount of the literature on leadership effectiveness is actually discussing managerial effectiveness. It is therefore not easy to define a set of qualities for effective managers and to identify those which are leadership attributes and those which are management attributes. For example, managers, because of their formal position in the organisational hierarchy, have a legitimate authority to demand the co-operation of subordinates. A manager who is also a strong leader will bring forth a willing and eager co-operation, releasing in others an energy to achieve goals that go beyond what is prescribed or even expected. An effective nurse manager must also be an effective leader, but separating the two concepts is difficult. Perhaps for this reason, Lippitt (1983) claimed that leadership is the worst defined and least understood personal attribute sometimes possessed by human beings. Even the conclusions of those who have done extensive research on leadership are contradictory, simplistic and ambiguous. But despite the lack of clear definition, leadership theory is widely read and utilised in formal organisations (Young and Hayne 1988). Nurses who aspire to be leaders and those who are expected to be leaders by virtue of their appointment to a nurse management position should be familiar with the literature on leadership theories.

From the vast volumes of research that have been devoted to understanding the concept of leadership, three basic approaches emerge. The first approach was leadership-trait theory, in which an attempt was made to identify those traits or characteristics that distinguished successful leaders from unsuccessful leaders. A universal list of traits has not been forthcoming, with only very modest correlations being found between identified traits and successful leadership. As one of the basic assumptions of this approach was the idea that 'leaders are born, not made', the lack of success indicated that leadership was a learned rather than an inherent skill.

When the trait approach did not provide the hoped-for results, researchers turned their attention to behavioural theory, seeking to explain leadership in terms of what leaders do. The aim of this approach was to identify critical behavioural determinants of leadership so that people could be trained to be leaders.

The most popular of the behavioural theories resulted from research which began in the late 1940s at Ohio State University. These studies identified two independent dimensions of leader behaviour which were labelled 'initiating structure' and 'consideration'. Initiating structure concerned establishing patterns of work, standards of performance, and time frames for goal achievement. Consideration concerned the leader's relationship with subordinates and a leader who ranked high on 'initiating structure' would be expected to be approachable, warm and friendly, and show respect to subordinates. Research indicated that leaders high in both initiating structure and consideration tended to achieve high subordinate performance and satisfaction more frequently than those who rated low on either or both of these dimensions. However, no one style provided an unconditional guarantee of performance effectiveness and work-group satisfaction. For further discussion of this approach see Stogdill (1974).

It became increasingly clear that the prediction of leadership success was more complex than the identification of traits or preferred leader behaviours. Situational variables had also to be considered, leading to the current interest in contingency based leadership. Contingency theory views leadership as a dynamic, two-way process of influence where not only leader characteristics are considered but also characteristics of the followers, the situation and the task. A number of theorists, including Fred Fiedler and Robert House, have proposed complex models to explain this contingency approach. But although it represents a significant advance in leadership theory, this approach has still fallen considerably short of a predictive model.

When commenting upon the extensive research on leadership, Alban Metcalfe (1982) claims that the individuals with whom one interacts are enormously varied, as are the situational features, organisational characteristics and a multitude of other factors. Thus it would be unrealistic to expect to develop a predictive model of leadership skills which could guarantee a successful outcome in every situation. In the final analysis, all leadership theories have one major concern, that of leadership effectiveness. The leader must achieve the goals required by the particular situation. Sometimes this demands concern for the task, sometimes concern for the people involved, and sometimes combinations of both (Altman, Valenzi and Hodgetts, 1985). In determining how to be a good leader, the manager must select an appropriate leadership style which takes into account the qualities and demands of the leader, the followers and the work environment.

Without doubt, leadership skills are important to managers. Peters and Waterman (1982), when analysing why some organisations were successful, found that one characteristic shared by successful companies was unusually strong leadership. The heart of management is dealing with people and co-ordinating the efforts of the work group in order to secure common goals. This must be the most urgent challenge of all managers. However, within the organisation some managers may have poorly developed leadership skills, while some strong leaders, even on appointment to a management position, may have few management skills. Thus, in the organisation, leaders can be considered to be both formal and informal. Formal leaders are those who have an appointed managerial position in the organisational hierarchy, their role being to lead a specified group towards the attainment of the organisation's goals. The informal leader, on the other hand, is appointed by the work group itself, usually as a result of some outstanding characteristic such as personality, job knowledge or experience. This individual tends to be a spokesperson for the group, the person to whom others go for advice and assistance. These informal leaders also lead the group towards objectives, and the nature of those objectives then becomes the point at issue. If the informal leader has objectives congruent with those of the organisation, then the manager has a strong ally, since the informal leader can have considerable influence over the group in terms of task achievement. However, if the informal leader has objectives which are not compatible with those of the nurse manager and hence the organisation, then the nurse manager has a potential problem and must take steps to defuse the influence of that person.

It is clear that leadership and management are not synonymous terms. The leadership role and the skills displayed by a nurse manager when interacting with a work group relate to only one of the roles which constitute a nurse manager's responsibility. Leadership is just one function, though an extremely important one, in a much wider range of daily activities. Nevertheless, leadership is a crucial component of the managerial role and skill as a leader will often make the difference between a competent nurse manager and an excellent one.

## 3.3 THE FIRST-LINE MANAGER

In organisations, different levels and types of managers are found. Table 1.1.1 identifies the levels of nurse managers and describes their responsibilities.

As the focus of this book is the first-line nurse manager, middle and top managers will be discussed only in so far as their role impinges on that of the first-line nurse manager.

It is only in recent times that the importance of the first-line managerial position of the nurse has begun to be recognised. Beaman (1986) describes the first-line nurse

TABLE 1.1.1:   Nurse managers and their responsibilities. Source: Douglass (1988)

| LEVEL | RESPONSIBILITY |
|---|---|
| Top Managers | Responsible for the overall operation of nursing services; establish objectives, policies and strategies; represent the organisation at community affairs, business arrangements and negotiations. Typical titles: Director of Nursing, Administrator, Matron. |
| Middle Managers | Usually co-ordinate the nursing activities of several units; receive broad overall strategies and policies from top managers and translate them into specific objectives and programmes. Typical titles: Assistant Director of Nursing, Supervisor, Co-ordinator. |
| First-line Managers | Directly responsible for the actual production of the nursing services; act as links between the higher level managers and non-managers. Typical titles: Charge Nurse, Shift Co-ordinator, Area Manager. |

manager as vital to quality client care and the fulcrum of managerial influence in the hospital. Barnum and Mallard (1989) see the first-line nurse manager as fulfilling one of the most critical and valuable roles in the administration of nursing practice by being the pivot which links nurse management to nursing care. Recent research in New South Wales indicates that this aspect of the role is also highly regarded (Duffield, 1989).

The role of the first-line nurse manager can be difficult and demanding because of this pivotal role between management and line staff — those who are actually delivering the client care. For this reason, first-line managers often find themselves in a position of conflict, caught between the demands of higher management and those of the clinical workforce. Higher management tends to see the first-line nurse manager as an extension of the workforce, while the workforce tends to see the first-line nurse manager as an extension of management. The potential for role ambiguity becomes apparent. It is therefore essential that first-line managers have very clear ideas about their role within the organisation in which they work as well as a wide knowledge of the management function.

## 3.4 THE TASKS OF THE FIRST-LINE NURSE MANAGER

As Stevens (1985) points out, nurse managers' tasks are discussed in two different ways: in terms of the nurse manager's skills required to complete the tasks, and in terms of the specific tasks themselves.

### 3.4.1. Management skills

Katz (1974) identified three basic types of skills needed by all managers. These are technical, human and conceptual skills.

Technical skill is the ability to use the tools, procedures and techniques of a specialised field. In nursing, it is the ability to perform 'hands-on' nursing care. Human skill is the ability to work with other people, either as individuals or in groups. It involves leadership, coaching, counselling, motivating and communicating. Conceptual skill is the mental ability to co-ordinate and integrate all the organisation's interests and activities. It involves such managerial tasks as long range planning, goal setting and forecasting needs. See Figure 1.1.1.

**FIGURE 1.1.1**:   Relative skills needed for effective performance at different levels of management.

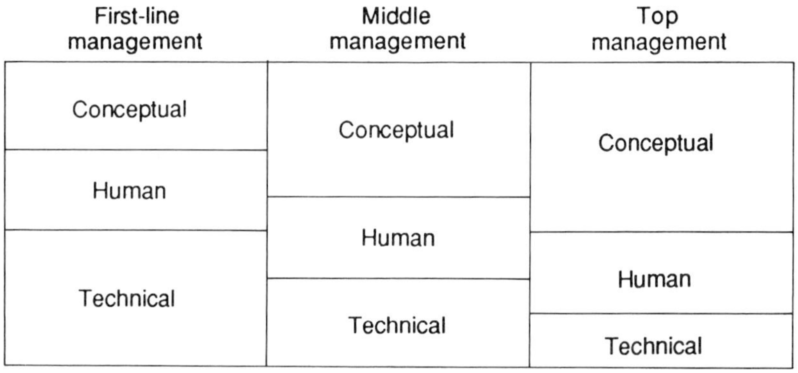

| First-line management | Middle management | Top management |
|---|---|---|
| Conceptual | Conceptual | Conceptual |
| Human | | |
| | Human | |
| Technical | | Human |
| | Technical | Technical |

Katz suggests that all three skills are essential for effective management, though their relative importance to the particular manager depends on organisational rank. Technical skills are of utmost importance to the first-line nurse manager since individuals in this position oversee the day-to-day work. This person, like managers at all organisational levels, also needs good human skills. Conceptual skills, however, are not a major requirement for this level of manager.

### 3.4.2 Management tasks

Many popular textbooks (for example Marriner-Tomey, 1988) present the management process as one which comprises five major functions: planning, organising, staffing, leading and controlling.

Planning is the first function and all other functions are dependent on it. It encompasses defining the organisation's goals, establishing an overall strategy for achieving those goals, and developing a comprehensive hierarchy of plans to integrate and co-ordinate activities.

Organising is the second managerial function. Having planned, the manager then assigns duties to personnel and co-ordinates employee efforts to implement the plans efficiently and effectively. To organise, the manager must consider what tasks need to be done, who is to do them, how tasks are to be grouped and who relates to whom in terms of authority, responsibility and decision making.

Staffing includes recruiting, selecting and developing staff to achieve the goals of the organisation. As soon as the organisation has identified its goals and has the people with the necessary skills to achieve them, leading then becomes the manager's most important function. Leadership is the process of influencing people to achieve goals and requires excellence in interpersonal skills.

Controlling is the final step in the management process. To ensure that operations are running smoothly, the manager must monitor the organisation's performance, comparing it with the previously set goals. If there are any significant deviations, it is the manager's job to make corrections and bring the performance on line.

This functional approach to the tasks of management has the advantages of clarity and simplicity. However, its relevance to the first-line management role needs to be explored. While these functions may describe the tasks of all managers, it is clear that some managers perform some functions more often than others. Top managers, for instance, are more likely to be involved in strategic planning than are first-line managers. Defining the first-line nurse manager's actual tasks on each of the functional classifications is not without difficulty. Beaman (1986) carried out a study in 10 hospitals in Los Angeles County, California to identify the tasks of first-line managers. Of all the tasks involved in first-line management, only 31 were selected by more than 50 per cent of the respondents as being common to the first-line management position in their particular hospitals. This indicates that the role of the first-line nurse manager can vary enormously between hospitals. It is unlikely that the situation would be any different in Australia. The implication is that in order to prepare for the management role, the nurse must have a broadly based preparation in management theory, strategies and techniques. As Barnum and Mallard (1989) point out, first-line nurse managers need to recognise that translating concepts and goals into concrete activities is a unique responsibility of their role.

# 4. MANAGEMENT THEORIES

A familiarity with the development of management thought can be extremely helpful for the first-line nurse manager in creating an individual management style. Although no single management theory can guide every action, drawing from the most applicable of these theories is useful in directing the nurse manager to appropriate action.

Management theories do not remain static. Since the introduction of the earliest principle of scientific management nearly a century ago, approaches to management have been marked by constant change and the development of several major schools of thought. The introduction of new theories does not, however, render previous theories invalid. Rather the effect is cumulative, adding to a body of knowledge and contributing further to an understanding of the managerial role in a complex changing environment, as well as offering the nurse manager guidelines for practice.

Broadly, management theories can be divided into four major approaches: scientific management, classical organisation, behavioural and quantitative.

## 4.1 SCIENTIFIC MANAGEMENT

Frederick Taylor (1856-1915) is generally accepted as the father of scientific management. Taylor conducted time and motion studies on workers to determine the most efficient way of completing a task. Workers were then trained in the new techniques and productive workers were rewarded with incentive wages. Other researchers in the scientific management school — which proclaimed the use of scientific method to define one best way for a job to be done — were Henry Gantt and the Gilbreths, Frank and Lillian. Scientific management developed a rational approach to solving organisational problems and also pointed the way for the role of the professional nurse manager. However, the basic assumption that workers are rational and interested only in higher wages became inappropriate as society changed.

## 4.2 CLASSICAL ORGANISATION THEORIES

Classical organisation theory began to receive attention around 1930. Henri Fayol (1841-1925), a French industrialist, studied the functions of managers and concluded that management was universal. All managers, he felt, had essentially the same tasks — planning, organising, issuing orders, co-ordinating and controlling. This model of management remains the keystone of management theory today, and readers will recognise the series of functions discussed earlier in this chapter. Fayol also developed principles of management. A believer in the division of labour, he argued that specialisation increased efficiency.

Max Weber (1864-1920), a German sociologist, developed the concept of 'bureaucracy', an organisational theory with an emphasis on rules rather than individuals, competence over personal favouritism, and clearly defined lines of formal authority with unity of command (a worker is answerable to only one supervisor). He provided a concise and rational guide for efficiently managing organisations.

Despite being a product of a different time, much in the classical organisational theories has endured. Their rational approach still has appeal for the manager overwhelmed by complexities. However, the depersonalisation and rigidity inherent in the principles of these theories can often create problems in today's organisations where lines of authority are frequently blurred.

## 4.3 BEHAVIOURAL APPROACH

The behavioural school emerged, in part, because managers found frustrations in the classical approach as people did not always follow predicted, rational behaviour patterns. There developed an interest in helping managers deal with the people of the organisation.

The major impetus for this line of thought came from a series of experiments conducted by Australian-born researcher Elton Mayo (1880-1949) and his associates from Harvard University. Mayo found that special attention (such as being selected by top management to participate in experiments) often caused workers to increase their efforts. This phenomenon became known as the Hawthorne Effect. The concept of 'social man', motivated by relationship needs and group involvement rather than management control, had to replace the economically motivated 'rational man' concept of the classical approach.

Since that time, many researchers have continued to work on the behavioural approach to management. Enormous contributions have been made to the understanding of factors which motivate individuals, how people work in groups, interpersonal relations in the workplace and what individuals seek to gain from their work. However, because human behaviour is so complex, many theorists have differed quite markedly in their recommendations to managers, often making it difficult for them to decide which advice it would be best to follow.

## 4.4 QUANTITATIVE APPROACH

Also called management science or operations research, the quantitative approach evolved from mathematical and statistical methods which were developed to help solve military problems of World War II. Quantitative techniques include the application of statistics and computer simulations such as linear programming to management decisions. This approach has contributed most directly to management decision making, particularly in the areas of strategic planning.

While the approach is widely used, especially in large organisations, it has never gained as much influence on management practice as has the behavioural approach. Many managers find the quantitative tools require specialist knowledge and that the abstract process of constructing quantitative models is too far removed from the reality of day-to-day managing.

# **5.** PLANNING

## 5.1 BASIS FOR PLANNING: MISSION, PHILOSOPHY AND OBJECTIVES

Planning is the foundation of good management and has its beginning in the mission, philosophy and objectives of the organisation. It is this basis that gives direction to all management planning, irrespective of management level. The organisation's mission, philosophy and objectives have just as much significance in guiding the decisions made by the first-line nurse manager as does top management.

### 5.1.1 Mission

The mission of the organisation is a statement that identifies why an organisation exists and its purpose, as distinguished from other similar organisations (Holt, 1987). It is important that the mission statement clarify the organisation's character. It may be considered that all health care organisations have the mission of 'delivery of care' or 'serving people'. However, different health care organisations may have other missions in areas such as education or research, or delivering care to people in a defined geographical region or with particular health problems. Documenting the purpose of the organisation in the mission statement characterises the uniqueness of that organisation.

Departments, units or other components of the organisation also need mission statements to explain their purpose. The nursing division, for instance, may have its own mission statement and the first-line nurse manager may wish to develop a specific mission statement for a unit. It is important that these departmental mission statements be congruent with those of the organisation.

### 5.1.2. Philosophy

Marquis and Huston (1987) define a philosophy as the set of values or beliefs that guide the actions of an organisation. It should be a statement that can be referred to as an explanation of why things are carried out in a particular way. A philosophy takes time and effort to prepare and should be a thoughtful reflection of the values of the group. The more the philosophy statement restricts itself to a clear expression of the collective concerns of the work group, the more meaningful the statement will be.

When developing a philosophy statement for a sub-unit of the organisation, it is most important to be able to begin the document with a statement similar to 'we are in accord with the philosophy of the organisation and support its beliefs and values'. As with the mission statement, congruence at all levels of the organisation is essential. An organisation, by definition, must be directed towards a common goal.

A philosophy therefore needs to be:

☐ written;

☐ communicated (placed in appropriate documents and displayed);

☐ recognised in the practice of members;

☐ a reflection of current values and a direction for future planning;

☐ updated periodically to reflect changes in attitudes and influences.

### 5.1.3 Objectives

Holle and Blatchley (1987) defined objectives as a series of desired outcomes needed to reach a pre-determined goal; an objective describes the results expected from a single activity. A goal is a desired or expected outcome. Goals generally have a long range time-frame or may be an ongoing activity. Objectives on the other hand, are much more specific. Some books, especially management texts (for instance Robbins, 1989) use the terms goals and objectives interchangeably. Nursing texts, probably because of experience in nursing process applications, make a clear distinction between the meanings of the terms.

If an objective is to be useful, it must be stated in terms of the results to be achieved so that it can be used as a basis for assessing the effectiveness of the process carried out (Cantor, 1973). Objectives must reflect the mission and the philosophy of the organisation.

Kron and Gray (1987) offer guidelines which can be used when stating objectives:

1. who is to perform the action or reach the expected outcome?

2. what is the expected outcome to be achieved?

3. what level of performance will be considered satisfactory and how will it be achieved?

4. when can the outcome be realistically reached?

5. is the objective consistent with the mission, philosophy, goals and objectives of the organisation?

6. if more than one objective is stated, are they listed according to priority?

It is the role of the nurse manager to provide accurate responses to these questions based on realistic assessments of the current situation.

### 5.1.4 Significance for planning

The mission, philosophy, goals and objectives are essential in providing the purposeful direction for planning at all levels of the organisation. It is critical that these documents are developed as operational tools and not meaningless 'management ornaments'. Trexler (1987) investigated the use and effectiveness of mission, philosophy, goals and objectives, in nursing departments in 27 American states. In this limited study she found a low level of relationship between the mission, philosophy, goals and objectives as defined in the documents and the actual nursing activity. Moreover, she found that most of the documents were both unachievable and stated in idealistic terms. The necessity for a realistic approach became apparent if these documents were to serve their intention as management planning tools. As Stevens (1985) points out, all too often these operational documents are seen merely as pieces of paper to have on file.

## 5.2 THE PROCESS OF PLANNING

'If you fail to plan you are planning to fail.'

'If you don't plan you may end up where you didn't want to be but will not recognise it because you didn't know where you wanted to be in the first place.'

All managers must plan. Planning is a part of every phase of management and an essential component of every manager's role. It is the basic process of defining objectives and determining how to achieve them. Reaching an objective entails making a plan about what has to be done. The plan must assign responsibilities and be communicated to those involved in its implementation.

Within the organisation, specific instances of planning can be categorised according to their time-frames and their associated organisational level. Long range or strategic planning most frequently covers more than five years and is considered to be the responsibility of top management. Intermediate planning has a time-frame of one to five years and is a function of middle management. First-line managers are involved in short-range planning (also called operational or tactical planning) which has a time-frame of less than one year.

Strategic planning is significant for the first-line nurse manager because it provides direction for the operational plans. Goals and objectives defined by the first-line nurse manager must be congruent with those defined by the strategic planning process. This is the method by which managers ensure that members of the organisation continue to head in the same direction, aiming to achieve the same goals.

One of the pitfalls for first-line nurse managers is acting without a plan. Because they can become so involved with the pressures of day to day activities, people and events, it is easy to become reactive rather than proactive. For this reason, it is essential that plans for first-line managers be adaptable and flexible enough to change when necessary. Once a plan has been established, the nurse manager must periodically review the situation and make any necessary revisions. Given the complexities of the Australian health care environment discussed at the beginning of this chapter, the need for flexibility becomes readily apparent.

Seven essential steps in planning may be defined:

1.  take a realistic look at the environmental influences which impinge upon the organisation. Try to accurately anticipate problems and opportunities;

2.  establish realistic goals and objectives. This should be done in the light of the mission, philosophy and objectives defined by the organisation as a whole as well as by the nursing division;

3.  develop alternative ways to handle and solve any problems and make the most of opportunities;

4. weigh up the advantages and disadvantages of each alternative to see which one is best;

5. decide which alternative(s) to follow;

6. implement the plan;

7. check the progress of the plan to make sure that objectives are being achieved. If the objectives are not being achieved, the fault may lie with the original plan (was it realistic?), or with the implementation (is the appropriate leadership style being used?). Be prepared to change a plan if necessary. It is much better to change a plan than to have no plan at all or to continue with a plan that fails.

Who undertakes the task of planning is a question which requires consideration. One approach is for the nurse manager to do all the planning. Although a time consuming exercise, plans can be altered quickly to meet changing situations. An alternative is for the nurse manager to plan, using suggestions solicited from subordinates. This fosters a feeling that they have made a positive contribution to the plan and thus they are more willing and likely to support it. However, the planning period becomes much longer and the group often feels the need to confer with the manager before any changes are made.

A third possibility is for 'bottom-up' planning, in which the subordinates plan and the nurse managers approve. The nurse manager's contribution to the plan becomes minimal. This process is time consuming and there is a danger of producing an unrealistic plan because the planners lack knowledge of the organisational constraints and other issues of which a manager should be aware. The nurse manager can also become very remote from the planning process.

The best approach depends on the circumstances and the individuals involved. It must be recognised that planning, irrespective of who is involved, demands a significant time commitment.

Kron and Gray (1987) suggest that a well developed plan should:

1. have a clearly worded objective, including expected results and methods for evaluation;

2. be guided by any policies and/or procedures affecting the planned actions;

3. indicate priorities;

4. develop actions which are realistic in terms of the available personnel, equipment and time;

5. develop a logical sequence of activities;

6. select the most practical method(s) for achieving each objective.

# 6. CHANGE THEORY

The changes in organisational, nursing and client variables outlined earlier can be classified as unplanned and external. First-line nurse managers have little direct control over them because they are external to the organisation and beyond their control. However change can also occur within the organisation. First-line nurse managers frequently have some input and control over these internal changes and indeed may even initiate them. In this case the change becomes planned change. Actions are directed towards solving a problem. The discussion which follows relates to planned change, the ways in which the first-line nurse manager can effect change at the internal (ward or unit and at times organisational) level. Planned change implies forethought on the part of the manager as to what the problem is, an analysis of the ways in which it can best be resolved, a selection of the best strategy to effect change and an evaluation of the effectiveness of this strategy.

The classic writer on change was Toffler in *Future Shock* (1970), which describes much of what influences workers in the health care sector at the moment. Toffler defined change as the process by which the future invades our lives; future shock is the shattering stress and disorientation which occur when individuals are subjected to too much change in too short a time (Toffler, 1970). A more classic definition of change is to substitute one thing for another, to experience a shift in circumstances that cause differences, or to become different from before (Douglass, 1988).

## 6.1 CHANGE MODELS

Many models have been used to describe the change process. The most commonly chosen is Lewin's Force-Field Model (1952). Lewin describes behaviour as a balance of two major forces: 'driving forces', which propel the individual along a desired path of change, and 'restraining forces', which inhibit change because they drive the individual in another direction. He describes three stages in the change process. The first stage is unfreezing, in which the forces which maintain the current equilibrium are disrupted; the second stage, moving, is implementing the planned change which will establish a new equilibrium; and the last is refreezing, in which forces which will maintain the new equilibrium are institutionalised either formally (using policies and procedures) or informally (through changed behaviour patterns) (Lewin, 1952). Inherent to this theory is the premise that change will not occur if the restraining and driving forces are balanced.

To use Lewin's theory, the nurse manager must identify both the driving and restraining forces involved in maintaining equilibrium. In order to then effect change the nurse manager may either increase the magnitude or number of driving forces, or decrease the magnitude or number of restraining forces. This can be achieved by adding a new driving force or by changing a force's direction or magnitude. It is easier for a nurse manager to implement change when the external climate is unstable or dynamic since equilibrium is less likely to be established or refreezing unlikely to be complete. The health care system provides such an example.

More recent writers equate the change process with the nursing process (Douglass, 1988; Sullivan and Decker, 1988; Young and Hayne, 1988; Gillies, 1989). In such a model, **assessment** incorporates the identification of the problem, data collection and analysis. Internal and external forces for change are identified, as are any constraints which may hinder change (unfreezing). **Planning** requires an identification of the goals of change, methods of achieving them, and a means of evaluating the success of each method. This is followed by a selection of the most appropriate strategy based on the information collected and analysed in the assessment and planning stages. **Implementation** requires the nurse manager to determine who is best able to undertake the necessary actions, to activate the plan one step at a time, and to co-ordinate the group's efforts directed at achieving the goals of change. The last step, **evaluation,** involves an assessment of the effectiveness of the planned change in resolving the problem or achieving the goals, as well as ensuring the introduced change is stabilised (similar to refreezing) or altered if ineffective in goal achievement.

As an example of the use of Lewin's model, consider a situation where the first-line nurse manager wishes to introduce primary nursing instead of client assignment on the unit to resolve two main problems, a decline in the quality of care and job dissatisfaction. Having identified the problem, the nurse manager must then collect and analyse the relevant data. In so doing the following driving and restraining forces are identified:

| Driving forces | Restraining forces |
|---|---|
| Pressure from the manager | Greater cost |
| Improved quality of care | Staff resistance |
| Greater job satisfaction | Desire for security |
| Greater staff responsibility | Loss of jobs for enrolled nurses |
| Increased staff autonomy | |

The next step is to determine the strength of each force identified. Status quo is maintained when the force strengths are equal. If the forces identified above are equal in strength, then change will not occur unless the nurse manager either increases the driving forces (in strength or number) or decreases the restraining forces (in strength or number). To assist with unfreezing, the first-line nurse manager might decide to increase the driving forces by soliciting support for the planned change from more senior nurse managers. Alternatively, the threat to the security of enrolled nurses could be diminished by determining where vacancies exist for this category of staff, so that appropriate transfers could be arranged later if so desired. A third possibility would be to diminish staff resistance through techniques described later.

Further information required in the assessment stage includes such aspects as who stands to gain (or lose), financially as well as in terms of status, position and control. In this way potential resistance and possible solutions and strategies for implementation can be identified. This information will be useful in 'selling' the change to staff at a later stage.

The next stage (planning) involves the identification of strategies to effect the desired change based on the information collected and analysed. The nurse manager must first of all convince staff that there is a need to change by suggesting that the quality of care is perhaps less than it should be, that job dissatisfaction has resulted in a significant loss of staff, or that perhaps staff are not as accountable for client care as they should be. Data to support these statements (for example results from the quality assurance programme) should be presented as this helps convince staff that change is necessary. The concept of primary nursing as a method of overcoming the problems described can be introduced using the support of driving forces mentioned earlier. The first-line nurse manager must be well informed about the positive and negative effects of primary nursing and be able to minimise the effects of the restraining forces. Staff from the unit should be involved in deciding how to organise the desired change as this will help decrease the inevitable resistance.

The next stage is implementation, whereby the strategies outlined in the planning stage are put into place. The nurse manager in conjunction with the staff must determine realistic goals, decide who will be involved in their implementation and what their functions will be, and establish an appropriate time-frame within which change must be accomplished. To effect a smooth transition to primary nursing a variety of strategies may be necessary, including information giving (such as supplying staff with articles supporting primary nursing); training and education if new skills are required; selection of new staff who wish to work on a primary nursing ward; and transfer of those staff who do not wish to remain on the unit when the system of care changes.

In the last stage, evaluation, the nurse manager must evaluate the process of change; to do this, measurable goals must have been identified and time-lines for achieving them established. The first-line nurse manager can then measure performance against a standard. Ideally the information collected should be quantifiable and might include, in the example given, evidence from the quality assurance programme that the standard of care has risen in the year over which change has been implemented; a decrease in staff turnover to less than 20 per cent in the year; greater staff and client satisfaction determined through a survey; remaining within budget for the subsequent financial year. Evaluation, to mean anything, should be undertaken only when equilibrium has again been reached. Therefore it would not be appropriate to evaluate the effects on the role of the first-line nurse manager of the transition to primary nursing immediately since it is estimated to take up to two years for changes to become evident (Shamian, Frunchak, Miller, Georges and Kagan, 1988).

## 6.2 OVERCOMING RESISTANCE TO CHANGE

In the example above it was mentioned that one of the strategies for decreasing the restraining forces (and assisting with unfreezing) was to diminish resistance. Human nature is such that most people desire constancy in their lives, and therefore any attempt to introduce change will inevitably meet with resistance from some staff. The strength of resistance to change is proportional to the staff member's emotional and economic stake in maintaining the status quo (Gillies, 1989). This must be remembered when endeavouring to introduce any change. Resistance should not always be viewed as a negative process since it may alert the nurse manager to aspects of the planned change which may not have been considered, such as an unforeseen outcome, poor planning, or failure to communicate the reasons and benefits of the proposed change effectively. Nevertheless, resistance related to an individual's perception that their position or stability in an organisation is threatened must ultimately be dealt with.

While it is impossible to eradicate resistance entirely, strategies can be employed to minimise or overcome its effects. Using the example described above, to introduce the planned change by reducing the strength of the restraining force (staff resistance), the first-line nurse manager must first be able to communicate with staff and seek their opinions in the decision-making process. Perhaps most importantly, the manager must be able to identify as many potential effects of the change on individuals as possible. These might include an alteration to the group's norms, particularly with the demise of enrolled nurses; perception that the workload would increase, or a belief that the change was being introduced for the wrong reason (perhaps to modify the role of the first-line nurse manager rather than enhance the quality of care). In this way responses can be predicted and dealt with.

The second important aspect which underlies much of what management is about is the principle of adequate communication with staff. Staff become alarmed when they are unaware of what is to happen to them, their positions or their security. A perceived threat to any of these aspects makes resistance more likely. A failure to communicate effectively increases the chances of misinformation being received, with a consequent lack of understanding of the real reasons for change, which potentially increases resistance. It should also be remembered that with any proposed change, some staff may have a very real fear of failure since their skills may not adequately equip them for the future as planned. The first-line nurse manager must explain as soon as possible the purpose of the change, the potential benefits and effects, as well as changes to positions or responsibilities. Staff who are involved in the decision-making process will be more committed to the planned change than those who are excluded.

The nurse manager should establish open group communication in which staff problems and concerns are identified and discussed. The benefits of the planned change need to be outlined for staff (and supported by the literature), highlighting such aspects as the increase in autonomy, job satisfaction and the quality of client care. Staff should discuss their perceptions of the new role which would evolve under the primary nursing model, while the nurse manager outlines the new role of the first-line nurse manager in such a model. Threats to security should be discussed and solutions sought. If new skills are required by staff, then an educational programme might need to be developed by the inservice department and the nurse manager should initiate this as soon as practicable.

## 6.3 THE FIRST-LINE NURSE MANAGER AS A CHANGE AGENT

In times of rapid organisational change it is important for the first-line nurse manager to provide leadership and direction for staff who are endeavouring to come to terms with a new and dynamic environment. More importantly, as a change agent the nurse manager must motivate staff to adopt the change by convincing them that their contributions will continue to be valuable and will probably be even more significant in a primary nursing model where nursing excellence is a cornerstone. Staff must feel that the nurse manager is communicating honestly and openly with them and that there is a feeling of trust between both parties.

The introduction of change may still have unexpected outcomes despite the best planning and skill on the part of the nurse manager. The leadership skills of the nurse manager are of paramount importance. It is important that the first-line nurse manager allow staff to express their concerns. To do this effectively, the ability to communicate is essential, not only at the individual level but also at the group level where skills in group dynamics are required. Group work will facilitate an acceptance of the planned change by introducing new group norms. The group will come to terms with the planned change and should be able to identify the benefits which will accrue to each member of staff and where possible, the problems for which as a group they should be able to find alternatives. Individuals most affected by the change must be supported.

## SUMMARY

The changes described in this chapter have provided an overview of the challenges facing first-line nurse managers today which may also prescribe the role they undertake. The result of these changes generally has been to increase the level of accountability and responsibility expected of the first-line nurse manager who must manage the clinical environment in order to achieve the major goal of the organisation, namely quality client care.

In order to function efficiently and effectively in such an environment, the first-line nurse manager must be prepared for the role with a thorough understanding of the principles that underpin the practice of management.

This chapter has discussed the role of the first-line nurse manager and introduced a theoretical basis for management and leadership. This discussion included planning, the function which serves as an essential basis of excellent management practice.

The implementation of change is a managerial process which is of critical importance to the role of the first-line manager. It is essential that the process be applied in an informed and systematic way. 'Complexity shock' refers to the sense of helplessness felt by someone confronting numerous and unpredictable changes with inadequate coping skills (Manez, 1978). A clear understanding of the role and responsibilities of the first-line nurse manager should prevent good nurses from becoming victims of the syndrome.

# BLUEFINCH CASE STUDY

Bluefinch Community Hospital is a hospital of 120 beds serving a community on the outer perimeter of a metropolitan area. The residents of Bluefinch are mainly young couples, families with young children, and elderly pensioners who have moved to the area because housing is much cheaper. Many residents commute to the city to work and for entertainment. Bluefinch Community Hospital does not provide intensive care services. It has a high dependency ward where patients may be stabilised before being transferred to the city. It has a busy Accident and Emergency centre as a major highway skirts the town and many residents of the area are prone to asthma and bronchitis at certain times of the year.

Robin Chua was appointed Deputy Director of Nursing at Bluefinch Hospital two years ago. Robin has a degree in Psychology which was completed while studying part-time and working in the coronary care unit of a major teaching hospital in the city. Shortly after taking up the position, Robin applied for, and was granted study leave, to undertake the Master of Nursing Administration Degree which is now nearing completion.

The Director of Nursing, Jo Pilocovitch, has been at the hospital 10 years and has a Diploma of Nursing Administration. Jo has not undertaken any further study since then except for fairly regular attendances at the annual conferences of the Health Executives and Nurse Administrators. These annual events have been viewed as pleasant social occasions which provide an opportunity for catching up with old friends and acquaintances. Jo is a member of the local golf club, and serves on the committee of the church, the Parents and Friends, and one of the service clubs which work for local charities in Bluefinch. The Chairperson of the Board of Directors of Bluefinch Community Hospital, Lesley Long, a solicitor, also belongs to these organisations.

Robin, partly as a result of the MNA studies, is trying to introduce some new practices to the hospital. Robin was very dissatisfied with some of the nursing care being delivered and felt that evidence was required to back up these feelings of dissatisfaction. Robin, some months ago, had begun collecting and analysing the figures of patient accidents, patient incidents, medication errors, needlestick injuries, wound and IV infections and pressure area occurrences with the help of the Surgical Ward nurse manager who is also studying at university. They are now feeding these results back to the ward staff and as a result IV infections are decreasing as are occurrences of pressure areas.

Formerly accident and incident forms had only been completed by staff if legal problems were likely to arise. The staff used to complain that it was just more paperwork. Since Robin has held a seminar for staff about the advantages of collecting data on performance indicators and dealing with problems at the ward level, there has been a marked improvement in the numbers of reports filed. However the Nursing Unit Manager of the Medical Ward is still resentful that the standard of care provided in that ward should be in any way questioned.

The collection and entry of data is eating into the time available for Robin's other duties, of which responsibility for quality assurance is only one aspect. Jo Pilocovitch does not see any value in collecting figures and considers that the occasional audit and discipline is all that is required for maintaining quality of care and that Robin would be better devoting more time to other administrative matters. Many of these administrative matters are dealt with on an ad hoc basis. There are no long-term goals for the nursing division or for the hospital. Robin also wants the nursing division to develop a strategic plan but Jo considers that a strategic plan is a waste of time. This is because Jo maintains that the government and the Department of Health are always changing their requirements and funding basis for the hospital and anyway the Hospital does not have one. Robin thinks that much could be gained by introducing the first-line nurse manager to ward budgeting and thinks this could be part of the plan for the nursing division.

On analysing the accident and incident figures for the previous six months, Robin found that Friday was the most common day of the week for reports to be sent in on each of the indicators and is surprised by this finding. Robin is not prepared therefore to discontinue data collection and analysis. Robin is also angry because Jo has refused to allow a Quality Assurance Committee to be established maintaining that Robin should be able to handle all that is required. Robin feels that representatives of the staff should be involved in decisions which are going to affect care delivery.

Additionally, both the CEO, Francis Brown, and Jo have been expecting Robin to deal with the resident medical officers' problems, and frequently also with problems that arise with general staff. The CEO, the DON and the Chairperson usually play golf together one afternoon a week and Robin feels that many decisions are made then rather than at executive meetings, and wonders what can be done about this situation.

Robin's present feelings of dissatisfaction have been further increased by feeling overworked and anxious that the improvements made at the hospital will be lost unless some of these delegated matters can be dealt with by those responsible for them.

---

1. How can Robin resolve these role problems?

2. How can Robin persuade the nursing division and the hospital to develop a strategic plan?

3. What should Robin's own strategic plan be?

Your answers should be based on theory and should not exceed 4000 words.

---

# REFERENCES

Adams, A., Donoghue, J., Duffield, C. and Pelletier, D. (1988), 'An exploratory study of attrition in a tertiary nursing programme', *Australian Health Review*, 11:4, 247-255.

Alban Metcalfe, B. M. (1982), 'Leadership: extrapolating from theory and research to practical skills training', *Journal of Management Studies*, 19, 3:295-305.

Alexander, J. W. and Bauerschmidt, A. D. (1987), 'Implications for nursing administration of the relationship of technology and structure to quality of care', *Nursing Administration Quarterly*, 11:4, 1-10.

Altman, S., Valenzi, E. and Hodgetts, R. M. (1985), *Organisational behaviour: theory and practice,* Academic Press, Florida.

Austin, T. W. (1981), 'What can managers learn from leadership theories?', *Supervisory Management*, July:22-31.

Beaman, A. L. (1986), 'What do first-line managers do?', *Journal of Nursing Administration,* 16,5:69.

Barnum, B. S. and Mallard, C. O. (1989), *Essentials of management concepts and practice,* Aspen, Rockville.

Bessant, J. and D'Cruz, J. V. (1989), 'When nurses and teachers strike: public perceptions of "the betrayal"', *The Australian Nurses' Journal*, 6:3, 26-33.

Brewer, A. (1982), Continuing education for health care workers in an era of high technological change: issues and questions, Bathurst: Mitchell C.A.E.

Brewer, A. M. (1983), 'Nurses, nursing and new technology: the implications of a dynamic technological environment', *School of Health Administration Publication* No. 47, Australian Studies in Health Service Administration, Sydney.

Burke, R. J., Weitzel, W. and Weir T. (1982), 'Effective management of day-to-day job performance: motivational strategies and work outcomes', *The Journal of Psychology*, 111:1, 35-40.

Butler, A. (1987), 'Market to recruit, manage to retain — an overview of effective marketing strategies', *Australian Health Review*, 10:3, 229-237.

Cantor, M. M. (1973), 'Philosophy, purpose and objectives: why do we have them?', in Stone, S. Firsich, S. C., Jordan, S. B. et al (1984), *Management for nurses: a multidisciplinary approach* (3rd edition), The C.V. Mosby Company, St Louis.

Carroll, E. and Dwyer, L. (1987), 'Causes of the nursing shortage in N.S.W.: a framework for discussion', *The Lamp*, 44:6, 17-21.

Davis, A. and George J. (1988), *States of health, health and illness in Australia,* Harper & Row, Sydney.

Douglass, L. M. (1988), *The effective nurse, leader and manager* (3rd edition), The C.V. Mosby Company, St. Louis.

Duffield, C. (1989), 'The competencies expected of first-line nursing managers — an Australian context', *Journal of Advanced Nursing*, 14:12, 997-1001.

Dunphy, D. C. and Dick, R. (1982), *Organisational change by choice,* McGraw-Hill, Sydney.

Farmer, E. (1978), 'The impact of technology on nursing', *Nursing Mirror*, 147:13, 17-20.

Gillies, D. A. (1989), *Nursing management a systems approach* (2nd edition), W. B. Saunders Company, Sydney.

Grant, C. and Lapsley, H. M. (1990), 'The Australian health care system 1989', *Australian Studies in Health Service Administration* No. 69, School of Health Administration, Sydney.

Hamilton, P. A. (1982), *Health care consumerism,* The C.V. Mosby Co, St. Louis.

Henry, B., Arndt, C., DiVincenti, M. and Marriner-Tomey, A. (eds) 1989, *Dimension of nursing administration,* Blackwell Scientific, Cambridge, Mass.

Hindle, D. and Scuteri, G. (1988), 'DRG production costs: one more dimension in management information for South Australian hospitals', *Australian Health Review*, 11:4, 320-332.

Hodges, L. C. (1987), 'Head nurses: their practice and education', *Journal of Nursing Administration,* 17:12, 39-44.

Holle, M. L. and Blatchley, M. E. (1987), *Introduction to leadership and management in nursing* (2nd edition), Jones and Bartlett Publishers, Boston.

Holt, D. H. (1987), *Management principles and practice,* Prentice Hall, New Jersey.

Huston, C. J. and Marquis, B. L. (1989), *Retention and productivity strategies for nurse managers,* J. B. Lippincott Company, Sydney.

Kast, F. E. and Rosenzweig, J. E. (1981), *Organisation and management: a contingency approach* (4th edition), Saunders, Philadelphia.

Katz, R. L. (1974), 'Skills of an effective administrator', *Harvard Business Review,* 52, 5:90-102.

Koontz, H., O'Donnell, C. and Weihrich, H. (1984), *Management* (8th edition), McGraw-Hill, Tokyo.

Kron, T. and Gray, A. (1987), *The management of patient-care — putting leadership skills to work* (6th edition), Saunders, Philadelphia.

Lewin, K. (1952), *Field theory in social science,* Tavistock Publications, London.

Lewin, K. (1953), 'Studies in group decisions', in D. Cartwright and A. Zander (eds.), *Group Dynamics: Research and Theory,* Row Peterson, Illinois.

Lippitt, G. (1983), 'Leadership: a performing art in a complex society', *Training and Development Journal,* March: 72-75.

Lumby, J. (1989), 'The new graduate's experience', *1989 Oration Conference: Management and the nurse clinician,* The New South Wales College of Nursing, Sydney.

Lundborg, L. B. (1982), 'What is leadership?', *Journal of Nursing Administration,* May: 32-33.

Manez, J. (1978), 'The untraditional nurse manager: agent of change and changing agent', *Hospitals,* 52:1, 62-65.

Marquis, B. L. and Huston, C. J. (1987), *Management decision making for nurses,* Lippincott, Philadelphia.

Marriner-Tomey, A. (1988), *Guide to nursing management* (3rd edition), The C.V. Mosby Company, St. Louis.

McClure, M. L., Poulin, M. A., Sovie, M. D. and Wandelt, M. A. (1983), *Magnet hospitals, attraction and retention of professional nurses,* American Nurses' Association, Kansas City, Missouri.

McFarland, G. K., Skipton-Leonard, H. and Morris, M. M. (1984), *Nursing leadership and management: contemporary strategies,* John Wiley, New York.

New South Wales Department of Health (1985), *Report of results from phone-in conducted February 1985 for nurses not currently employed in the nursing workforce,* Australian Government Printing Office, Sydney.

New South Wales Department of Health (1986), *Public hospital nurses award 1986 ministerial reference case,* Circular No. 86/308, Australian Government Printing Office, Sydney.

New South Wales Department of Health (1988), *Annual Report 1987-1988,* Australian Government Printing Service, Sydney.

Palmer, G. R. and Short, S. D. (1989), *Health care and public policy, an Australian analysis,* Macmillan, Sydney.

Pelletier, D., Adams, A., Donoghue, J. and Duffield, C. (1989), 'The functions of a nurse: perceptions held by university students of nursing', *Australian Health Review,* 12(3), 43-55.

Pembrey, S. (1984), 'Nursing care: professional progress', *Journal of Advanced Nursing,* 9:6, 539547.

Peters, T. J. and Waterman, R. H. (1982), *In search of excellence,* Warner, New York.

R.A.N.F. (1987), *What you need to know about your new career structure,* Royal Australian Nursing Federation, Perth.

Robbins, S. P. (1989), *Management concepts and applications* (4th edition), Prentice-Hall, Englewood Cliffs, New Jersey.

Shamian, J., Frunchak, V., Miller, G., Georges, P. and Kagan, E. (1988), 'Role responsibilities of head nurses in primary nursing and team nursing units', *Journal of Nursing Administration,* 18:5, 7.

Stevens, B. J. (1985), *The nurse as executive* (3rd edition), Aspen, Rockville.

Stogdill, R. M. (1974), *Handbook of leadership: a survey of theory and research,* Free Press, New York.

Stoner, J. A., Collins, R. R. and Yetton, P. W. (1985), *Management in Australia,* Prentice-Hall, Sydney.

Sullivan, E. J. and Decker, P. J. (1988), *Effective management in nursing* (2nd edition), Addison-Wesley Publishing Company, Sydney.

Toffler, A. (1970), *Future shock,* Random House, New York.

Trexler, B. J. (1987), 'Nursing department purpose, philosophy, and objectives: their use and effectiveness', *Journal of Nursing Administration,* 17, 3:8-12.

Vogt, J. F., Velthouse, B. A., Vox, J. L. and Thames, B. H. (1983), *Retaining professional nurses, a planned process,* The C.V. Mosby Co, St. Louis.

Weisman, C. S., Alexander, C. S. and Chase, G. A. (1981), 'Determinants of staff nurse turnover', *Medical Care,* 19:4, 431-443.

Young, L. C. and Hayne, A. N. (1988), *Nursing administration, from concepts to practice,* W. B. Saunders Company, Sydney.

# CHAPTER 1.2

# Organisational structures and their effects on communication

CHRISTINE DUFFIELD AND JANE STEIN-PARBURY

On completion of this chapter the reader will be able to demonstrate an understanding of:

1.  organisational variables which may affect communication processes;

2.  the unique nature of health care organisations;

3.  the ways in which health care organisations may be structured;

4.  the effects of organisational structures on communication processes and information flow;

5.  ways to facilitate communication flow in an organisation.

The previous chapter described the milieu in which nurse managers are expected to function. Another important factor which influences the role and functions of the first-line nurse manager is the formal structure of the organisation in which he or she must operate. Since competent management involves effective communication, it is important to understand structural variables which can impede or promote communication within the organisation.

The purpose of this chapter is to describe the variety of organisational structures found in health care institutions and the ways in which key organisational variables associated with these structures can have an impact on the communication processes. The relationship between organisational structure and communication is reciprocal; the organisational structure affects the functioning of communication, and communication affects the functioning of the organisational structure. This chapter focuses on the former relationship.

Understanding the relationship between organisational structure and its inherent communication system is necessary for a first-line nurse manager for a variety of reasons. This understanding can be used to enhance communication flow within the existing structure; to develop strategies to overcome communication difficulties caused by that structure; and to influence organisational design so that it will help improve communication effectiveness.

# 1. THE PURPOSE OF STRUCTURE IN AN ORGANISATION

Organisations have three major functions. They have an economic function because they make a productive contribution to the economy. They have a political function because their internal order is based on power and authority. And they have a social function by which human needs such as the need for status, prestige or friendship are fulfilled (Drucker, 1951). An organisation is simply a group of individuals who have come together to achieve a common goal. An understanding and sharing of this goal is dependent on communication processes within the organisation. The formalised way in which these individuals are connected socially and politically is designated by the organisational structure.

An organisation is structured in a particular way to achieve its specific goals. To achieve these goals, which must be congruent with the organisation's mission statement, resources need to be dispensed in an orderly way so that the necessary services can be provided (Beyers, 1984). The organisational structure facilitates the process of resource allocation in several ways. It details the reponsibilities of staff members' attempts to ensure co-ordination between services; clarifies the functions of each sub-unit; identifies where decisions are made and by whom; and outlines formal lines of communication (Brooten, 1984; Douglass, 1988). The relationship between an organisation's structure and its functions is obvious since resource allocation and control are detailed within the structure's budget and documents. The structure, and therefore the functions, of the particular organisation are most frequently represented diagrammatically in the form of an organisational chart.

## 1.1 GENERAL EFFECTS OF ORGANISATIONAL STRUCTURE ON COMMUNICATION

The central feature and primary purpose of communication within organisations is information flow and processing. The communication of information is necessary for the purposes of planning, decision making, evaluating productivity and monitoring the quality of work. The manner in which information is transmitted, perceived and interpreted in an organisation influences organisational effectiveness. The communication of information needs to be both effective and efficient. Effectiveness relates to the sharing of meaning and is dependent upon clarity and sufficiency of information. Ambiguous or insufficient information decreases the effectiveness of communication by obscuring meaning. Efficiency refers to the least amount of resource expenditure necessary to achieve the desired outcome. When information processing is inefficient because it takes an inordinate amount of time, or gets bogged down in the system, this can affect task performance and job satisfaction (Schermerhorn, 1989). Access to information within the organisation may be equated to control and power. These characteristics are often attributed to those 'in the know' because information can be intentionally withheld or intentionally ambiguous for the purposes of gaining or maintaining control.

The organisational structure affects communication in a formal sense by clarifying authority channels and creating 'positional communication' (Redfield cited in Pace, 1983). The content of messages and the manner in which they are transmitted throughout the organisation are often dependent upon the relationship between the position of the person sending the message and the position of the intended recipient. For example, memoranda from superiors to subordinates are frequently couched in prescriptive language, conveying the way superiors view themselves in relation to subordinates. However, positional communication which is based on the formalised structure does not account for all communication in an organisation (Daniels and Spiker, 1987). It refers only to communication which is required by the structure. The head of the radiology department in a large metropolitan teaching hospital may need to communciate to first-line nurse managers the policies and protocols which have been established for patients undergoing specific procedures. He or she may also choose to communicate informally with these same managers regarding the workability of these procedures. Similarly, a member of the medical profession will need to communicate with the nurses on the ward regarding changes in treatment regimens or to determine their views on the client's progress. In this way the information necessary to co-ordinate care between both professional groups can be shared. However, this communication is not usually formalised on the organisational chart, despite its obvious importance for the organisation to achieve its goal of quality patient care.

The way the organisation is structured indicates who has the information, the ways in which this information is accessed and shared, the channels through which the information passes, and the predominant mode of transmission. Although the raw material of communication is information, meanings attached to and derived from the content of the information are bound by the context in which communication occurs (Daniels and Spiker, 1987). The organisational structure is a critical factor in determining this context. An organisation's structure helps to shape the perception held by employees about the importance of their work, their motivation to work as a group and, perhaps more importantly, the distribution of resources and therefore the distribution of power. As an example, in a health care setting, an organisational chart may contain several management layers above the nursing division. Under these circumstances it is difficult to believe that the provision of nursing care is central in achieving organisational goals. A chart such as this also implies that nurses at the ward or unit level have little direct communication with decision-makers, and furthermore, have minimal involvement in decisions which may affect their work at the unit or ward level. The individual's positon relative to where decisions are made also influences communication in terms of the amount and type of information received.

## 1.2 FUNCTIONAL CHARACTERISTICS OF ORGANISATIONAL COMMUNICATION

Before exploring various organisational variables and structures, and their impact on communication, it is necessary to describe some basic characteristics of organisational communication and their relationship to organisational structure. Formal organisational structures affect communication within the organisation primarily in terms of access to information and involvement in decision making. Structures determine whether information flow is centralised or decentralised (Northouse and Northouse, 1985). Channels of communication and the direction of communication flow are most important when evaluating the effects of an organisational structure on communication within that organisation. Other factors, such as managerial style of communication, are also important, but are not reviewed here.

Channels of communication are those avenues or routes through which messages are transmitted in an organisation. They can be formal or informal. An organisational chart prescribes the formal communication channels which are frequently referred to as the 'chain of command'. This formalised system includes reporting responsibilities and accountability. These formal channels flow in a downward, upward and lateral direction.

The type of information disseminated along these channels is characteristic of each channel. Directives often come from the top of the organisational structure and are disseminated along the formal lines of authority. This is the downward flow of information along the structural lines of the organisation. For example, a new method or procedure to be followed in a hospital is sent from nursing administration to each nursing unit via the first-line nurse manager. It is then expected that this new procedure will be adopted by staff at the unit level.

Downward flow often involves information giving, directing and evaluating, all of which can be viewed as prescriptive. The general climate of dominance and submission which pervades downward communication is one of its potential drawbacks because this climate affects the perception of meaning (Daniels and Spiker, 1987). In addition, it is usual for messages flowing downward to be in the form of written communication, which does not allow immediate feedback for clarification. Another potential problem of downward flow is that gatekeepers may receive information but fail to pass it on. This can also occur in upward flow.

Upward flow is the transmission of information from subordinates, those lower on the organisational chart, to superiors, those in a higher position. This form of communication often provides those higher up in the organisation with information which has been sought, as well as requests for clarification in the form of information or feedback. The last use, feedback, is perhaps the most important aspect of effective communication. The major drawback of an upward flow of communication is that subordinates may not be honest with superiors out of fear of reprisal or the need to create a favourable impression (Northouse and Northouse, 1985). Thus, upward communication is frequently filtered and altered before the message is sent.

Lateral or horizontal communication occurs between equals within the organisational hierarchy and does not necessarily relate exclusively to the formal structure. The purpose of this type of communication is not only to inform but to co-ordinate and integrate various organisational activities. It is also one of the means by which people within organisations request and receive support, thus meeting socio-emotional needs of employees. This latter function makes lateral communication unique within the organisational structure. Early discussions of organisational communication frequently ignored this form of communication because it did not fit within the formalised organisational structure (Northouse and Northouse, 1985). Reliance on horizontal communication may not make decision-making and information flow more efficient, but it may enhance effectiveness (Daniels and Spiker, 1987).

Informal communication within an organisation occurs irrespective of the organisational structure and its positional relationships. Informal channels are formed by clusters of people within the organisation who communicate for reasons other than job title or placement on the organisational chart. Informal channels include, but are not limited to, the 'grapevine', and may be sanctioned within the organisation although not part of its formal structure. Information obtained on the grapevine involves what someone else heard or said rather than what was announced by authorities (Pace, 1983). Information transmitted in this manner is often accurate but may be incomplete (Pace, 1983; Northouse and Northouse, 1985; Thompson, 1986; Daniels and Spiker, 1987).

# 2. ORGANISATIONAL VARIABLES AFFECTING THE STRUCTURE OF COMMUNICATION PROCESSES

A variety of organisational variables may affect the nature of management within a given organisation. They do so because of the effects they may have on communication processes, motivation, satisfaction, conflict, resolution and leadership (Kerfoot and Johnson, 1987). Characteristics such as size, complexity, patient mix and specific purpose all influence the ways in which managers function and communicate in health care delivery systems. While many of these variables are not usually amenable to change by nurse managers, nor for that matter by any managers, they are nevertheless important to consider when discussing organisational communication, if for no other reason than to understand the environment in which management is performed.

## 2.1 AGE OF THE ORGANISATION

The age of the organisation determines to some extent the nature of the work conducted within; the classification of staff which undertakes specific tasks; the ways in which this work is allocated and by whom; and the functions of each level of managerial staff. For example, a newly-built organisation will have none of the pre-existing policies, procedures and duty statements which the longer standing organisations will have established. In particular, with no set boundaries as to the classification of employees, one of the first tasks which will need to be undertaken is that of establishing functional delineations between the professions or workers. The uncertainty associated with not knowing the specific work of the organisation in its early development is of particular significance. Once the work has been clearly delineated, the manager must then determine the most efficient and effective method of allocating tasks to work groups, thereby defining the structure of the organisation, the communication processes and the managerial levels necessary to co-ordinate the activities. Older organisations, on the other hand, will have more established work patterns and communication processes, at both the unit or micro level and the macro administrative levels. As a result, newer organisations may appear to be more flexible in their early development, permitting, for example, a novel approach to the development of communication networks. In contrast, older organisations may appear to have firmly entrenched communication channels which cannot be altered. However, it must be assumed that to some extent these communication channels and processes have proved successful or they would not have survived the test of time.

## 2.2 ORGANISATIONAL COMPLEXITY

Health care organisations are complex open systems, characterised by countless interdependent sub-systems (Young and Hayne, 1988). In a work environment such as this, employees have specific roles and tasks to perform, all of which are directed at contributing to the achievement of the organisation's main goal. As the means by which each work group arrives at this goal differs, interdependence is necessary to ensure co-ordination between the various activities of each group. Appropriate communication channels are needed to facilitate an integration of these functions between groups.

A complex organisational environment which exists in most hospitals and health care agencies also requires more accurate and plentiful communication than may otherwise be the case. Formalised and highly developed communication processes may be established in an attempt to meet these requirements. However, decision making in a highly complex organisation is usually more effective if decentralised, since the information required to make a decision may reside further down in the chain of command. Accessing this information can be time-consuming and difficult, especially if gatekeepers or other barriers to effective communication are present.

## 2.3 SIZE OF THE ORGANISATION

The size of the organisation affects management functions and therefore communication patterns. The basic role of nursing managers at all levels remains the same, irrespective of the size and complexity of the organisation (Gugenheim, 1979). However, the scope and dimension of these tasks changes, as does the opportunity the manager has to delegate to others (determined by whether or not there is anyone else to delegate to). Hence the first-line nurse manager in either a 100 or 500 bed hospital may be required to prepare a budget, but the nature of that budget and the support available to assist with budgeting will vary.

The impact of size and information flow on an organisation is fairly obvious. The more employees there are, the more difficult it is for them all to report to the one supervisor. Thus, the larger the organisation, the greater the amount of information flow which is needed, vertically and horizontally, in order to achieve its work (Charns and Schaefer, 1983). To accommodate this flow, an appropriate organisational structure needs to be developed which will enhance and expedite the flow of information. It is likely that larger organisations will have more divisions and subdivisions to facilitate information flow, but all too frequently these divisions create their own barriers to effective communication, unless appropriate methods of integration are in place. Informal communication channels may become significant in facilitating information flow in this instance.

Importantly, as the size of an organisation increases, so does the level of stress among staff (Kahn, Wolfe, Quinn and Snoek, 1964). One of the essential features of communication is listening, which means an ability to accurately perceive the message that is being sent (Young and Hayne, 1988). Stress undoubtedly interferes with this process. An increase in stress levels therefore requires greater skill in communication on the part of managers to overcome the inability of the other party to listen.

## 2.4 COMMUNITY SERVED

The health needs of a particular community can and should influence not only the services offered by health care agencies, but also the way in which these services are structured in the parent organisation. For example, it makes little sense to have a hospital with an infrastructure to support large numbers of operating theatres and an accident and emergency department capable of dealing with major trauma, when the client population consists mainly of elderly residents. Resources need to be allocated to the services required by the community and this allocation then determines the structure within an organisation. It may be more appropriate in the community described above to have an organisation with many nurses, physiotherapists, occupational therapists and social workers who provide less intensive and medically oriented therapies. The greater the mix of staff, the more complex becomes both the co-ordination between staff and the organisational structure necessary to facilitate this co-ordination. The more complex the organisation, the greater the need for accurate and plentiful communication. Again communication processes can only be facilitated when a suitable formal structure is in place.

## 2.5 ORGANISATIONAL CULTURE

Perhaps one of the most pervasive influences on managers and professional practitioners within an organisation is the nature of the organisation itself. Charns and Schaefer (1983) believe that although the performance of the organisation is highly correlated with the quality of the workers it employs, the organisation itself has a significant impact on the performance of the workers. An organisation is a social system and as such has behaviours specific to it or its structure (Smith et al., 1982). An organisation's culture derives from socially learned behaviours and values which are adopted by new members in the organisation. As Peters and Waterman (1982) found in their study, the concept of organisational culture is important in developing the desired organisational values in workers. In this way organisational performance can be enhanced.

A well defined and explicit organisational culture can make the difference between a mediocre company and an excellent one. Health care organisations should be no different. The organisation's culture or its values can be expressed in many ways. Perhaps one of the most common is the symbolic representation of office size or location. If the director of nursing has a very small office removed from the other senior executives, the impression given is that nursing is unimportant to the organisation's activities. This impression filters down through the nursing division as well as through-out the organisation, perhaps manifesting in poor quality nursing care, an inability to recruit outstanding nursing staff, and high rates of staff turnover.

Understanding an organisation's culture can be enhanced by studying the human communication within it. Rules observed in the communication activities may reveal underlying cultural values. How people are addressed is one example. Are doctors referred to by their proper title and surname while nursing staff are called by their given name? This transmits messages regarding the value system. Communication in the organisation helps to shape values and is also the means by which values are shared.

## 2.6 ORGANISATIONAL PHILOSOPHY, GOALS AND OBJECTIVES

An organisation's stated philosophy formally prescribes the ways in which goals and objectives should be achieved. While the goal of two organisations of comparable size, (one a teaching hospital and the second a non-teaching hospital), may be the same (to provide quality patient care), the ways in which each approaches this goal could vary. The teaching hospital with its educational philosophy may encourage knowledge development through research and ongoing staff education, as a means of improving the quality of patient care delivered. On the other hand, the non-teaching hospital may believe that the provision of quality care depends very much on servicing the needs of the particular community, and therefore may view the establishment of a palliative care unit as most important in achieving its goal.

The philosophy of the nursing division, and indeed all divisions within the organi-sation, should be determined by the overall organisational philosophy. Therefore, if an organisation has a strong belief in staff development and research, this should be reflected in the philosophy espoused, not only within the organisation's structure but also within the nursing structure. An examination of the organisational chart should indicate the presence of both education and research positions to which all staff have access.

It is possible that the stated philosophy may not match the organisational culture as described earlier. For example, a philosphy may espouse the belief that patients come first within the health care delivery system. However in reality, because the needs of the organisation come first, under-staffing occurs as a result of drastic cost cutting. In this situation, a conflict exists between that which is idealised in the stated philosophy and that which is real in the culture.

## 2.7 THE NATURE OF HEALTH CARE ORGANISATIONS

There are a variety of characteristics which, although not specific to health care organi-sations, when combined do create a unique environment. These characteristics determine to some extent the structure and therefore the communication processes within the organisation. The most obvious characteristic is the crisis nature of the work undertaken within the organisation, particularly for those in the professions of nursing, medicine and allied health. Coupled with this factor is the high emotionality associated with the health problems which may interfere with communication effectiveness by creating an environment in which there is little time for feedback. The round-the-clock need for care, often of a critical nature, is another overriding factor, since managers are obliged to ensure service provision even in their absence. An appropriate organisational structure is one which provides for adequate after-hours support.

As mentioned earlier, complex organisations require formal channels of communication which are embodied in an hierarchical fashion. The complexity and size of most hospitals have ensured that overdeveloped hierarchies have traditionally been the norm. Under these circumstances, information flow may be restricted and highly formalised, with the decision-making authority centralised at the top. The potential problems outlined previously with regard to downward and upward communication may be realised. Burnout, the result of employees feeling their contribution to the organisation's work or purpose goes unnoticed, is increasingly evident among workers in these organisations, particularly those in the nursing profession. The more formal and developed the organisation and the more critical the nature of the work, the more necessary co-ordination of services and effective communication become.

Health care organisations are unique in that decisions need to be made regarding both patient care and the administration of the organisation (Thompson, 1986). At times organisational values and goals may conflict with those of the professions. Nursing staff may perceive that the organisation is stifling professional standards and values in order to support organisational goals. For example, the quality of patient care may be perceived to be of secondary importance to the running of the organisation in an entrepreneurial manner, particularly when budgetary cuts are imposed. This conflict between organisational and professional values may result in communication conflicts within the organisation.

# **3.** ORGANISATIONAL STRUCTURES: AN OVERVIEW

Within an organisation there are usually multiple divisions and layers, depending on variables such as the size and age of the institution. One of these divisions will invariably relate to nurses and the work of nursing. While the overall structure of the organisation may determine the ways in which this division operates, there are many alternative ways in which it can be structured.

This section will provide an overview of some of the organisational structures found within the health care sector and the effects of each on communication patterns. It is important to consider for each where the nursing division is located and how each structure will affect the role of first-line nurse managers through the relevant reporting mechanisms.

## 3.1 THE BUREAUCRACY

The most common organisational structure is the bureaucracy, first described by Max Weber. A bureaucracy of today can be defined as '... a method for administering a government or business through departments (bureaux) and their subdivisions' (Ford, Armandi and Heaton, 1988). Colloquially, any organisation of a substantial size is referred to as a bureaucracy.

The bureaucratic model of organisation was perceived by Weber to be far superior to any others. There were two main features of his model. The first was leadership style which refers to the social relations within an organisation; the way superiors, subordinates and peers interact. The second was structure, the formal aspects of a bureaucracy which he described as encompassing:

☐ a hierarchy of structure;

☐ a division of labour;

☐ delegated authority to undertake functions;

☐ a formalised structure enshrined in written rules and regulations;

☐ personnel appointed to positions because of their competency (Lansbury and Spillane, 1984; Ford et al., 1988; Young and Hayne, 1988)

**FIGURE 1.2.1**:  Pyramidal model

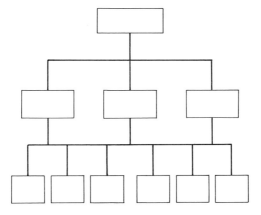

Figure 1.2.1 indicates a clear link between the structure of a bureaucratic organisation and the communication patterns which emerge. A formalised structure such as that depicted above indicates clearly that communication occurs between superiors and subordinates along the vertical axis with little horizontal communication, except at the

upper echelons of management. In this model the higher the position in the hierarchy, the more involved is the individual in planning and decision making and the greater their degree of control. Decision making is largely centralised and outcomes rather than processes are emphasised (Brooten, 1984). This pyramidal structure is based on the theory that as work and the conditions under which it is performed become more complicated, comprehensive and significant to an organisation, then decision making should be shifted upward (Moore and Simendinger, 1979).

Since the focus of this structure is on authority and responsibility, communication can be viewed as a tool for management control and the co-ordination of organisational processes (Daniels and Spiker, 1987). In a classical bureaucratic structure, decision making is centralised near the top and this may restrict information flow. Downward communication may be filtered in a patriarchal 'we know what's best for you to know' fashion. Upward communication can become highly filtered because of mistrust of the hierarchy and/or a lack of access to decision-making power. If an organisation which is structured in this classical way is also enormous, a feeling of disenfranchisement may develop among those in the lower ranks, and a perception that available information is neither adequate nor relevant may prevail. Enormous organisational size may also produce information overload for those at the top. Another difficulty is that the emphasis in this structure is on vertical communication, perhaps minimising the role of horizontal communication and ignoring the informal channels. Generally speaking, in the classical bureaucratic structure, efficiency of communication may occur at the cost of effectiveness (Northouse and Northouse, 1985).

The bureaucratic model also fails to take into account the external environment in which the organisation must function. The dynamic health care environment described in the previous chapter, combined with the complexity of health care organisations described in this chapter, place demands on an organisational structure to be efficient. A bureaucracy is therefore inappropriate because of the difficulties of communication within it. An organisation's structure needs to facilitate lateral communication and be co-operative, non-hierarchical, decentralised and flexible (Barnard cited in Lansbury and Spillane, 1984).

Many of the challenges faced by the health industry have a parallel in other organisational structures in Australia. Dunphy (1982) documents clearly the economic, social and technological forces facing society. He reaches the simple yet significant conclusion that the only certain characteristic of the future is that it will be substantially different from today. He believes that bureaucracies as they currently exist will continue to be unable to cope with the ever-increasing rapidity of change. To be able to deal with the issues, organisations will need to have a flexible, flattened structure with an emphasis on participative and educated managers who manage rather than control. Such a move inevitably leads to further horizontal subdivision within an organisation.

## 3.2 DEPARTMENTALISATION

It is clear from the previous discussion that the dynamic nature of health care and the increased size of organisations have necessitated a move to departmentalisation, which essentially means further subdividing the organisation. Lawrence and Lorsch (1967) noted that as organisations increase in size they begin to differentiate, but at the same time the need for supervision increases. Mintzberg (1983) suggests four benefits of dividing an organisation into departments. These are that a system of supervision becomes possible as like-minded groups are joined; resources are shared within the group; the quality of the group's efforts can be judged by the quality of the common product; and the work group becomes cohesive. He sounds a note of caution, however. While departmentalisation may facilitate co-ordination within the group, intergroup conflict may occur in the battle for limited resources. Conflicts of this kind may impede information sharing. Therefore, due consideration needs to be given to the most appropriate subdivision for the particular organisation.

### 3.2.1 By function

The traditional structure of health care organisations has usually included a division along functional lines. Specialists from the same discipline are divided according to function, for example nursing staff, medical staff and administrative staff each reside in a different division (Figure 1.2.2). Within each of these functional units there are usually further subdivisions. Thus the nursing division could be divided into staff in gastroenterology, cardiology and neonatology, to name a few. Such a division is logical, and simple to organise. It limits duplication of services since all the specialists associated with a particular skill type, for example nursing, are grouped together rather than scattered throughout the organisation. As a result, this type of structure has the advantage of providing ample opportunity for groups to acquire highly developed technical or professional skills. Career development is also facilitated since members of the functional group possess the knowledge and skills necessary for that particular division and can progress upwardly when vacancies arise. Supervision of staff is easy as managers are familiar with the work being performed.

Communication within a functional division is enhanced since it is likely that those performing similar duties will share beliefs and meanings. Communication is facilitated downwards and upwards throughout the division.

There are a few disadvantages of a division by function. Notably, different functional divisions may not share the same view of reality by virtue of their functional orientation and different perspectives. Members of one division may become narrow in their perspective, use specialised language (for example, medical versus nursing diagnoses) and follow certain communication rules in their interactions. Moreover, members of different departments may not share a common language and ground rules for communication interactions. This is particularly true if functional divisions must also compete for limited resources, which is frequently the case between the medical and nursing divisions. All these factors have the potential to interfere with the sharing of meaning and effective communication between members of different divisions.

A further disadvantage is that there may be little formal interchange between staff in different functional divisions. Again this may have an adverse effect on communication patterns. There may be little communication between divisions such as medicine and central administration, except at the more senior levels where the positions are all on the same line. In large organisations this type of structure has a further disadvantage in that the director of the division has a much more difficult task in co-ordinating work efforts than he or she would in a smaller organisation. While senior managers may have highly developed expertise in their particular speciality (for example, nursing), they may lose the breadth of knowledge necessary to manage a large and usually complex division. Another phenomenon seen in Australian health care institutions is the difficulty in moving from one functional group to another, for example nurses moving into mainstream management.

**FIGURE 1.2.2:** Functional division

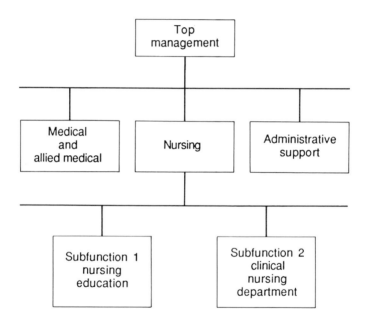

### 3.2.2 By programme or project

In order to overcome the problem of ineffective communication or service duplication, the project organisation was developed (Figure 1.2.3). This structure is topical at the moment and has been proposed frequently in New South Wales as the desired configuration for the Area Health Board structure. It involves organisation into programmes, for example, mental health services or women's health. In this structure, all of the expertise required to deliver the product to a specific target population and attain specific goals is contained within one multidisciplinary team. The team, which may comprise nurses, doctors and allied health, paramedical and administrative staff, reports to the programme director, who is often a representative of one of the disciplines within the team. A structure such as this usually follows from a functional division when the organisation's size or complexity increases (Dunphy and Dick, 1982).

**FIGURE 1.2.3:** Programme division

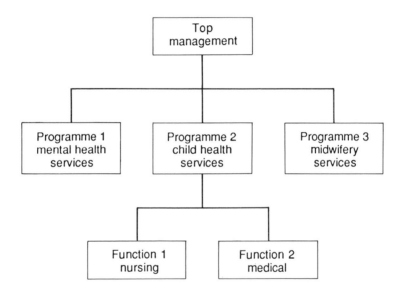

An obvious advantage of this approach is that the manager of the product team is responsible for co-ordinating all work efforts directed at achieving a suitable quality product, rather than a discrete service such as nursing or medicine. This approach overcomes one of the difficulties associated with a separation of employees by function. Team work is facilitated and managers can determine whether the quality of the final product (the outcome) is satisfactory. For such a structure to work effectively, persons selected to co-ordinate teams or programmes must have general management skills, since they are no longer relying solely on the technical skills and specific knowledge needed to manage a division of like-minded individuals. Instead they are responsible for a multi-disciplinary, multi-skilled team.

A disadvantage of this structure is that while duplication of services directed at a target population is overcome, duplication along divisional lines may occur instead. For example, a team directed at the care of persons with a mental illness will require a social worker, as might three or four other project teams, each with a different specialist focus and each necessitating the employment of several specialist social workers. On a different note, the nurses working in the mental health team may lose their affiliation with the nursing division, resulting in 'de-skilling' and a lack of familiarity with changes in nursing practice and professional issues. A further disadvantage (as perceived by senior managers) is that heads of teams usually have a great deal of autonomy and authority. As a result, senior management may lose control of the activities conducted within the organisation by employees who would usually report to them. For example, the senior nurse manager would have little control over the work of nurses in such a model since they report to a team leader. Lastly, while information flow may be effective within a programme, it may be impeded across programmes, depending on the size, complexity and decision-making authority within the organisation.

### 3.2.3 By territory or location

This model occurs more frequently as a structure for a large organisational framework rather than within a specific institution, and as a result is seen less often in health care organisations. In this structure an organisation is divided according to different geographical locations (Figure 1.2.4). For example, several buildings in a particular health care complex could be organised according to location, Block A, Block B and so on. The advantage of such a structure is that each location or building is self-contained. However this can also lead to the disadvantage of a duplication of services and positions, and therefore of resource consumption, between locations. For example, there may need to be a director of nursing at each location with a more senior nurse manager to co-ordinate nursing services overall (for example a principal director of nursing). Similarly, social workers, dieticians and other personnel may be required for each location, resulting in further duplication. The communication between locations is usually minimal and frequently occurs only at the senior levels of management.

FIGURE 1.2.4:   Division by location

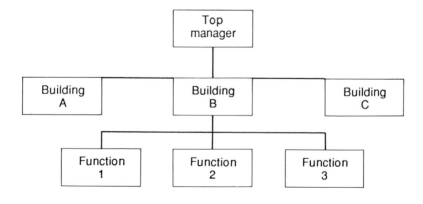

## 3.2.4 Matrix organisation

The last organisational structure to be discussed is the matrix, or multiple command system (Figure 1.2.5) (McClure, 1984). This structure is particularly suitable for complex organisations which must function in a dynamic environment. The matrix is a two dimensional model in which work and responsibilities are grouped according to two different dimensions (diagrammatically displayed along horizontal and vertical axes), often according to function and programme (Dunphy and Dick, 1982; Charns and Schaefer, 1983). This structure combines the programme and function form of departmentalisation. There are two hierarchies involved in decision making, one responsible for a specific programme, the other responsible for a specific function. Programmes are frequently service oriented, while functions often have a professional orientation. Such a model overcomes many of the difficulties associated with a classical bureaucratic model, particularly when used in the nursing division. For example, it eliminates layers of administration, rules and regulations are less rigid and individual nurses are able to rely more on their own professional judgement than on that of superiors (Johnson and Tingey, 1976). A movement away from task orientation by nursing staff is also facilitated. This has the potential for decreasing conflict between professional and work environment values, thereby enhancing job satisfaction.

**FIGURE 1.2.5:**  A matrix

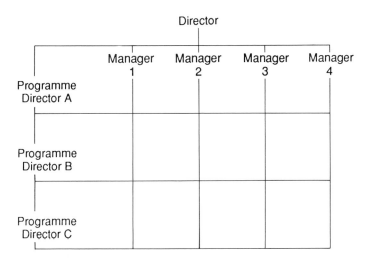

The matrix model overcomes another of the difficulties associated with the bureaucratic model by facilitating not only vertical but also horizontal communication, thus emphasising flexibility and co-ordination between services or units. This model has as a major goal the devolution of decision-making to the level at which specialist knowledge is most usually found, and an increase in the amount of communication between staff.

The matrix model may be used throughout the organisation or alternatively within a particular division, for example a nursing division (Figure 1.2.6). If a matrix structure is used throughout an organisation, the health care agency may become divided into a series of teams with a manager in charge of each. The organisation can be divided into large multi-disciplinary teams using programme organisation or different geographic sites, or alternatively into smaller multi-disciplinary units such as a unit or ward. The latter places first-line nurse managers in the ideal position to co-ordinate and integrate all the services and facilities at their disposal. All personnel required to provide services to a particular client population report to this first-line manager who directs and co-ordinates nursing, medical, paramedical and ancillary services. Staff continue to report to their own respective department head in an administrative sense. Herein lies one disadvantage of the matrix structure, the potential conflict that arises in reporting to two superiors. Such a system engenders conflicts of dual allegiance (Schermerhorn 1989). A high demand for co-ordination is placed upon the communication system, and clear role differentiation between functional and programme heads is vital.

**FIGURE 1.2.6:**   Matrix structure in a nursing division

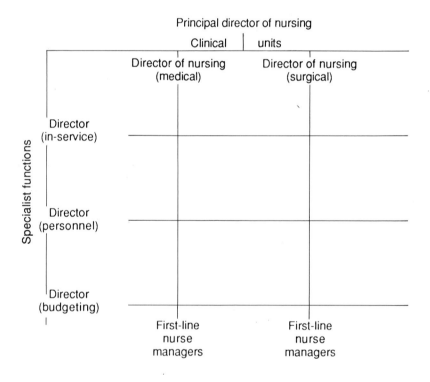

Irrespective of whether the entire organisation or just the nursing division is structured in this way, use of the matrix model provides nurses with a greater opportunity to expand their role in co-ordinating patient care (Moore and Simendinger, 1979).

# 4. ENVIRONMENT AND ORGANISATIONAL STRUCTURE

Burns and Stalker (1961) endeavoured to explain the link between environmental considerations and organisational design and structure. They studied 20 industrial firms in the United Kingdom, concluding that there were two different types of organisations, 'mechanistic' and 'organic'. The mechanistic structure is highly bureaucratic and therefore has centralised decision making, rules, procedures, a precise division of labour, narrow spans of control and formal methods of co-ordination. The organic structure, on the other hand, is decentralised, has fewer rules, regulations and procedures, a less precise division of labour, wider spans of control and less formal methods of co-ordination (Schermerhorn, 1989). In a stable environment a mechanistic structure is more appropriate, while in an unpredictable market where flexibility is required, the organic structure is more suitable.

The work of Burns and Stalker was extended by Lawrence and Lorsch (1967). While Burns and Stalker determined that an organisation must be capable of responding to the environment, Lawrence and Lorsch found that in large organisations individual departments must also be responsive. They concluded that departments or subsystems within organisations develop a structure which is related to the certainty of their own environment, and thus there may be variations throughout the organisation. For example, nursing units which are technologically dependent and have patients requiring frequent monitoring and observations, require less consultation by superiors with staff in decision making. On the other hand, those wards with varying patient diagnoses function better with a structure in which horizontal participation in decision making is the norm (Alexander and Bauerschmidt, 1987).

Lawrence and Lorsch defined two terms in their study, 'differentiation', which was the degree of difference between sub-systems in the organisation, and 'integration', the level of co-ordination between sub-systems. The more uncertain the organisational environment, the greater the need for differentiation between sub-systems. The greater the degree of differentiation, the greater the need to co-ordinate the activities which occur within.

Peters and Waterman (1982) noted that those organisations which were considered excellent and innovative were those which were loosely organised, relied heavily on informal communication and were capable of rapid responses to customer demands and needs. Peters and Waterman refer to 'structural fluidity', a means by which excellent companies function because they are unimpaired by tight organisational constraints. They contrast this concept with the adhocracy described by Toffler (1970) which is a structure where nobody is really clear who performs which function. Overnight an organisation may change, resulting in different jobs, responsibilities and reporting mechanisms. As described by Peters and Waterman, the result may be that 'nobody does anything'. However, in their experience excellent companies were able to take advantage of this type of structure through the use of a large and informal open communication system. Informality, intensity and the use of physical structures to facilitate communication are the features of excellent companies.

Kramer and Schmalenberg (1988a, 1988b) applied the characteristics of excellence, as developed by Peters and Waterman, to a selected sample of magnet hospitals in the United States. These hospitals demonstrated the same communication characteristics of informality, spontaneity and encouragement for innovation as found by Peters and Waterman. Information flowed freely and continuously in these institutions. There was both perceived and real access to management and trust in management's responsiveness to the identified work needs and problems. Decentralised decision making prevailed and this 'radical decentralisation' is cited as the 'major force in helping these magnet hospitals develop into institutions of excellence' (Kramer and Schmalenberg, 1988b:17).

The elements of communication found in magnet hospitals are similar to those characteristics of an organic structure described by Burns and Stalker, (1961). The importance of adequate and effective communication to an organisation's functioning becomes clear. Excellence is fostered in institutions with a structure that ensures information flow is adequate and accurate. These institutions rely on and use informal channels, and provide ready access to management in the process. Circumstances such as these create a climate of openness, trust and responsiveness. The emphasis on informal communication in these excellent or magnet organisations cannot be ignored. Informality and flexibility promote responsiveness and adaptation to a changing environment. An organisation too reliant on formal channels along structural lines may be limited in its efforts to respond to a changing health care delivery environment.

# 5. INTEGRATING FUNCTIONS

A number of organisational variables associated with institutions in the health care sector have been discussed. Variables such as the nature of the work of providing care for sick clients; the size of most organisations, which necessitates departmentalisation; and the scarcity of resources, indicate that there is a need for great co-ordination. To maintain effectiveness, organisations must have a means by which functions can be integrated. This can be achieved through either vertical or horizontal co-ordination, and ideally by both.

## 5.1 HIERARCHY OF AUTHORITY

The hierarchy of authority, or chain of command as it is referred to, is depicted in the organisational chart and identifies to whom each member of staff reports. Ideally a staff member should report to only one superior. This is the case in all structures described except the matrix structure. Referral of a problem upwards facilitates co-ordination since by virtue of their position, superiors have a different perspective of the organisation. Similar units should be placed together so that as few levels of the hierarchy as possible need to be contacted for these like-minded units to communicate. For example, in a nursing division, units which are similar functionally, such as intensive care, burns, coronary care and perhaps accident and emergency, should report to the same superior. This individual will co-ordinate the flow of information between these units and facilitate integration between them.

## 5.2 SPAN OF CONTROL

The span of control is the number of staff members who report to each superior and between five and seven is frequently quoted as ideal for any manager. However this depends on a variety of factors such as the similarity and complexity of tasks, geographical spread in the organisation, group size and subordinate characteristics (Ford et al, 1988; Schermerhorn, 1989). The wider the span of control, the fewer levels will appear in the organisation's structure. A tall hierarchy, as in the classic pyramidal bureaucracy, is slow to respond and does not enable information to flow quickly throughout the organisation. Generally, the flatter the structure and therefore the greater the span of control, the more rapidly will information be disseminated. Adequate and accurate information can lead to more effective problem solving and decision making.

## 5.3 DELEGATION

Associated with the span of control is delegation, which is an important managerial tool for allocating work, authority and responsibility to employees. The wider the span of control, the greater the number of staff a manager has for the purposes of delegation. Weighed against this factor though is the fact that the more staff there are to whom work must be delegated, the less supervision the manager will be able to provide. This necessitates the selection of autonomous employees who are capable of working with little direct supervision. A small span of control enables the manager to delegate tasks while still providing a great deal of supervision. A delegation of tasks by managers facilitates the participation of staff in decision making, provides staff with information, and also ensures that more employees are familiar with the functioning of the organisation.

Delegation has another advantage for a manager. By allocating responsibility for certain functions to other members of staff, the manager is required to process less information. Managers who are unable or unwilling to delegate are at risk of suffering from information overload, especially in a classical bureaucratic structure. Delegation also places a greater responsibility for communication within an organisation on the employees. It is no longer seen solely as the responsibility of managers.

## 5.4 DECENTRALISATION VS CENTRALISATION

The other difference in structure which affects the complexity of co-ordination and integration by nurse managers is the degree to which decision making is permitted to be undertaken at the various levels of management. In other words, do senior managers make all the decisions or is this process to some extent decentralised? At the unit level, are first-line nurse managers allowed to determine and control their own budget and staffing or is this responsibility held by the senior managers?

Decentralisation is not a new idea: it was first discussed in the 1960s. Its goal is to ensure that decision making occurs where the work is actually being undertaken (McClure, 1984). The effect of this process is obvious. Accountability for actions extends beyond the senior management level, with employees at all levels being responsible for decisions directly related to their work. There are two components of decentralisation, the communication aspect and the delegation aspect (Dessler, 1986). The link between communication and decentralisation centres on the degree to which employees must continue to channel their communication through the head of the organisation. The more decentralised an organisation, the greater the likelihood that the knowledge required to make decisions will reside at the lower levels and the more involved managers at the workface will be in the communication process. Perhaps even more important is that information flow will be multi-directional. On the other hand, placement in the organisation too far away from centralised authority could result in feelings of alienation, especially if the position held carries a degree of responsibility. In this way organisational structure affects accessibility to the decision-making authority, and therefore, the integration and co-ordination of information flow.

# 6. HORIZONTAL CO-ORDINATION

The classic bureaucratic structure provides little opportunity to co-ordinate functions horizontally, except at the senior management levels. Similarly, the subdivisions described earlier, such as by function, programme and location, also provide little opportunity for horizontal communication between each subdivision, except at the top. However, there are methods for facilitating horizontal co-ordination. For example, the use of staff managers as advisers to line managers will ensure that information passed on is consistent. This same principle applies to the use of highly specialised staff such as clinical nurse consultants, who can provide technical knowledge and expertise wherever it is required. Along this same line, the use of specialist teams such as palliative care and geriatric assessment teams also integrates functions throughout an organisation. Another method of horizontal co-ordination seen increasingly in nursing divisions is the use of personal assistants to directors of nursing. By delegating much of the routine administrative work to their assistants, senior nurse managers have more time for complex problem-solving, while the administrative assistants ensure that information is disseminated and similar advice is given throughout the nursing division. Dessler (1986) also advocates the use of a liaison person and committees to facilitate horizontal integration.

Horizontal communication is plagued by difficulties related to territoriality, specialisation and lack of effort (Daniels and Spiker, 1987). Information may not be shared because of 'turf' battles, lack of shared experiences and an unwillingness to invest time and effort in resolving these differences. These difficulties need to be addressed before attempts are made to increase horizontal communication. One of the most successful methods of overcoming these difficulties and ensuring horizontal co-ordination is the use of informal communication networks. Informal systems of communication will not make up for information inadequacies within the formal structure. However a variety of information sources, both formal and informal, enable managers to keep abreast of what is happening. Information communication methods such as the grapevine need not be feared, since people talking to each other about their work is a sign of active engagement and involvement. (Pace, 1983; Northouse and Northouse, 1985; Thompson, 1986; Daniels and Spiker, 1987). Lack of an active grapevine within an organisation could indicate apathy. Knowing what is being discussed on the grapevine provides useful information for the first-line nurse manager. Often, however, managers are not included in grapevine discussions between staff. One solution to this is for the manager to give out more information, thereby enabling greater reception of it. This suggestion is based on the assumption that managers are left out because they don't give out information (Thompson, 1986). Another suggestion is for managers to send accurate information along the grapevine. The rationale here is that since the grapevine exists anyway it can be put to some use.

# 7. A FINAL NOTE ON ORGANISATIONAL COMMUNICATION

As was seen throughout this chapter, organisational structure determines some parameters within which an organisation can operate. This includes certain rules about the flow of information. While organisational structures cannot prevent people from communicating on a personal level (informal), they do prescribe authority and reporting relationships in the formal channels. This can limit or enhance the communication interaction in a prescriptive way. Interpersonal communication has two dimensions, the content dimension and the relationship dimension. The former refers to the information in a message as displayed through language, while the latter details the relationship between participants in the interaction (Northouse and Northouse, 1985). These two dimensions are inextricably connected. Organisational structure affects the relationship dimension of communication interactions in particular by defining status and power differences. For example, a comment such as 'I want to see you today' would have a different meaning if it came from a superior than if it came from a colleague. The content remains the same but the power and status relationship between the two participants is different, thereby affecting the interpretation of the message. If top management sends a memorandum to all employees suggesting a voluntary alteration in work practices, it is unlikely that it will be interpreted as a suggestion. It will more likely be interpreted as a mandate, however 'veiled' may be the message. The interpretation of the message content in these examples pertains to the relationship dimension of human communication.

The most appropriate climate for effective organisational communication is one which is flexible, allowing channels to be accessed easily and freely by those who need to do so. Rigid adherence to the hierarchy and the formal chain of command can result in faulty decision making by restricting the flow of information in the organisation. It also places high information processing demands on those at the top who may suffer information overload as a result. Decentralisation of decision making is one way to promote an effective climate for organisational communication. Through decentralised decision making, accurate and adequate information is shared with those affected by the decisions. Involving the people who will be most directly affected by the decision encourages a sense of influence and control, as it conveys the message that workers in the organisation are capable and competent. The general climate of openness and trust which is likely to result can positively affect communication within the organisation.

However, all communication occurs within a context and these general guidelines do not account for situational variables. Decentralised decision making is best for large organisations, together with flattened hierarchies, flexible administration and participative managers. There is a danger that a philosophy of control, if firmly entrenched, will prevail despite change in the formal organisational structure. Belief systems operating within an organisation may be resistant to change.

Ways of dealing with these effects can include:

☐ improving communication with staff by providing adequate and accurate information;

☐ increasing upward communication;

☐ using informal channels;

☐ developing feedback systems.

# SUMMARY

The formal structure of an organisation affects and is affected by communication within the organisation. Some structures are more likely to limit information dissemination while others may enhance it. Inherent in all organisational structures is the need to co-ordinate activities and integrate various functions. This places high demands on the people within the organisation to share information in an effective and efficient manner. Information flow along structural lines accounts for part of the communication within organisations, the formal communication channels. In addition, an awareness and use of informal channels assists with information flow and enhances overall communication.

# DRYANDRA CASE STUDY 1

Dryandra Base Hospital is located in Dryandra, a city which serves as the commercial centre of a thriving rural area some 300 kilometres from the state capital. The town has excellent educational and recreational facilities. There are two high schools, a number of primary schools, and a private school which caters for all grades. In addition there is a new university. There are two dams in close proximity, one of which is available for water sports, and the snowfields are within three hours' drive. The population of the Dryandra region is approximately 170 000 with about 32 000 being resident in Dryandra city.

Dryandra Base Hospital is a 300 bed hospital with a recently established day surgery unit, a psychiatric unit, a regional geriatric assessment unit, a regional developmental disabilities unit and rehabilitation unit in addition to the usual facilities for the care of accidents and emergencies. The wards in the hospital care for acute medical, surgical, orthopaedic, paedriatric, obstetric and gynaecological patients. Community health services are also co-ordinated from a separate Community Health Centre located within the hospital's grounds.

Adjacent to the Dryandra Base Hospital are the Dryandra Nursing Home and Hostel with 30 beds each. There is also a private nursing home and hostel in the large Dicksonia Retirement Village situated in one of the outlying suburbs as well as a number of other small private nursing homes scattered throughout the town.

Another major hospital situated in Hakea, an affluent suburb of Dryandra, is the Hakea Private Hospital which has taken over much of the elective surgery in the town. The Hakea Private Hospital has also recently obtained a lithotripter as there are now two urologists among the town's 54 general practitioners and specialists.

The Director of Nursing at Dryandra Base Hospital is Lesley Linum, who returned to Dryandra after a number of years absence. Lesley had served as an Assistant Director of Nursing for three years at a 200 bed hospital in another state prior to completing a Master of Nursing Administration degree. Lesley has been the DON for the past year but is only now beginning to feel comfortable in the position which is just as well considering the events of the past week.

Last Monday at the Executive Meeting the Chief Executive Officer, Radna Razneuth, a Master of Health Administration graduate, had announced that a letter had been received from the Regional Office notifying them of the formation of Area Health Services. Dryandra was to combine with the smaller towns of Cordyline and Psoralea to form the Dryandra Area Health Services. Both Cordyline and Psoralea have their own hospitals, Cordyline with 64 beds and Psoralea with 32. There is also a small Community Health Centre in each town providing the usual services.

Radna asked Lesley and the Director of Medical Services, Tsui Lei, to submit their plans for the reorganisation of the nursing and medical services on an area wide basis being mindful of the functions of the Area Health Boards as outlined in the Government report on the restructuring of health services. They were also asked to submit their plans for implementation and their timeline for the project.

Prepare Lesley's plan for the reorganisation of the nursing services on an area wide basis.

1. Describe how you intend to implement the plan.

2. Provide a realistic time frame for implementation of the reorganisation.

# REFERENCES

Alexander, J. W. and Bauerschmidt, A. D. (1987), 'Implications for nursing administration of the relationship of technology and structure to quality of care', *Nursing Administration Quarterly*, 11:4, 1-10.

Beyers, M. (1984), 'Getting on top of organisational change, Part 1. Process and development', *The Journal of Nursing Administration*, 14:10, 32-39.

Brooten, D. A. (1984), *Managerial leadership in nursing*, J. B. Lippincott Company, Philadelphia.

Burns, T. and Stalker, G. M. (1961), *The management of innovation*, Tavistock, London.

Charns, M. P. and Schaefer, M. J. (1983), *Health care organisations, a model for management*, Prentice-Hall, New Jersey.

Daniels, T. D. and Spiker B. K. (1987), *Perspectives on organisational communication*, Wm. C. Brown, Iowa.

Dessler, G. (1986), *Organisation theory, integrating structure and behaviour* (2nd edition), Prentice-Hall, New Jersey.

Douglass, L. M. (1988), *The effective nurse leader manager* (3rd edition), The C.V. Mosby Company, St. Louis.

Drucker, P. F. (1951), *The new society*, Heinemann, London.

Dunphy, D. C. and Dick, R. (1982), *Organisational change by choice*, McGraw-Hill, Sydney.

Ford, R. C., Armandi, B. R. and Heaton, C. P. (1988), *Organisation theory, an integrative approach*, Harper & Row, New York.

Gugenheim, A. M. (1979), 'Health care leaders examine role of nursing service administrator', *Hospitals*, 53:2, 109-111.

Johnson, G. V. and Tingey, S. (1976), 'Matrix organisation: blueprint of nursing care organisation for the 80s', *Hospital and Health Services Administration*, 21:1, 27-39.

Kahn, R. L., Wolfe, D. M., Quinn, R. P. and Snoek, J. D. (1964), *Organisational stress: studies in role conflict and ambiguity*, John Wiley and Sons, Sydney.

Kerfoot, K. M. and Johnson, J. E. (1987), 'Assessing the organisation', in K. W. Vestal (ed.) *Management concepts for the new nurse*, J. B. Lippincott Company, Sydney.

Kramer, M. and Schmalenberg, C. (1988a), 'Magnet hospitals: part I', *Journal of Nursing Administration*, 18:1, 13-24.

Kramer, M. and Schmalenberg, C. (1988b), 'Magnet hospitals: part II', *Journal of Nursing Administration*, 18:2, 10-19.

Lansbury, R. D. and Spillane, R. (1984), *Organisational behaviour: the Australian context,* Longman Cheshire, Melbourne.

Lawrence, P. R. and Lorsch, J. W. (1967), 'Differentiation and integration in complex organisations', *Administrative Science Quarterly,* 12:1, 1-47.

McClure, M. L. (1984), 'Managing the professional nurse Part 1: The organisational theories', *The Journal of Nursing Administration,* 14:2, 15-20.

Mintzberg, H. (1979), *The structuring of organisations: A synthesis of research,* Prentice-Hall, New Jersey.

Mintzberg, H. (1983), *Structure in fives: designing effective organisations,* Prentice-Hall, New Jersey.

Moore, T. F. and Simendinger, E. (1979), 'The matrix organisation: its significance to nursing', *Nursing Administration Quarterly,* 13:2, 25-31.

Northouse P. G. and Northouse L. L. (1985), *Health communication: a handbook for health professionals,* Prentice-Hall, New Jersey.

Pace, R. W. (1983), *Organisational communication: foundations for human resource development,* Prentice-Hall, New Jersey.

Peters, T. J. and Waterman, R. H. (1982), *In search of excellence,* Harper and Row, New York.

Schermerhorn, J. R. (1989), *Management for productivity* (2nd edition), John Wiley and Sons, New York.

Smith, M., Beck, J., Cooper, C. L., Cox, C., Ottaway, D. and Talbot, R. (1982), *Introducing organisational behaviour,* Macmillan, London.

Thompson, T. L. (1986), *Communication for health professionals: a relational perspective,* Harper and Row, New York.

Toffler, A. (1970), *Future shock,* Random House, New York.

Young, L. C. and Hayne, A. N. (1988), *Nursing administration from concepts to practice,* W. B. Saunders Company, Sydney.

# Staffing: the human resource challenge

SUSANNE ROSBROOK

After reading this chapter, you should be able to:

1. identify influences both external and internal to the organisation which affect the development of the nursing staff plan;

2. distinguish between differing modes of nursing care delivery, by reference to their basic underlying philosophies;

3. understand the difference between methods for determining the number and mix of staff required;

4. describe methods used in the allocation and rostering of staff;

5. discuss the role of the nurse manager in dealings with the human resource functions;

6. recognise the importance of shaping the work environment and work practices to reflect the value placed upon these resources.

How managers structure the work and the work force within their areas affects the efficiency and effectiveness with which the organisation's mission is achieved. As well, such structuring reflects the extent to which the stated nursing philosophy is used to guide nursing practice. Where the manager views staff as the catalysts in the provision of nursing services, rather than as ingredients in the manufacture of this product, staff participation in defining the work environment and practices is actively encouraged. Many approaches to the structuring of the work and of the workforce are possible, and the methods adopted within each nursing service setting should reflect the values of staff working within that area. This develops a climate in which trust and staff responsibility for accounting for patient care outcomes can thrive.

As has been identified elsewhere in this book, the quality of any organisation's products depends not only upon good organisational structuring, but also upon the reliability of its operations and the commitment of its employees. The values and beliefs reflected in the organisation's philosophy and mission statements should also be incorporated in all policies underlying its operations. These then establish the organisation's priorities in the management of all the resources available as it seeks to provide a high quality product which meets the general public's needs and expectations.

Within a service industry, the most vital organisational resource consists of the individuals who provide the services. This is recognised by the increasing tendency to alter the name of staff or personnel departments and practices to more accurately reflect the value placed on human resources. No longer are workers conceived of as being only a part of a machine-like production process, the continuation of which is unrelated to the individuals who are part of the production line. They are now recognised as being the actual determinants of the quality and quantity of the service provided, as Yuill et al (1978:20) clearly state:

> Astute managers know that their subordinates have positive power to carry out their tasks. The manager may order, threaten or cajole, but unless dynamic man is willing to actively perform his tasks there will be no effective work.

Structuring the human resource functions and patterns within an organisation or unit, so that organisational goals are achievable, requires adoption of a future-oriented, comprehensive and integrative perspective. Not only is the manager looking to ensure that the right number and type of people are available at the right time and place to undertake the work required to fulfil organisational needs, but also to ensure that the practices and approaches of employees to their work reflect commitment to the organisational mission, values and beliefs. Management practices which recognise the value of employee contributions to the achievement of the organisation's goals enhance the probability that employees' expectations of the work and work environment will be met. Where these expectations are met, Friss (1981:14) identifies that 'employees are more likely to be satisfied, to remain with the organisation and to stay active within the profession'.

Schuler et al (1988:10) identify the five main functions and activities of human resource management as being 'planning for human resource needs; staffing the personnel needs of the organisation; appraising and compensating employee behaviour; improving employees and the work environment; [and] establishing and maintaining effective working relationships'. In nursing, terms frequently used when referring to these functions and activities include the following:

☐ establishing a staffing plan, designing and describing jobs and positions within the organisation and specifying the preferred skill mix;

☐ recruiting, selecting and assigning appropriately skilled individuals to these positions to ensure the right numbers and types of individuals are available at the right time and place to fulfil organisational needs;

☐ undertaking performance appraisals, and providing rewards (both monetary and non-monetary) appropriate for the performance and positional level occupied;

☐ providing orientation, in-service training and staff development, conducting quality assurance and related activities and seeking means to develop the organisation to meet the expectations of those both within and outside the organisation;

☐ seeking to establish role relationships which, as well as enabling monitoring of activities, provide support, assistance and guidance within work teams at all levels of the hierarchy, and promote job satisfaction, worker motivation and commitment to achieving nursing and organisation goals.

# **1.** INFLUENCES ON THE DEVELOPMENT OF A STAFFING PLAN

More and more, nurse managers are being called upon to substantiate their staffing plans, and demonstrate how the components will help achieve effectiveness, efficiency, cost benefit and specified quality outcomes. The challenge is to specify a plan which maximises the opportunities and minimises the constraints associated with achieving nursing's identified mission.

The objectives of any health care organisation, its nursing division and the service units within it, describe in specific terms what is to be achieved — the goal or purpose of practice. As the means of achieving the goal cannot be separated from the goal itself, these objectives include both those relating directly to the provision and outcomes of nursing care and those related to the practitioners who provide that care. In efficient and effective provision of nursing services, these objectives are achieved simultaneously.

Objectives relating to the staffing of nursing organisations are developed within the environment of the experiences, expectations and beliefs of those both within and without the particular organisation.

Some of the **external** influences arise from:

☐ the Government, which directly regulates many activities through legislation as well as less directly (but far more obviously) through the economic boundaries prescribed;

☐ the general community, members of which have (often unstated) expectations of what a health care organisation provides;

☐ the general workforce, with expectations of what form the relationship between employer and employee should assume in Australia. These expectations are to some extent moulded by the formal Industrial Relations system which, through its approval of Industrial Awards and Agreements, establishes specific conditions of employment binding on both employers and employees within various workplaces;

The influences **internal** to the organisation include those arising from:

☐ the administrators, who seek to define what the terms economy, effectiveness and efficiency mean within this particular setting or organisation;

☐ the health care workforce, many of whom have been socialised as 'professionals', and so have expectations about what the provision of health related services entails, and the relationships which should exist between those providing such services;

☐ the actual consumers of the health care services provided, who seek to reconcile the experience with their previous expectations;

☐ the culture of the organisation, which is expressed not only formally in its philosophy, statements of desired outcomes, authority relationships and operational documents, but also informally in how the shared, collectively accepted values and meanings of those within an organisation shape actual relationships and practices.

The combination of experience and expectations about the nature of the work and of the workforce underlies the development of the staffing plan. Staffing is the largest and most crucial aspect of management in a service industry. The staffing plan should be a document flexible enough to guide current human resources practices within the organisation, as well to enable adaptation as changes occur as a result of influences from both the internal and external environment. In addition the plan components should help substantiate requests for resources, and account for the manner in which the abilities and qualities of staff members will help achieve the organisation's goal.

In meeting the challenge of developing such a plan, the goals of the nursing service are not the only issue to be considered. At least some of the environmental opportunities and constraints which influence the extent to which any plan is realistically attainable must be identified. This requires the identification and analysis of such areas as the numbers and levels of personnel which are currently or potentially available to the organisation; methods by which appropriate personnel can be attracted, selected and recruited to, and retained and developed within, the organisation; the extent to which current legal, industrial relations, economic and mind-set factors predetermine how the objectives may be achieved; how 'quality patient care' is defined in this service setting; and the degree and type of technology considered appropriate for achieving such quality.

Consideration of such information, as Graham et al (1987:14) point out, can enable the nursing organisation's philosophy and mission to be:

transformed into a positioning statement that articulates a "vision" for the department of nursing and provides a framework when planning to thrive rather than merely survive in today's changing and competitive health care environment ... (thus enabling) nurse executives to empower staff to respond proactively to change and prepare for the future.

The most obvious outcome of this is the delineation of the 'who', 'what' and 'why' of nursing in this setting; the expectations associated with this are expressed in the job descriptions or position statements which identify what is expected of the individual nurses. The manner in which these expectations are expressed — the extent to which the statement of expectations focuses upon outcomes or processes of care provision — will reflect the model selected for delivery of nursing care services.

# 2. NURSING CARE DELIVERY MODELS

Nursing literature is replete with descriptions of various modes by which the delivery of nursing care services may be organised. It includes descriptions of functional nursing, team nursing, modular nursing, total patient care nursing, primary nursing, case nursing, and case management nursing. As a generalisation, these different modalities reflect the extent to which the service has adopted one of the two differing philosophies on how total patient care needs can be met.

The two philosophies are 1) that the completion of all tasks related to patient care will ensure that patients' needs for care are met; and 2) that one nurse's adoption of responsibility for planning and providing the total care of a patient will result in all of that patient's needs for care being identified and met. The first of these underlies task-based nursing practice, the second patient-based practice.

The task-based approach to the provision of nursing services is a result of accepting the 'scientific management' rationale — that maximum efficiency, economy and effectiveness result from the standardisation of overall processes into tasks which can be undertaken by a team of workers, each member of which, through repetition, gains proficiency in performing a limited range of tasks. The advantages and the disadvantages of this approach are outlined in Table 1.3.1. Table 1.3.2 contains a summary of the advantages and the disadvantages associated with using a patient-based approach to the provision of nursing services — one nurse being responsible for meeting the total nursing needs of a patient in a one-to-one relationship, the nurse remaining with the patient until the services are no longer required. Behaviourist theories provide justification for using this approach.

Given the constraints on the hours of work which can realistically and legally be expected of one nurse, variations upon case-nursing assignment within organisations usually result in an emphasis upon one nurse planning the care required, and delivering this care while actually with the patient. Assistant or associate nurses then continue to implement the care plan whenever the case-nurse is absent.

Although it must be realised that the style, focus and ability of individual nurses influence the actual type of care received by patients, examples of the components of some of the nursing care delivery systems which may be adopted follow.

## 2.1 FUNCTIONAL OR TASK NURSING

In functional or task nursing, the emphasis is on completion of tasks for all patients within the total nursing unit. Delegation of tasks to individual staff members who subsequently document completion of the tasks is the essential component of this system.

TABLE 1.3.1: Advantages and disadvantages of task-based nursing

| ADVANTAGES | DISADVANTAGES |
|---|---|
| Task-based nursing is extremely efficient in getting all the work done in the shortest possible time. | Staff concentrate on task completion, not meaning or appropriateness of the task — promotion of care rituals. |
| It is the most economical way to deliver nursing services which meet the minimum identified health care standards with as few personnel as possible. | Personnel provide services at an identified standard — there may be no challenge to improve the level or quality. This perpetuates the myth that 'nursing shortages' determine practice. |
| As staff are assigned specific tasks on the basis of their qualifications, experience and competence, there is efficient use of all levels of staff. | It reduces desire or opportunity to attempt innovations in practice as task relationship to patient outcome is obscured. |
| Workload is determined by what can realistically be expected of one nurse in one working day. | Variations in patient acuity are perceived as affecting the available amount of a worker's time for task completion, not as the time available to provide services to individual patients. |
| Part-time staff can be easily assimilated into the system. | Frequently part-time staff are assigned the most mundane tasks as other staff are less knowledgeable about their abilities. |
| Learners can develop proficiency in performing the specific tasks, and staff development is achieved through training in, and the development of proficiency in, the performance of each specific type of task. | Task orientation reduces vision of nursing practice to the series of hurdles which must be overcome before the nurse is a professional/ specialist in the area. |
| There is a checklist of care for evaluation and co-ordination purposes. | There is no responsibility for care planning, as assessment and planning is related to the task. |
| It provides a degree of security for patients and staff as job descriptions are highly specified and narrowly defined with each nurse responsible and accountable for the completion of the identified tasks. | The fragmentation of care causes difficulty for patients' families, and co-workers, in determining whom to approach about what aspect of care. |
| Staff, patients and their families know what the normal operating routines are, and the times when activities should occur. | Patients have to conform to strict routines in provision of care. |
| As many different nurses are in contact with the patient, any gross care deficiencies are likely to be identified and addressed. | Although each nurse is responsible for own actions, all nurses are not responsible for identifying problems which occur with the patients. |
| Ideally, the nurse in charge of the unit is accountable for all aspects of the planning, delegation, supervision, co-ordination and evaluation of the work undertaken, and of the total care outcomes. There is a central and identifiable focus of responsibility, authority and communication for the activities of the unit. | The role of the nurse in charge is fragmented — role confusion can occur, time is spent on acting as an information gatherer and disseminator, delegating and supervising tasks, rectifying omissions and errors, rather than on total care outcomes of individual patients (managing nurses, rather than nursing). |

TABLE 1.3.2: The advantages and disadvantages of case-based nursing

| ADVANTAGES | DISADVANTAGES |
| --- | --- |
| It is extremely efficient in ensuring that the actual needs of each patient are identified and addressed, saving on provision of unneeded services. | Concentration on patient needs can obscure the desirability, necessity or ability of the organisation to actually meet these needs — potential also for nurse frustration at being unable to meet the identified needs, and increased patient dependency upon the nurse as the provider of all that is required. |
| It is the most economical way to deliver high-quality nursing services as only staff able to provide all aspects of patient care are employed. More time is spent on direct patient care activities and less on supervision, teaching, waiting for instruction and other ancillary activities. | A total complement of staff with the desired skills and abilities may not be available. Even if it is, not all nurses are able to practise at the same level of autonomy, requiring provision of ancillary support services. Frequently requires resocialisation of nurses to ensure ability to function independently is developed. |
| Nursing time is used to meet the care needs of the patient resulting in greater economy. | Patient acuity may be such that the demand upon the nurse could be too low or too high for the economical and realistic employment of one nurse. |
| As staff are assigned specific patients on the basis of their qualifications, experience and competence, there is efficient use of all staff. | Changes in patient conditions denoting deterioration may not be observed where these are outside staff member's area of expertise — resulting in extended nursing care requirements. |
| Learners can develop proficiency in interpreting patient needs, learn to appreciate the total care requirements of the patient, and how to organise their own workload. Such learning is usually fostered by placing the learner as an assistant to the case-nurse, or through preceptorship arrangements. | The learners may not be aware of their own limitations and may not seek advice when needed. As the learner is at what Benner identifies as the 'beginning practitioner' level, an absence of the lists and sequence of tasks to be performed can engender feelings of insecurity, especially as not all experienced nurses have the same preceptor abilities. Potential to perpetuate the 'apprenticeship' training aspect of education of nurses. |
| It provides a degree of security for patients and staff as each is able to develop an ongoing relationship with the other. Patients' families and co-workers know whom to approach to discuss the patient's care. | Job descriptions are global and evaluation of performance focuses on the appropriateness of the planning and on patient outcomes, a more difficult process than focusing on how tasks are performed. |
| Patient satisfaction is increased as the nurse is able to conform with the habits and customs of the patient. | Family and visitors would be unaware of the basis for a flexible routine, thus feeling that they are intruding, or that the nurse is not working. The nurse may have to work extended hours to provide the care needed to conform with the patient's own time schedule. |
| Each nurse is responsible both for own actions and for identifying the problems which occur with the patient, and for seeking appropriate assistance. | As no different nurses are in contact with the patient, and only one is responsible for planning the nursing care to be implemented, deficiencies in care may be overlooked. |

TABLE 1.3.2: The advantages and disadvantages of case-based nursing (continued)

| ADVANTAGES | DISADVANTAGES |
|---|---|
| Ideally the role of the nurse making such assignments is one of guidance and advice, which enables others to draw upon his/her experience. More time is available to know the abilities of the nurses, know what is happening overall, and to apply management techniques such as communication, leadership, and the estimation and appropriate deployment of resources — to manage nursing, rather than the individual nurses. | The nurses in charge may feel threatened at having to hand over responsibility for the delivery of care to the nurses, based on the perception that they will not know what is happening, or that they do not know the capabilities of their staff. As some nurses feel unable to use their initiative although given the opportunity to do so, much time and effort can be directed to coaching and attempting to develop the confidence of the nurses. Frequently those in charge find themselves caught in the dilemma of being expected to manage nursing, but in fact having to manage nurses. |

## 2.2 SPECIALISED OR SPECIALTY NURSING

With specialised or specialty nursing, the provision of services is related to each nurse's area of expertise and specialty. It is frequently associated with the provision of progressive patient care services and the patients' 'progress' through the various specialty units as their care needs alter. Assessment of the extent to which such special care needs exist underlies this system, and the nurses' areas of practice and concern can be affected by how specialty is defined.

## 2.3 TEAM NURSING

Team nursing may be either task or patient oriented. The unit staff is divided into teams and a particular group of patients is assigned to each team. It is postulated that, as fewer nurses interact with each patient, this system encourages caring for each patient as an individual. However, the leadership ability of the team leader and the mix of skills and qualifications within the team frequently lead to task allocation or specialisation within the team, whether wholly or only for those tasks which are beyond the capabilities of certain team members. Use of nursing care plans and team conferences are essential components of this system.

## 2.4 MODULAR NURSING

Modular nursing further breaks down the overall patient care load into smaller teams caring for smaller modules of patients. Adoption of this system, which Stevens (1980:91) considers 'permits closer monitoring of care than is the case in team nursing, probably decreasing the percentage of errors and increasing the chances that patient needs will be identified', is frequently dictated by the geographical layout of the unit. This system may include each two or three member team being the primary care planners for some patients from admission to discharge, and acting as an associate team in the delivery of care for other primary team patients within their case load (Gillies, 1989:235).

## 2.5 PATIENT ASSIGNMENT OR TOTAL PATIENT CARE

With patient assignment or total patient care, 'the professional nurse is assigned a number of patients to whom she provides all the care needed while she is on duty' (Halloran, 1983, cited in Kron and Gray, 1987:13). The number of patients is determined by the level of their care needs, and includes those special circumstances where one-to-one care is needed. Although care is not fragmented during the time the nurse is on duty, generally no one person is responsible for co-ordinating each patient's care across shifts or throughout the patient's stay (Kron and Gray, 1987:13). Complete adoption of this system is only possible where all staff have the knowledge, ability and qualifications to deliver the total care required by the individual patients.

## 2.6 PRIMARY NURSING

Primary nursing extends an identified nurse's responsibility for individual patient assessment, care planning, delivery and evaluation from during the shifts she works to the entire period until that patient's discharge.

> Theoretically, the quality of care is assured by the continuity of her interaction with her clients throughout their hospitalisation and immediately thereafter.
>
> (Marram et al, 1976:2)

When the primary nurse is not on duty, the planned care is implemented by associate nurses, each of whom would also be the primary nurse for other patients. Thus the quality of care actually provided depends not only on the practical skills of the primary nurse, but also on the accuracy of forecasting and clarity of direction contained in the nursing care plans.

## 2.7 NURSE-MANAGED CARE

The nurse-managed care model, Stillwaggon (1989:21) suggests, 'builds on primary nursing but frees the nurse from institutional contraints'. Generally, the descriptions of this system assume that nurses involved are self-directed professional individuals who have the maturity to work flexible hours as required to provide care when needed and when acceptable for 'their' patients. A further assumption apparently underlying this in a hospital setting is that there will be what McClure (1984:13) terms 'blue collar nurses' who work regular duty hours and assume the 'professional' nurse's patient responsibilities in their absence. This appears to limit use of this system to those nurses in clinical specialist or consultant roles, or to non-institutional settings.

## 2.8 CASE MANAGEMENT

Case management models further seek to move 'the care delivery process beyond the traditional discipline boundaries of time or shift and geographic or unit orientation' (Olivas et al, 1989:19). In community health settings, multi-disciplinary case management models are common, and care delivery is co-ordinated by either the person with greatest expertise in the case area, or by the person who was the patient's first point of contact with the system. Models proposed within acute care settings generally recommend that nursing services act as co-ordinator, both in recognition of nursing's continual contact with patients, and as a means of increasing nurses' job satisfaction.

Matthews (1987:59) considers the most important influences upon the method of organising and delivering patient care in the individual service setting to be:

☐ staffing levels;

☐ ratio of qualified nurses;

☐ ward design, for example, Nightingale, race-track, small rooms;

☐ patient turnover;

☐ type of patients nursed in the ward.

The components of this list indicate that not only expectations but also local working conditions must be considered when seeking to convert the 'vision' in the positioning statement into a reality.

# 3. DETERMINING STAFFING NUMBERS

A number of approaches can be used to determine the number of staff and the levels of experience and qualifications required on either a daily or annual basis. These approaches vary in design sophistication and in the degree to which they provide 'hard data' to substantiate decisions on staff requirements. Variables underlying this process include the number of patients requiring nursing services, the amount and level of services they require, and the manager's ability to accurately predict future nursing workload.

In service organisations, personnel salaries represent the principal item of budget expenditure, and it is often necessary to justify staffing decisions on economic grounds. However, imbalances between the numbers or mix of staff and their workload can also be costly in terms of worker dissatisfaction. Gillies (1989:237) notes that:

working in a chronically understaffed unit leads to frustration, fatigue and disillusionment. Working in a chronically overstaffed unit leads to boredom and excessive interpersonal friction. Working in a unit that is alternately under- and over-staffed produces irritation, uncertainty and confusion. Working in a unit that has an improper mix of personnel creates role confusion, communication problems and time waste ... (while) nursing personnel are demoralised if their immediate work group suffers frequent changes of membership.

There is no magic formula which will enable a nurse manager to calculate accurately the optimal numbers and mix of staff needed to provide appropriate care for all patients within an area at all times. Outlined below are some of the more common approaches used in attempts to ensure that the staff available is appropriate to meet the care needs of the everchanging patient population. Both the stated philosophy of the nursing division and the mode of nursing chosen to structure the delivery of nursing care will assist the manager in identifying which approach, or which combination of approaches, should underly the staff planning process. Examples of how these approaches can be applied are shown in the figures for this chapter.

## 3.1 TRADITIONAL APPROACH

The traditional approach, so called because it identifies the staffing traditionally associated with a nursing service or area, provides a subjective and descriptive identification of what staffing is required. On the basis of experience gained through trial and error, judgements can be made on what constitutes the most appropriate number and mix of staff to provide the required services (Halloran and Hadley Vermeersch, 1987:26). As it is developed from knowledge of local conditions, including knowledge of geographic layout of work or variations in patient acuity, this can be a very effective method of estimating staff requirements both overall and for particular circumstances (Figure 1.3.1). However, it lacks any perceived scientific basis or rationale, and other methods must be sought to validate staffing decisions made using this approach.

FIGURE 1.3.1:   Using historical data to calculate nursing staff requirements

### OUTCOMES OF VARIOUS METHODS OF CALCULATING STAFFING REQUIREMENTS BASED ON HISTORICAL DATA
[ All Care Hour figures used are hypothetical, not based on any recommended by any authority ]

This example refers to a 30 bed unit which experienced 1582 admissions in the last year, resulting in 9490 occupied bed days. The patient census varied between 18 (on 20 days) and 31 (on 12 days). Staffing of this 30 bed unit is traditionally held constant at 10 per day, each of whom works an 8 hour shift.

The AVERAGE LENGTH OF STAY was: $\dfrac{\text{Occupied bed days}}{\text{Admissions}} = \dfrac{9490}{1582} = 6 \text{ days}$

The AVERAGE DAILY CENSUS was: $\dfrac{\text{Occupied bed days}}{\text{Days of year}} = \dfrac{9490}{365} = $ 26 patients

TOTAL AVAILABLE BED DAYS were: number of beds x days in year = 30 x 365 = 10 950 available bed days

AVE. OCCUPANCY RATE of the unit was: $\dfrac{\text{Occupied bed days}}{\text{Available bed days}} \times 100 = \dfrac{9490}{10\ 950} = 86.7\%$

DAILY AVERAGE NHPD:

$$\dfrac{\text{daily average available nurse hours}}{\text{(Number of staff x hours worked per day x days worked per year/days in year)}}$$
$$\text{daily average census of patients}$$

$$= \dfrac{(10 \times 8 \times 365 + \text{additional float hours} - \text{short staff hours})/365}{26}$$

$$= \dfrac{(29\ 200 + 0 - 0\ /\ 365}{26}$$ = 3.08 av. nursing hours per patient day

Variations in DAILY NHPD: $\dfrac{\text{number of nurses x hours worked}}{\text{number of patients}}$

At minimum census $\dfrac{10 \times 8}{18}$ = 4.44 NHPD.

At maximum census $\dfrac{10 \times 8}{31}$ = 2.58 NHPD.

PRODUCTIVITY INDEX: $\dfrac{\text{average daily NHPD}}{\text{daily NHPD}}$ x 100

Productivity at minimum census

$\dfrac{3.19}{4.44}$ x 100 = 71.8%

At maximum census

$\dfrac{3.19}{2.58}$ x 100 = 123.6%

DAILY AVERAGE NHPB: $\dfrac{\text{daily average available nurse hours}}{\text{number of beds}} = \dfrac{10 \times 8}{30}$

= 2.67 nursing hours per patient bed

VARIABLE DAILY STAFFING: $\dfrac{\text{daily patient census x average NHPD}}{\text{number of hours each nurse works per day}}$

(for Av. NHPD: 10 nurses)

at minimum census: $\dfrac{18 \times 3.08}{8}$ = 7 nurses required

for maximum census: $\dfrac{31 \times 3.08}{8}$ = 12 nurses required

## 3.2 NURSING HOURS PER PATIENT DAY (NHPD)

Nursing Hours per Patient Day (NHPD) statistics provide one means of identifying outcomes of staffing practices (Figure 1.3.2). These statistics, by dividing the nursing hours available by the number of patients in a unit, reflect what staffing ratio currently exists in the service or units by providing some measure of hours of care available for each patient (Reid and Melaugh, 1987:4). But it does not identify whether the ratio of nursing hours to patient is appropriate to produce the level of care required, nor the appropriateness of the personnel providing such care. If developed from the viewpoint that the work performed is appropriate to provide the required standard of care of the 'average' patient in the organisation or unit, the results obtained can be useful for quantifying existing staffing practices or for forecasting future needs.

FIGURE 1.3.2:   Using patient data to calculate nursing requirements

### OUTCOMES OF VARIOUS METHODS OF CALCULATING STAFFING REQUIREMENTS BASED ON PATIENT-NEEDS DATA *
[ All Care Hour figures used are hypothetical, not based on any recommended by any authority ]

USING PATIENT CLASSIFICATION: (On average census)

| | Type/ Category | No. of patients | Category Av. NHPD | Total care hours required |
|---|---|---|---|---|
| by type of diagnosis | | | | |
| | Medical | 10 | 3.5 | 35 |
| | Surgical | 8 | 4.0 | 32 |
| | Critical Care | 1 | 10.0 | 10 |
| | Paediatric | 3 | 4.5 | 13.5 |
| | Maternity | 1 | 2.5 | 2.5 |
| | Nursing Home | 3 | 4.0 | 12 |
| | TOTAL | 26 | | 105.0 |

Nursing staff required:

$$\frac{\text{Total care hours}}{\text{hours per nurse day}} \quad = \quad \frac{105}{8} \quad = 13 \text{ nurses required}$$

## USING PATIENT PROFILE CLASSIFICATION:

| | Type/<br>Category | No. of<br>patients | Category<br>Av. NHPD * | Total care<br>hours required |
|---|---|---|---|---|
| by prototype | | | | |
| | 1. Minimal care | 7 | 2.00 | 14.00 |
| | 2. Average care | 7 | 3.08 | 21.56 |
| | 3. Above average | | | |
| | care | 11 | 4.15 | 45.65 |
| | 4. Maximum care | 1 | 6.16 | 6.16 |
| | TOTAL | 26 | | 87.37 |

Nursing staff required:

$$\frac{\text{Total care hours}}{\text{hours per nurse day}} \quad = \quad \frac{87.37}{8} \quad = 11 \text{ nurses required}$$

\* Calculations relate to the same information as in Figure 1.3.1. Figures derived from formula proposed by Schmied (1977, cited in Rowland and Rowland, 1985:153), wherein patients requiring minimal care are considered to require 65% of average daily hours; those requiring average care 100%; above average care 135%; and maximum care 200% respectively.

## BY USING PATIENT CARE NEED CLASSIFICATION

| | General Care Needs | | | | | | Technical care needs | | | TOTAL*<br>HOURS/ |
|---|---|---|---|---|---|---|---|---|---|---|
| Care Needs<br>Name | Diet | Fluids | Mobility | Hygiene | Elimination | Safety | Medication | Treatment | Teaching | POINTS |
| 1. . . . . . . | | | | | | | | | | |
| 2. . . . . . . | | | | | | | | | | |
| ^\V | | | | | | | | | | |
| 25. | | | | | | | | | | |
| 26. | | | | | | | | | | |
| ^\V | | | | | | | | | | |
| Indirect Care<br>Allowance + | | | | | | | | | | |

* TOTAL CARE
HOURS/POINTS

Some factor\* denoting the time to complete each procedure, multiplied by the frequency of repetition, is entered into all applicable squares in the matrix.

+ Where the hours are being calculated per need, this allowance is included in the patient column.
  If hours are calculated per patient, this allowance is included in the needs columns.

\* Depending upon the system used, these factorial times may be expressed in actual minutes/hours of care required, or in points which represent periods of time, and must then be converted to actual times. As examples of the latter, in the GRASP system, 'the time values are expressed in tenths of hours' (Meyer, 1984:53), while the PETO system uses patient care units each equalling 7.5 minutes of nursing care (Polland et al 1970, cited in Stevens, 1980:106).

It provides a constant single figure measure of activity both within and across vary-ing settings and has frequently been used as a de facto measure of hours of care associated with nursing different types of patients. Thus, figures such as the 'average' medical patient requiring four hours of nursing care per day, or the 'average' intensive care patient requiring 12 hours, are established. When this figure is multiplied by the expected daily average within the area, staffing requirements can be projected. Similarly, it can be used as a measure of productivity. Variations between actual daily and average daily workload figures reflect peaks and troughs in workload within a unit, or in aver-age figures between different organisations, allowing efficiency conclusions to be drawn. The validity of many of the resulting conclusions is frequently questioned because little is known of the variability of nursing dependency of the patients in each ward or unit.

## 3.3 NURSING HOURS PER PATIENT BED

Nursing Hours per Patient Bed statistics calculate the nursing hours available in a unit per number of beds within that unit, and identify a potential minimum quantity of nurs-ing time available, rather than the actual amount. Staffing decisions are made on the basis of the 'minimum acceptable staffing at maximum occupancy' (Hancock and Fuhs, 1984:22), with no consideration being given to different degrees of bed occupants' acuity (Figure 1.3.1).

In addition to sharing many of the flaws associated with NHPD measurement, its validity is frequently questioned on the basis of 'how much nursing care do beds need?'. The resultant staffing regimen is typically based on 'maximum workload condi-tions and "fixed" staffing to wards and shifts' (Bennett and Duckett, 1981:435). However, this approach can be used in conjunction with an admissions policy to achieve equita-ble distribution of patients (and by association workload) across different units of one organisation, thus rationalising use of resources.

## 3.4 PATIENT CENSUS

Using the patient census approach, it is considered that by specifying a set ratio of nurs-ing staff to occupied patient beds, staffing can be varied to accommodate peaks and troughs in workload, and that nurses can be distributed across areas to ensure each has an equitable workload (Figure 1.3.1). Areas can be staffed for the care required at minimum census and additional staff provided for periods when more beds are occupied. However, as Gillies (1989:238) points out, '. . . in any hospital, the average daily census is roughly the product of the average admission rate times the average length of stay'. This approach ignores that, even where the census is stable, variations in nursing workloads and activities frequently relate to both the admission rate and the length of stay of individual patients. As the census is generally taken only once a day, the figure can grossly misrepresent the number of patients who actually receive nursing care within a unit. Furthermore, there is no recognition that one group of patients can have far higher care needs than another group of a similar category and number.

## 3.5 PATIENT CLASSIFICATION SYSTEMS (PCS)

Patient Classification Systems (PCS) seek to provide an objective method of determining staffing requirements by quantifying patients' care needs and converting these into the number of nurses required to meet these needs (Figure 1.3.2). Jenkins (1983:8) identifies that 'all nurse staffing methodologies use some quantification or estimation of time required to provide the care for the particular categories within the classification system'.

Three types of patient classification systems are in common use: classification primarily according to medical diagnosis, age and sex; classification into the 'typical prototype' category which most closely describes the patient's characteristics; and classification based on a range of patient 'factors' — some range of nursing care indicators identified as distinguishing between care-time requirements of different patients.

Classifying patients by phases of illness, or by type or classification of illness, is demonstrated in its most rudimentary form by unit/ward placement within a multi-department hospital. Example of these include classification into intensive care, intermediate care, convalescent care units; or as maternity, medical, surgical, obstetrics, etc, cases. Differing hours of care required are associated with the different types of patients, allowing determination of staff required to meet the needs of patients within this setting. More sophisticated designs seek to associate specific amounts of nursing time with each category within the diagnostic-related groupings (DRGs) system. Such groupings are based not only on medical diagnosis but also upon age of the patient and the presence of complications or other diseases. Gillies notes that 'the major difficulty in determining the amount of nursing time required to care for a patient in each diagnostic category is the fact that patients generally require different types and amounts of care at different stages of illness' (1989:243), and this reduces the utility of adopting this approach in varying day-to-day unit staffing. However, calculating the 'average nursing time per patient' within each specific DRG for the total care episode (admission), and the number of admissions within each group, can assist in forecasting total staffing requirements.

Prototype classification classes patients by resemblance to one of the descriptions of typical patients within an area.

> The classes relate to the acuity of illness and care requirements, such as minimal, partial, moderate or intensive. The variables entering into the patient classification systems generally relate to the capability of a patient to meet his physical needs to ambulate, bathe, and feed himself.
>
> (Rowland and Rowland, 1985:153)

The typical patient in each of the care categories is defined after consideration of those characteristics of the patient population served which most accurately predict the variations in nursing requirements. Projected staffing can be based on the average number in each category over a period, while daily staffing requirements can be adjusted on the basis of the actual numbers present.

Further accuracy in quantifying patient care needs can be achieved by using a number of salient indicators to identify the frequency or complexity associated with providing certain aspects of care for patients within the unit. Meyer (1984:52) says that 'of the hundreds of possible direct nursing activities, on average 40 to 50 will account for 85 per cent of the nursing time provided to any given patient'. Average care times associated with providing each factor category are aggregated to identify the total required nursing care hours. Alternatively, the nursing care hours individual patients will need can be calculated.

In addition to these identified direct care hours, an allowance for indirect care activities must be included. Bell and Storey (1984:57) calculated the contingency allowance at 4.25 to 5 per cent per shift.

## 3.6 NURSING INTENSITY

Seelye (1982:196) considers that 'the mix of nurses in terms of qualifications and experience may be as important as the number of nurses'. Benner (1984) describes individual variations in performance between those with the same qualifications, from beginner to expert level. Various nurse classification systems have been proposed to enable quantification of the tasks staff with different levels of preparation can complete so that the cost-benefit of employing the differing levels can be determined. Prescott and Phillips (1988:17) discuss one approach where:

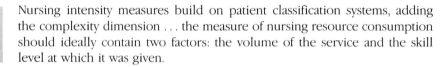

> Nursing intensity measures build on patient classification systems, adding the complexity dimension . . . the measure of nursing resource consumption should ideally contain two factors: the volume of the service and the skill level at which it was given.

Another proposal, a method of converting contributions of other staff into '"trained nurse equivalent" hours available, rather than "pairs of hands" available', is described by Storey and Bell (1985:42). As registered nurses can provide care to meet all levels of patient need, some authors (for example Donovan and Lewis, 1987) have identified cost-benefit results from the use of an all registered nurse staff, although results of studies in this area have not been conclusive. Rowland and Rowland (1985:142) emphasise that no guidelines have been established 'for determining the proper skill mix for each unit'.

## 3.7 BUDGET ALLOCATION

Many articles identify how to develop a staffing budget, based on previous experience, projected patient classifications, nurse rostering practices, or anticipated DRG case mix.

The nurse manager may not know the basis upon which the allocation of monies has been determined, or the allocation received may differ from that requested (Figure 1.3.3). If using the budget allocation to determine staffing mix and level, a total for on-costs (those relating to shift penalties, annual leave loadings and other payments which raise salaries above the base award levels for each category) should be subtracted to enable identification of the actual monies available for wages. It is then useful to consider the numbers and salaries for the coming year of 'stayers' within the unit/organisation so that the amount of money remaining after these salaries have been paid can be determined. After specifying the minimum level/s of staff desired to replace the likely 'leavers', the salaries associated with these are identified, and the remaining monies divided by these salaries to determine the number of such staff which could be employed.

**FIGURE 1.3.3:**  Using budget allocation to calculate annual nursing staff numbers

METHODS OF CALCULATING STAFFING REQUIREMENTS
BASED ON BUDGET ALLOCATION

Using historical salary data:

TOTAL FTE NURSES            =            total budget allocation
                                         average annual nurse salary

[ where average annual nurse salary    =        total salary budget last period                    ]
                                                number of FTE nurses employed in this period       ]

Using projected data:

TOTAL FTE NURSES            =            total budget allocation

                            (less) historical 'on-costs' of penalty rates, allowances, leave loading, etc.

                            (less) salary and next year's level of those who appear likely to remain for year

                            =            budget available for replacement staff
                                         average salary of preferred mix of replacement staff

                            =            number of replacement staff at this mix
                                         (add) number of 'stayers'

                            =            annual FTE equivalent nurses of preferred mix
                                         which can be employed on this budget allocation

Alternatively, the average staffing cost per patient, per patient day or per patient category, can be calculated. The anticipated number of patients within an area is averaged and staff numbers determined by dividing the budget allocation for the projected period by that average cost. In either calculation, by playing 'what if' games — varying the possible combinations of levels and mix of staff and relating these to the budget figure — optimum numbers and mix of staff in light of monies available can be decided. A system such as that proposed by Nauert et al (1988:28), allows for monitoring nursing costs and subsequent adjustment of staff numbers and mix (Figure 1.3.4).

**FIGURE 1.3.4:** Using daily staffing to calculate weekly and annual nursing staff requirements

### CALCULATING WEEKLY AND ANNUAL FULL-TIME EQUIVALENT (FTE) STAFF BASED ON DAILY STAFFING DATA

Calculations relate to the same information as in Figure 1.3.1. In addition, it is assumed that the award nominates that all staff work a 38-hour week and receive 6 weeks' annual leave.

Weekly FTE STAFF:

$$\frac{\text{total nursing hours required per week}}{\text{1 nurse's available hours per week}}$$

$$= \frac{\text{10 nurses per day x 8 hours per shift x 7 days per week}}{\text{38 hours per week}}$$

$$= \frac{560}{38} \qquad = 14.74 \text{ (say 15) staff per week}$$

[ Where different numbers of staff are employed on different days of the week, this alters the total hours required ]

Annual FTE STAFF

$$\frac{\text{total nursing hours required per year}}{\text{1 nurse's available hours per year}}$$

$$= \frac{\text{10 nurses daily x 8 hour shifts x 365 days per year}}{\text{38 hour week x 46 2/7 weeks per year} \quad (46\ 3/7\ \text{weeks})}$$

$$= \frac{29200}{1759} \quad = 16.6 \text{ FTE staff per year} \qquad \begin{array}{l}\text{In leap year} \\ (366\ \text{days})\end{array}$$

## 3.8 GEOGRAPHIC COVERAGE

Staffing in some areas often cannot be justified solely on the basis of existing patient workload. The use of a NHPB approach highlights the necessity to consider what Larter (1982:164) refers to as:

those other factors broadly labelled as readiness to serve — the need to provide a minimum of staff at all times in specialised areas such as labour and delivery, critical care, the emergency room, and so on regardless of whether the number of patients justifies this staffing.

Similarly, where an award specifies a minimum number per (specific) shift, the staffing must reflect this. Seelye, although presenting no definite guidelines for staffing differently designed patient care areas, nevertheless states that 'when the layout is considered, decisions (on staffing) tend to be made on commonsense assumptions by local managers on local evidence' (1982:197). The effect of geographical influences is particularly obvious when staffing in domiciliary nursing settings is considered.

## 3.9 AWARD SPECIFICATIONS

In some areas, as well as specifying hours of work and holiday and sick leave entitlements, the industrial award covering staff within the organisation also specifies the minimum number of staff per patient load or specified shift, the maximum mix of skill levels, specific study leave requirements and other determinants of staff establishment. Where there is agreement between management and employees that some alteration to these conditions is desirable for both parties (for example length of shifts within overall weekly hours of work), such agreements can be accepted by the union concerned. Any such agreement which substantially alters the conditions of employment set out in the award, and which either the employer or the union (as the representative of the employees) wishes to make legally binding on both parties, can be registered as an industrial agreement by the appropriate industrial tribunal or commission.

## 3.10 CONVERTING DAILY STAFFING TO ANNUAL REQUIREMENTS

Some of the above approaches provide details only for daily required figures. These can be converted to annual full-time equivalent staff requirements by dividing the estimated number of patient care days or hours by the annual number of hours one nurse is actually available to work. In some organisations, an allowance for sick leave is included in determining this figure, but possible long-service, maternity or other long-term leave is generally ignored.

Numbers of managerial, supervisory and consultative staff to provide support and co-ordination for patient care services also need to be determined. It must be established whether these are five- or seven-day week positions, full-year or able to be left vacant during periods of the incumbents' absence, so that the overall staffing required to provide these services can be identified.

# 4. ROSTERING AND ALLOCATING STAFF

Even once an appropriate number and mix of staff has been determined, the nurse manager is still faced with the major task of ensuring that sufficient nurses are available to provide the care required *when* it is required. The process underlying rostering sounds simple — all that is required is to identify staff requirements for each shift and allocate staff members to meet the requirements.

However, as anyone who attempts this discovers, the process is complicated by several factors including:

1.  nurses' hours of work are restricted on a daily, a weekly and an annual basis, either by the award for full-time staff, or by the employment agreement for those employed part-time;

2.  24 (hours in day) is easily divisible only by 12, 8, 6, 4, 3 and 2;

3.  7 (days in week) is not evenly divisible by any number;

4.  in most areas, nursing and patient care activities are not spread evenly across all hours of the day, days of the week, or weeks of the year;

5.  different nurses perform at different levels;

6.  different annual leave (and frequently study leave and sick leave) entitlements apply to different staff members. Even where similar entitlements apply, the extent to which the individual employees claim these varies.

## 4.1 IDENTIFYING SHIFT NUMBERS

An analysis of activity patterns within an area provides information not only on what work is performed when and by what level of staff but also on where peaks and troughs in the workload occur. Where patient care activity remains relatively constant across all hours of the day — as in an intensive care area — obviously available staff must also remain constant. Other areas where activities vary by time of day and/or day of week should reflect this in the percentage of staff members allocated to each day and shift. Thus, the desired number of personnel and mix of skills at different periods across the week can be identified and written into the staffing policy.

Wherever reasons are sought for shortages or excessive turnover of nurses, one of the major reasons given relates to dissatisfaction with how hours and days of work are determined, with particular reference to areas such as inflexibility of schedules, perceived unfairness in the allocation of shifts, and lack of personal control in choosing the pattern of hours and shifts to be worked. These dissatisfactions are especially evident where staffing practices are not in accord with nursing's stated philosophy.

## 4.2 SPECIFYING WORK PATTERNS

The traditional pattern of apportioning hours to periods of duty since the advent of the 40-hour work week has been five eight-hour days per week. Even with the recent reduction in work hours in some states, this pattern is frequently followed until the nurse has accumulated sufficient reduced week hours to enable a full day to be deducted from the normal week's work. This enables definition of three equal shifts within each 24 hours. Alternative patterns described in Braddy (1987/88:73) include the 4–40 pattern of four 10-hour work days followed by three days off; the 7–70 pattern of seven 10-hour work days followed by seven days off; the 3–36 pattern where three 12-hour work days are followed by four days off; and even a 2–32 pattern where only two 16-hour periods are worked in the week. Some organisations use different patterns for different shifts or personnel. Each pattern has its own attendant advantages and disadvantages which should be carefully considered before any changes are made in the system currently in use in the organisation.

## 4.3 ALTERNATIVE ROSTER FORMATS

Possible formats for rosters, whether these be individual or group based, include fixed or permanent rosters where the same days and shifts are worked each week; rotating rosters where the work hours are rotated through the different shifts; cyclical rosters where a work pattern of shifts across differing days of the week and/or different weeks is repeated permanently; cyclical rotating rosters where personnel are rotated through all shifts and across all work days as identified in a fixed permanent pattern; and flexible rosters where personnel are assigned to rostered periods either at their request or on the scheduler's judgement of how best to fill the gaps.

## 4.4 RESPONSIBILITY FOR ROSTER PREPARATION

The responsibility for assigning staff to certain periods of work can be centralised within nursing administration, decentralised to the manager of the unit or work team, or devolved to the nurses themselves. At whichever level the responsibility lies, guidelines to facilitate roster preparation must be specified. Kron and Gray (1987:149) state that some of the guidelines that underlie rostering are:

1. a qualified person must be in charge at all times on every unit;

2. scheduling of staff duty time must include enough people to provide adequate patient care 24 hours a day, seven days a week;

3. time on duty must be planned according to institutional policies;

4. time schedules should be planned . . . preferably one month in advance, and changed only in emergencies;

5. staffing requirements must be flexible and adjustments must be made as necessary.

Centralised rostering, by dint of depersonalisation and the scheduler's ability to consider staffing throughout the organisation, offers a higher possibility of ensuring fairness and consistency in allocation across all work areas and decreases repetition in roster development. However, unit or team managers are accountable for the care provided within their area and have greater knowledge of the abilities of their staff. A decentralised system facilitates the scheduling of individuals by reference to their experience and skills, as well as rostering of individuals to concurrent shifts to ensure development and maintenance of cohesive and complementary work groups. Perhaps the most cogent argument for decentralised rostering is that advanced by Stevens (1980:111):

> the head nurse is the one who will have to live with the schedule; she should have the right to make it.

The system most likely to overcome complaints about inflexibility of schedules, perceived unfairness in the allocation of shifts, and lack of personal control in choosing the pattern of hours and shifts to be worked is self-rostering. Within criteria specifying the number and mix of personnel for each work period, and, at least initially, guidelines to ensure equity in staffing the least preferred shifts, 'nurses on a unit collectively decide and implement the monthly work scheduled' (Rowland and Rowland, 1985:169).

# 5. THE MANAGEMENT CHALLENGE

Donley and Flaherty (1989), in discussing how expansion in demand for nurses' services in areas outside acute-care hospitals has resulted in shortages in the nursing workforce, explain that nurse managers

> ... hold key information about staffing patterns, control the personal and work environment, influence the development and execution of budgets, and plan the ratio of nurses to nurse helpers. They can be significant forces in influencing the organisational climate and the work environment (1989:186).

How work and work relationships are structured affects the outcomes not only for the patients but also for staff, the manager and the organisation.

As a result of the hospital based training of nursing students who formed the bulk of the workforce but few of whom were subsequently retained on staff, nurse service organisations have tended to view nurses as replaceable resources. With the predominantly female nature of the nursing workforce

> hospitals adjusted to social forces that were described as marriage and child rearing; employment by another hospital; employment in other health settings; a return to school; movement along a career path to teaching, management or primary care; or a change in career

with the expectation that only a few of those recruited would remain within the organisation (Donley and Flaherty, 1989:186). Management practices were developed upon consideration of how best to control use of such a transient and inexperienced resource, and the structuring of work reflected this orientation.

Nursing students now receive pre-service education in tertiary educational settings and are no longer the predominant component of the nursing workforce. Economic forces have resulted in patients being treated in hospitals only when actually ill, and in an increased demand for provision of patient care in other nursing service settings. The more intense the care needs of patients, the greater the need to recruit and retain qualified and experienced nurses. However, the ensuing change in the nature of the workforce is frequently not reflected in changes in prevailing management practices, nor in a recognition of the changing nature of nursing itself.

Kramer and Schmalenberg in their study of 16 magnet hospitals where nursing staff shortages '. . . were generally not reported or observed' (1988a:13) concluded that these hospitals were

> infused with values of quality care, nurse autonomy, informal, non-rigid verbal communication, innovation, bringing out the best in each individual, value of education, respect and caring for the individual, and striving for excellence (1988b:17).

These values cannot be demonstrated in organisations which consider nurses as replaceable (and hence expendable) resources.

A reorientation in defining the nature of the human resource is therefore required. Instead of considering individuals as a raw resource in the process of providing nursing services, they should be recognised as the catalysts in the process of converting knowledge, skills and technology into desired patient care outcomes. Once the catalytic role of practitioners is recognised, nurse managers are no longer faced with the problem of how best to manage nurses, but can address the challenge of how best to manage nursing, and how to utilise available opportunities to the maximum benefit of nursing.

# 6. ANALYSIS FOR CHANGE

The search for the most appropriate way to structure nursing to facilitate nurses' practice commences with an examination of the current situation. This enables identification of the full range of linkages that co-ordinate practice patterns within the organisation or department. Wilson and Firestone (1987:19) identify two types of linkages: bureaucratic and cultural. The bureaucratic linkages, the formal rules procedures and authority relations are 'designed to control the behaviour of organisation members . . . and establish constraints and opportunities on what, where, to whom and for how long' employees provide services. 'Cultural linkages work on the consciousness (of staff) by clarifying what they do and defining their commitment to the task.' They derive from the collective values by which organisational members interpret their surroundings, and which they use to guide their regular daily activities (19–20).

To understand how an organisation's philosophy, its purpose or function, structure, communication patterns and control techniques influence current practices, an organisational analysis such as that described by Gaynor and Berry (1977:17–22) can be undertaken. From the results of such an analysis those practices which should be continued and strengthened can be identified, as well as those which should be discarded and replaced. As this process is intended to introduce changes which will recognise and reward nurses for their active role in nursing (not to promote the view of nurses as being one of its ingredients), the staff themselves should be encouraged to participate in identifying the factors which facilitate and those which constrain their approach to and behaviour at work.

Hilmer (1985:17–18) notes that

> most Australians can and want to make worthwhile, lasting contributions through their work. To be a creative, innovative individual working with others towards a common goal is considered more rewarding than simply doing a job because you are told to do it. However, in order to work together in an environment which will allow everyone to make an individual contribution often required the establishment of a different attitude towards work — a new mindset.

To allow these outcomes to eventuate, the successful manager should establish the following six conditions within the workplace: a trusting environment; widespread experimentation; a driving purpose; a positive approach; real jobs; a network of teams (Hilmer, 1985: 14–15).

In establishing these conditions, showing nurses that their involvement in structuring their own working environment and practice is valued will encourage and sustain alterations in all parties' attitudes to work and the work setting. The manager who, by the recognition of individuals' personal worth, generates staff commitment to seeking and exploiting opportunities to achieve self- or group-identified goals, and establishes a climate wherein participants are trusted and encouraged to seek better ways of achieving the organisation's overall goal, helps others to excellent performance. Such excellence is reflected in the effectiveness, efficiency, economy and apparent ease with which the organisation's purpose is fulfilled.

# 7. CONCLUSION

Many different approaches to the structuring of nursing work and of the nursing workforce are possible. The selection of a particular approach depends upon how the values and beliefs contained within the organisation's philosophy and mission are reflected in its policies and practices, and in the priorities established to manage utilisation of its available resources. In seeking to choose the most appropriate means of promoting effective and efficient provision of high quality patient care, the manager should determine the predominant values of practitioners within the specific service area. Knowing whether the emphasis is on team work, individualism, security or a 'vision of nursing as it could be' will assist the manager to select the most appropriate way of organising the delivery of nursing services in this setting, or identify areas where staff development will be needed before structural change can be implemented.

Where changes in behaviour are expected within the work environment because of changes in the way work is structured, managers must seek to develop different expectations and attitudes both in themselves and in the members of staff. Literature supports the view that, when individuals see their work contributions as being meaningful and significant in achieving the desired outcomes, their commitment to striving towards achieving excellence is enhanced. By recognising the valuable role each nurse plays in fulfilling the organisation's mission, the nurse manager is recognising the importance of the human resources entrusted to their care.

In managing nursing and seeking to achieve the desired high quality patient care outcomes, the nurse manager is responsible for the development and retention of highly productive, internally motivated nurses who find their work satisfying and challenging and are committed to achieving the goals and promoting the values of the organisation. How work and work practices are structured can either constrain or facilitate efforts to achieve successful outcomes.

# CORELLA CASE STUDY

Corella District Hospital is a 120 bed hospital serving the population of a large country town and the surrounding district. The town of Corella is situated on the slopes of the Great Dividing Range and is close to the coast and a number of popular tourist resorts.

It is the commercial centre of a rich grazing and dairying district. There is also a large timber mill as forestry work is carried out in the mountains. The town has a direct air service to the city twice daily, and is on the railway line. There are two municipal pools, two golf courses, several squash centres and tennis complexes and a large number of playing fields with most sports catered for adequately.

Corella Hospital has 343 beds made up of four recently converted Nightingale wards of 30 beds each used for general medical and surgical patients; an orthopaedic and an obstetric ward of 30 beds each; an oto-rhinolaryngology and opthalmology ward of 10 beds; new paediatric, psychiatric and rehabilitation units of 30 beds each; recently renovated ICU, CCU and accident and emergency wards of 10 beds each and a day surgical ward of 20 beds. In addition there are six humidicribs/cots in the special care nursery and seven beds in the recovery ward. There are four operating theatres also and an extensive outpatients department. The hospital has 442 EFT nursing staff funded positions.

The Chief Executive Officer of Corella Hospital is Alex Kandici, who is in the mid-

30s and has been at Corella for the past three years. During this time Alex has persuaded the Health Department to convert the hospital management information systems to fully computerised systems. Alex was able to do this by indicating in the submission that several positions could be saved in 12 months' time, through the change to computerisation. The submission had also indicated the achievements that could be expected through increased efficiency. Alex had also been instrumental in encouraging the local Lions, Apex and Rotary Clubs to combine their efforts and raise the money that was required for the renovation of the ICU, CCU and A and E units. The staff were therefore not surprised to find that Alex had been appointed the new Area Chief Executive Officer.

Among the first to congratulate Alex was the Director of Nursing, Sala Tanner. Sala has been at Corella for four months following the completion of the Master of Nursing Administration Degree. Previously, Sala had been the DON of Lorikeet Hospital, one of the hospitals in the region, which is now to be included in the Corella Area Health Service along with Cockatoo and Galah Hospitals which serve two of the smaller holiday resorts on the coast.

Sala and Alex have known one another for some years, both through work and university associations, and get along well together. Sala has had some difficulties though, in relationships with the Director of Medical Services, Dr Frigett. However, Sala feels that these problems will gradually be overcome as they get to know one another better. Many people, in fact, find it difficult to get along with Dr.

Frigett who has been described as "a pompous ass", "an overbearing prig", and someone "who wants everything done yesterday".

Over the past two years there have been a number of other changes taking place at Corella. The School of Nursing has gradually been reduced with the final group of hospital trainees graduating two weeks ago. This has meant a change in the composition of the workforce at the hospital from younger students to a fully registered mature age workforce who are more assertive with their demands for hours to suit their family and other commitments. The present staff also appear to be less tolerant of the hierarchical nursing division structure and recently requested more say in the decisions affecting nursing staff.

Sala would even say that there was some degree of alienation present in the workforce as evidenced by their lack of commitment to the nursing profession. Very few staff showed any interest in their professional associations, or in attending continuing education courses if they were not paid for by the hospital or occurred out of work time. Sala finds this difficult to understand as nursing has been the major interest in her life, and full participation in nursing associations and conferences has been part of that interest, occupying many hours both on and off duty.

There have also been difficulties in attracting and retaining nurses at Corella since the closure of one of the large factories recently. Hence greater use has been made of agency staff. This has not helped the financial position of the hospital. The simple nursing dependency system that was used by the nursing staff to calculate their workload was discontinued 12 months ago when the previous DON lost the Deputy DON who was responsible for collating the dependency data. These difficulties have led to the closure of two of the 30 bed wards and restrictions on the amount of elective surgery carried out. This has created tension with the doctors and there have been several articles in the paper on the cut-back in services.

The nursing staff have also expressed concern following the announcement of the introduction of area health services. Some of the Community Health Staff were employed by the Health Department and are wondering whether they will change to being employees of the Area Health Board and how this will affect them. There have also been numerous rumours circulating about the administrative and staff changes that might take place under the new Area Health Boards.

At a recent meeting of the Medical Advisory Committee, the Visiting Medical Officers decided to make a formal complaint to the Board, with copies to the Regional Director and the Minister of Health, objecting to the budget received by the hospital. This was 1 per cent less than last year and did not allow for inflation, the growth in the population of the region of 6 per cent due to the opening up of the Beaunest Estate, and the work generated by the new VMOs and the opening of the new wards.

Alex and Sala are concerned because Corella Hospital is due for accreditation in 12 months' time. It is the third time the hospital has applied for accreditation and following the last accreditation the surveyors made a number of recommendations. The recommendations included that the hospital should implement an approved nursing dependency system and should set up a safety committee. There appeared to be large numbers of back injuries among the nurses and numerous patient falls with little identifiable action being taken. The surveyors had also recommended improvements to the orientation programme and commented on the limited inservice lectures being given to nursing staff both in number and variety.

## QUESTIONS

1. In 3000 to 4000 words, describe the actions Sala Tanner should take to alleviate the problems facing the nursing division of Corella Hospital and Area Health Service. Give a time frame for the implementation of any changes considered and provide a rationale for your decisions.

2. Explain why a safety committee is necessary. What would be the terms of reference for the proposed safety committee? What would be the appropriate positions to be represented on the committee?

3. As nurse manager of the medical unit with the greatest number of back injuries and patient falls, prepare a report for the Director of Nursing on the ways in which you intend to reduce this problem being mindful of other factors mentioned which may also have a bearing on this problem.

# REFERENCES

Bell, A. and Storey, C. (1984), 'Assessing Workload by a Nursing Study', *Nursing Times,* August 22: 57-59

Benner, P. (1984), *From novice to expert,* Addison-Wesley, Menlo Park.

Bennett, T. R. and Duckett, S. J. (1981), 'Operations Research and Nurse Staffing', *International Journal of Bio-Medical Computing,* 12: 433-438.

Braddy, P. (1987/88), 'Scheduling alternatives for Administrators', *Nursing Forum,* 2: 70-77.

Donley, R. and Flaherty, M. J. (1989), 'Analysis of the Market Driven Nursing Shortage', *Nursing & Health Care,* 10(4): 183-187.

Donovan, M. I. and Lewis, G. (1987), 'Financial Management Series — Increasing Productivity and Decreasing Costs: the value of RNs', *Journal of Nursing Administration,* 17(9): 16-18.

Friss, L. (1981), 'An Expanded Conceptualisation of Job Satisfaction and Career Style', *Nursing Leadership,* 4(4): 13-22.

Gaynor, A. K. and Berry, R. K. (1977), 'Observations of a Staff Nurse: an organisational analysis', *Nursing Dimensions,* Fall: 17-22.

Gillies, D. A. (1989), *Nursing Management: a systems approach,* 2nd edition, W. B. Saunders: Harcourt Brace Jovanovich, Philadelphia.

Graham, P., Constantini, S., Balik, B., Bedore, B., Hooke, M.C., Papin, D., Quamme, M. and Rivard, R. (1987), 'Operationalising a Nursing Philosophy', *Journal of Nursing Administration,* 17(3):14-18.

Halloran, E. J. and Hadley Vermeersch, P. E. (1987), 'Variability in Nurse Staffing Research', *Journal of Nursing Administration,* 17(2): 26-32.

Hancock, W. M. and Fuhs, P. A. (1984), 'The relationship between Nurse Staffing Policies and Nursing Budgets', *Health Care Management Review,* Fall: 21-26.

Hilmer, F. G. (1985), *When the luck runs out,* Harper & Row, Sydney.

Jenkins, E. (1983), 'Nurse Staffing Methodologies: the relationship between quality and cost', *Australian Journal of Advanced Nursing,* 1(1): 6-11.

Kramer, M. and Schmalenberg, C. (1988a), 'Magnet Hospitals: Part I — Institutions of Excellence', *Journal of Nursing Administration,* 18(1): 13-24.

Kramer, M. and Schmalenberg, C. (1988b), 'Magnet Hospitals: Part II — Institutions of Excellence', *Journal of Nursing Administration,* 18(2): 11-19.

Kron, T and Gray, A. (1987), *The management of patient care: putting leadership skills to work,* 6th edition, W. B. Saunders, Philadelphia.

Larter, M. H. (1982), 'Creative Staffing', in Marriner, A. (Ed.) *Contemporary Nursing Management: issues and practice,* C.V. Mosby, St Louis: 161-179.

Marram, G., Flynn, K., Abaravich, W. and Carey, S. (1976), *Cost-effectiveness of primary and team nursing,* Contemporary Publishing, Wakefield.

Matthews, A. (1987), *In charge of the ward,* 2nd edition, Blackwell Scientific, Oxford.

McClure, M. L. (1984), 'Managing the Professional Nurse. Part 2: applying management theory to the challenges', *Journal of Nursing Administration,* 14(3): 11-17.

Meyer, D. (1984), 'Manpower Planning: One — an American approach', *Nursing Times,* August 22: 52-54.

Nauert, L. B., Leach, K. M. and Watson, P. M. (1988), 'Finding the Productivity Standard in Your Acuity System', *Journal of Nursing Administration,* 18(1): 25-30.

Olivas, G. S., Del Togno-Armanasco, V., Erickson, J. R. and Harter, S. (1989), 'Case Management: a bottom-line care delivery model. Part 1: The Concept', *Journal of Nursing Administration,* 19(11): 16-20.

Prescott, P. A. and Phillips, C. Y. (1988), 'Gauging Nursing Intensity to Bring Costs to Light', *Nursing and Health Care,* 9(1): 17-22.

Reid, N. G. and Melaugh, M. (1987), 'Nurse Hours Per Patient: a method for monitoring and explaining staffing levels', *International Journal of Nursing Studies,* 24(1): 1-14.

Rowland, H. S. and Rowland, B. L. (1985), *Nursing administration handbook,* 2nd edition, Aspen, Rockville.

Schuler, R. S., Dowling, P. J. and Smart, J. P. (1988), *Personnel/human resource management in Australia,* Harper & Row, Sydney.

Seelye, A. (1982), 'Hospital Ward Layout and Nurse Staffing', *Journal of Advanced Nursing,* 7: 195-201.

Stevens, B. J. (1980), *The nurse as executive,* 2nd edition, Nursing Resources, Wakefield.

Stillwaggon, C. A. (1989), 'The Impact of Nurse Managed Care on the Cost of Nurse Practice and Nurse Satisfaction' (Financial Management Series), *Journal of Nursing Administration,* 19(11): 21-27.

Storey, C. and Bell, A. (1985), 'A Useful Pair of Hands?' *Nursing Times,* March 27: 40-42.

Wilson, B. L. and Firestone, W. A. (1987), 'The Principal and Instruction: combining bureaucratic and cultural linkages', *Educational Leadership,* September: 18-23.

Yuill, B., Polites, G. and Smart, J. (1978), *Personnel management in Australia,* 3rd edition, John Wiley & Sons, Brisbane.

# CHAPTER 1.4

# Education and the nurse manager

MARJORIE CUTHBERT

This chapter aims to:

1. provide the nurse manager with an understanding of the different types of education required for professional development;

2. define the key concepts associated with professional nursing education;

3. define the role of continuing education as a means of transmission of the philosophy and vision of the employing agency;

4. discuss the expectations of the patient, the employer, the employee, professional bodies, and the education agency relating to professional education (eg ACHS, Colleges of Nursing, Nursing Registration Boards, Professional Groups, Universities Private agencies, and Consumer groups);

5. identify methods of planning career paths and the requisite professional education and development required;

6. increase awareness of the relationship of education to quality patient care and issues of professional accountability.

---

This chapter addresses specifically the relationship between continuing professional education, nursing management and patient care within the context of health care organisations (whether public hospitals, private hospitals, specialist hospitals, nursing homes or community health centres). It focuses on the responsibilities of the registered nurse manager who is employed to supervise staff and manage both patient care and the environment in which the patient or client is dependent. It suggests ways that nurse managers can build on their individual levels of educational expertise as part of a management strategy. The goal of this approach is twofold: to assist with the performance and job satisfaction of both the nurse manager and staff and thus lead to positive patient outcomes. Other aspects considered in relation to staff education are the orientation of staff, maintenance education, remedial education, and the continuing professional education needs of the nursing staff on the unit. The second objective is to assist with patients/clients needs for education. Aspects considered here are orientation of the institutionalised patient, assessment of prior knowledge, planning and design of the teaching process, evaluation of the effectiveness of teaching.

Briefly, orientation refers to the introductory education and socialisation provided to staff when they enter a new work situation or to patients or clients entering a new environment. Maintenance education (Stevens, 1985:390) refers to the education required to maintain little used skills at a reasonably high level or needed when new equipment is introduced to the work situation. Remedial education (Stevens, 1985:390) is the education required to remedy gaps in professional knowledge or skills. It can also include the learning of new skills when a nurse moves into a new position or returns to nursing after a period of absence. Continuing professional education includes both staff development and inservice education. It can assist nurses in progressing professionally in their chosen career path, or increase general knowledge, or update skills in the specific area of their nursing practice.

The belief that education is primarily for the school aged and that on completion of a formal qualification or skills training programme there is no necessity to continue with professional education, is outmoded. Due to the rapid technological changes that our society has experienced it is necessary for individuals to keep learning so as not to be disadvantaged in their work environment. A possible outcome of falling behind in professional knowledge in nursing practice could be litigation. This aspect is discussed further in chapter 1.5.

The term 'continuing professional education' also covers a number of other terms such as adult education, lifelong education, and on-the-job training. Adult education is described by Jarvis and Gibson (1985:31) as being broader in scope than continuing professional education. He views adult education as encompassing 'liberal, general or vocational' studies undertaken in an educational institution or in a more informal community setting. Jarvis' views on adult education have implications for the nurse manager. Continuing professional education should be seen as part of an individual's broader adult education which continues over the life-span of the individual (Jarvis 1985: 51-52). The relevance of any form of education depends on the individual's learning needs at that point in time. Stevens (1985:390) describes the process as getting up, catch[ing] up, stay[ing] up, mov[ing] up, and moving out.

On-the-job training is directly related to the development of expertise required for a specific job or task. This utilises teaching skills such as task analysis (Mason, 1984, pp. 31, 250) and the demonstration method, and is usually conducted on a one-to-one basis or in small groups. Demonstrations are often provided in on-the-job training by preceptors who are very experienced nurses who have participated in a training programme and are prepared to work alongside new graduates to assist them adjust to the workplace (Puetz, 1983:92). The aim of the training programme is to equip preceptors with the necessary teaching skills required to assist the new staff members (Benner, 1984:278).

Ongoing training and professional development are now considered as essential for increasing productivity in Australian industries (Federal Government Training Guarantee

Bill, 1990). There are many benefits to be derived from encouraging professional development in nursing for the individual, the organisation and for patient care. These benefits will be considered under the discussion of the various types of continuing professional education.

# 1. DEFINITION OF TERMS

A review of the literature indicates confusion in the terminology relating to staff education so some definitions are provided:

1. **orientation** is the process of assisting personnel to adjust to a new environment. This occurs with a change of role, or department, or a position in a new organisation.

2. **inservice education** is education usually given within an institution in order to maintain infrequently used skills, such as fire safety and cardio-pulmonary resuscitation; to update skills when necessary, for example when a new document such as a nursing history chart is introduced; and to ensure acquisition of new skills and knowledge when new equipment or nursing procedures are to be implemented.

3. **continuing education** is carried out external to the health care service and includes workshops, seminars, conferences, specialty courses such as oncology nursing, and post-graduate courses such as Bachelor of Advanced Nursing and Master of Nursing Administration. Continuing education provides specific development to those people already working in a field related to the content of the programme, ie nursing, clinical practice, management or education.

4. **staff development** is concerned with developing the potential of the individual for the benefit of the organisation or the individual at some future time. For example, those nursing unit managers displaying leadership or executive potential are encouraged to serve on committees, relieve in higher positions or attend advanced management courses in order to develop the skills and confidence required to apply for senior positions.

# 2. ORGANISATIONAL CULTURE

The culture of an organisation is determined to a large extent by the philosophy and mission of the organisation. The philosophy usually reflects the beliefs and values of the board and executives and the mission defines the purpose of organisation.

Implementation by middle managers is dependent on their acceptance of the beliefs and values expressed in the philosophy and their understanding of the mission. Middle managers such as the nursing unit manager or team leader in the community health setting must not only have accepted the values but also be committed to their implementation in practice.

The commitment of the individual to the organisational philosophy is derived in a number of ways. The first approach is through the selection process. At interviews the nurse applicant must demonstrate a similar set of beliefs and values to those of the organisation. If the organisation has a strong belief in continuing professional development of staff, then the applicants must have demonstrated evidence of ongoing commitment to their own professional education.

Such evidence would include subscriptions to relevant journals, attendance at workshops, seminars and conferences (not necessarily in the organisation's time) participation in research activities, and the practical implementation of research findings.

The applicant at interview would also ascertain the likelihood of continued support in these endeavours. The organisation with a commitment to professional development of staff would have in place a continuing education programme. The culture would be one of active acceptance and encouragement of staff attendance at external seminars, conferences, inservice courses and further education through tertiary institutions.

Each organisation develops its own set of 'norms'. These are behaviours judged by the organisation members to be acceptable according to their own particular standards. These norms may cause approval or disapproval of certain behaviours in certain circumstances. In some organisations continuing education may be the preserve of executives and long-standing employees only. This is a limited application of a philosophy which encourages education as a reward for long service rather than a right for all employees.

Although a philosophy may strongly reflect a recognised need for ongoing education there may be problems of access. It may be possible for only those on day duty to attend. Education may not be provided for evening duty or night duty staff. We believe it is possible to provide education for those working on all shifts.

All ongoing education has budgetary implications. This again reflects the strength of commitment to the value of education for all employees. Any programme of continuing professional development requires an appropriate budget allocation and a strategic plan. The plan should assess the strengths, the weaknesses, the opportunities, and threats likely to affect any educational programme, using 'force-field analysis' (Craig, 1978:42–45). An educational plan should also consider the following questions: what proportion of the overall organisation budget can be allocated to education? Is it to be restricted to the one per cent demanded by legislation as discussed below, or is it to be proportionally larger than this? What are the 'on costs' or additional costs associated with provision of this education such as educators' salaries, photocopying, electricity, cleaning, clerical staff, printing and travel?

# **3.** FEDERAL GOVERNMENT TRAINING GUARANTEE BILL, 1990

The Federal Government introduced the above legislation in 1990 in an attempt to improve the knowledge base 'of Australian employees and their flexibility in their work environment'. Each organisation with an annual payroll of $200 000 or more is required to commit one per cent of their annual payroll for training purposes. This amount will rise to 1.5 per cent by July 1992.

Employers failing to meet these minimum requirements will be forced to pay a Training Guarantee Charge which will be distributed to each state for new training activities. The one per cent–1.5 per cent spent on training attracts a tax deduction. However money paid into the Training Guarantee Charge Fund will not be tax deductible.

For programmes to be acceptable under the Act they must 'constitute an eligible training programme of particular expenditure' (44(1) p. 23). For programs to be eligible they must be specifically structured with objectives designed 'to develop, maintain or improve employment related skills of employees'. The aims of the programmes are to increase the productivity of the Australian workplace and in manufacturing to allow Australian products to compete with those manufactured overseas. (Training Guarantee Bill 1990 Explanatory Memorandum: 20).

Allied to the concept of increasing production through education is the concept of Total Quality Management or TQM (Sprouster, 1987). TQM changed the face of Japanese manufacturing after World War II. Dr Edwards Deering, who introduced the TQM concept to Japan, believed that 'quality cannot be inspected-in, it must be built-in' (Sprouster, 1987 p. 48). The general philosophy is that the workers are the people best able to identify and deal with production problems. Participative management is the keystone. TQM was introduced in Australia in 1984 under the auspices of the Federal Government and Enterprise Australia in the endeavour to improve the quality of Australian products and again make them more competitive both at home and abroad. The key to both programmes is education and its importance to improving both productivity and quality cannot be overstressed.

When introducing TQM to nursing we aim at continual improvement of nursing care through improved management and communication processes and continual improvement in nursing knowledge and skills. This is explained in more detail in the chapter on evaluation systems for nurse managers.

# 4. MANDATORY VERSUS VOLUNTARY EDUCATION

Mandatory continuing professional education has been described as 'compulsory continuing education for all practitioners of a particular profession in order to retain or renew their licences to practise'.

Continuing professional education may be made mandatory by law, as for employers with the Training Guarantee Act 1990; for employees by membership requirements of professional associations; or less formally by employers' expectations of employees. At this stage of development of the nursing profession in Australia continuing professional education remains a voluntary activity for all members of the profession. It is therefore the responsibility of all nursing professionals to maintain their own level of continuing professional education. Nurse employers may keep either formal or informal records of continuing professional education seminars, conferences, courses and workshops that their staff attend. Employers in some fields of the profession require details of continuing professional education attendance for consideration for career advancement. Under the new legislation in Australia, employers now are required to maintain records of their employees' participation in continuing education and inservice sessions. However there are a number of issues associated with mandatory continuing professional education.

The concept of mandatory continuing professional education is based on the belief that professionals lack the motivation to voluntarily attend continuing professional education programmes. It also reflects the notion that provision of education and associated costs is the responsibility of the employer rather than that of the employee, or a shared responsibility.

In regard to how adults learn, this form of external motivation may only act to decrease the individual's level of motivation. Making continuing professional education compulsory may lead to the result that the professionals may resent the experience (Cooper, 1973: 16–17). Houle (1981) suggests that to force attendance may actually discourage self-initiated and self-directed learning.

Other issues are the relevance and quality of the continuing education programmes offered to professionals. Little attempt has been made to assess individuals' learning styles when continuing professional education is made compulsory. There is a danger in offering programmes of only a technical nature to the exclusion of non-technical subjects. Several states in America have made it mandatory for nurses to participate in continuing education programmes, and various bodies such as the Joint Commission on Accreditation of Hospitals (JCAH) have specified where the emphasis is to be placed. JCAH specified continuing education be directed to discharge planning to improve the turnover of patients (Betz, 1983). There is also a danger of courses aimed at the majority.

A further issue relates to whether or not it is necessary to have a body to accredit courses, their administration and content. In NSW the College of Nursing has recently assumed the role of accrediting body in that state for nursing colleges while within universities the Academic Board accepts the responsibility. This issue highlights the level of administration that would be necessary for the implementation of mandatory continuing professional education. Perhaps a cost analysis is needed to measure whether the expected gains would be offset by the expenses associated with the process of making continuing professional education compulsory. Conversely, the outcome of a well managed, non-mandatory continuing professional education programme conducted in conjunction with a needs analysis and effective programme evaluation could be preferable.

# 5. STANDARDS AND NURSE MANAGEMENT

In Australia standards for continuing education and staff development are written by the accrediting body for health organisations, The Australian Council on Healthcare Standards (1990) based on those of the professional nursing association the Royal Australian Nursing Federation (1983), now known as the Australian Nursing Federation. Graduating nurses from university courses will also be required to meet the Australian Nurse

Registering Authorities competencies (ANRAC, 1991).

While the ACHS standard (Nursing Division Standards Staff Development and Education, ACHS, 1990) is clear and easy to follow, this is one standard where some major changes have occurred in the ACHS criteria, particularly in relation to the resources allocated to staff development and education of nursing staff. The RANF (1983) standard specified in criterion 1.2 that:

> the role [of co-ordinator] is the sole function where the qualified nursing staff establishment is 100 or above, or the role is incorporated in the job description of another nursing position where the qualified nursing staff establishment is below 100.

See also RANF criterion 3 (1983) which specifies a ratio of 1:150 educators to qualified nursing staff. This is in marked contrast to the present situation which was negotiated when nurse education was transferred to CAEs. RANF criterion 5 also stipulates that a separate budget allocation is required. The present ANA (1987) standard 6 — Staff Development states:

> there is a staff development programme for all nursing personnel to facilitate and encourage continuing development of each individual as a professional practitioner.

Both ACHS and RANF criteria include orientation to clinical areas but the ACHS criterion 5.3 states that 'there is an orientation programme for all newly appointed nursing staff and for those new to specific areas . . .' If one remembers Benner's (1985:21) findings that a nurse reverts to a novice or advanced beginner when allocated to work in an unfamiliar area, then from both the patients' point of view and the nurses', orientation in new clinical areas could be considered essential.

Often in our hospitals nurses are asked to plug gaps in rosters and work in a new clinical area without any orientation to the unit. Agency nurses also work in areas constantly with limited orientation. Sub-section 5.3 (g) states that the orientation will include 'identification of individual learning needs' while 5.3 (h) states that provision of 'information about safety procedures to be followed' is required. How many agency nurses or nurses who are transferred from their regular wards to work in a new area determine where the emergency equipment is kept, what are the special procedures which are used for that patient population, what are the particular preferences of the attending doctors and so on. In fact if each nurse rostered to a ward for a short time were to do these important activities there would be very little patient care time left. Is it possible that this lack of orientation is why very few nurses accept the challenge to become expert in a number of areas and so few nurses are prepared to work in more than one or two wards? These issues are all vital considerations for the nurse manager whose responsibility it is to ensure that standards are maintained in the ward or unit and appropriate educational programmes for staff are provided within budget limitations.

The setting of standards and the advantages and limitations of the ANRAC competencies are discussed in much more detail in two recent publications by the Department of Employment Education and Training (Gonczi, Hager and Oliver, 1990; Masters and McCurry, 1990).

# **6.** THE CONTINUING EDUCATION DEBATE

Generally, the aim of continuing education and inservice programmes is to maintain or increase competence for practitioners, keep them up-to-date with new developments in their fields of expertise and avoid obsolescence, especially in an era of increasing specialisation. The ACHS standard 5.5 (c) also includes 'supports and encourages nursing investigation and research' while standard 5.5 (e) supports the promotion of courses outside the institution. Del Bueno (1976) argues that courses provided by hospitals or health services must be designed with one aim in mind, to improve performance in a particular area and that course objectives should be specific performance objectives with the content reflecting these objectives. Evaluation can determine the effectiveness of the course in improving skills of staff members.

In recent years there has been an increasing trend within hospitals to purchase high technology equipment. Jones (1982: 232–233) claims that 'the medical profession is particularly addicted to high-technology solutions to problems' and later that hospital

> management faced with a choice of heavy investment in capital equipment such as scanners, or employing more nurses to provide intimate personal contact with patients, may well choose the first option, which may not always be to the patient's benefit.

Brewer (1983) also sees technological development changing the organisational structures and processes of hospitals and thus making the work environment more complex, while at the same time emphasising the therapeutic approach and down-grading the traditional caring approach of nursing. She sees a need therefore for training and educating new types of nursing personnel. This need was also expressed by Heimstra (1976) who used the analogy of the physicist's notion of 'half-life' and suggested that the 'half-life' of the competent practitioner, from the time of entry to the nursing profession, was approximately five years.

Occupational half-life is based on the assumption that new developments, techniques, and/or knowledge evolve in a short period of time, so that a person becomes roughly half as competent to do the job for which his or her initial training was intended (Heimstra, 1976:8).

In recent years there has been a shortage of nurses with specialist skills and nurses prepared to work in specialties such as intensive care and operating rooms in major metropolitan hospitals. 1984 saw the establishment of a Task Force by the New South Wales Department of Health to investigate the difficulties within the profession at that time — high turnover and absenteeism levels, shortage of specialist nurses and problems with recruitment and retention of registered nurses. Two of the many recommendations were that:

The Department (of Health) investigate ways of increasing the output from post-basic clinic specialty courses and of retaining appropriately qualified nurses in the workforce in the short term and development strategies for meeting the need for increased training capacity in the long term in consultation with the higher education sector

and that:

An investigation be made of methods to ensure that nurses in the workforce have adequate exposure to continuing education particularly in areas where there is increasing utilisation of more sophisticated equipment and drugs.

The results of this study are also supported by the Report of the Committee of Enquiry into Nursing in Victoria (1985:202, 249). The results of the Victorian enquiry indicated strong dissatisfaction with the lack of educational programmes in hospitals and the quality of the educators. This dissatisfaction was most marked in metropolitan regional and specialised hospitals (222). Again nurses in these hospitals were particularly dissatisfied with training provided for new equipment (223). In other words they felt a need for provision of maintenance education.

In the Marles report (1988:236) many nurses also expressed a view that mandatory contining education should be essential for maintenance of the right to practise nursing.

However, inservice and continuing education problems are not restricted to nurses working with the new technology. Professor Styles (1983), at the International Nursing Conference in Brazil, considered that the most pressing problem facing nursing was inadequate leadership and stressed that energies in continuing education should be 'concentrated at the highest levels'. These recommendations have direct implications for continuing education for registered nurses working at all levels in different types of organisations in Australia. Recent research by Duffield (1989) into the role of first line managers identified the competencies considered essential for this position. Postgraduate courses have now been put in place to meet these identified needs. However this is a long term problem. At the beginning of the eighties King (1981) reported that of the 53 per cent of nurses who completed a survey into learning needs, 19 per cent considered that in the previous 12 months they had felt unprepared in situations or tasks involving procedures and equipment, 9 per cent in management situations and 7 per cent in interrelationships. There have also been claims made that inservice and continuing education programmes in Australia are failing to meet the needs of the majority of nurses (McClelland, 1985; Marles, 1988).

An American writer (Kubat, 1976) considered that several factors may have been operating within the nursing profession in the US at that time which may have worked against nurses' entry into appropriate forms of continuing education. In her study of registered nurses, Kubat outlined five major points in this regard:

1. a decreasing inclination by nurses to read professional journals, attend professional seminars and maintain membership in relevant professional associations;

2. a failure to recognise current changes in knowledge and practice;

3. lack of interest in gaining a broader knowledge or skill base though self-directed or formal continuing education programmes;

4. lack of personal initiative;

5. a desire to maintain the status quo.

A similar criticism, that nurses were not interested in undertaking continuing education, was made by a speaker at the 1987 annual conference of the College of Nursing Australia in Hobart. However at that conference there were over 400 nurses present and while the numbers at this conference increase each year it is not generally known whether those present find the lecturers satisfy their continuing education needs or whether other aspects such as informal networking and trade displays play an important role. In New South Wales and in Victoria the Colleges of Nursing have both markedly increased their continuing education programmes, extended them to country areas and introduced distance learning courses. There are now a number of Masters courses in nursing offered in Australia which have far more applicants annually than there are places available. This indicates a belief that higher education is desirable and that professional nurses are prepared to undertake it.

Graeme Rawson (1986:33) in his study on the continuing education needs of health service administrators found the Directors of Nursing (DONs) surveyed considered that personal and inter-personal skills such as:

1. leadership abilities;

2. staff motivation;

3. performance evaluation;

4. personnel administration;

5. public and media relations;

6. dealing with conflict; and,

7. stress management

were most important in the successful performance of their DON duties. The areas in which DONs feel they have a personal need for continuing education are

> preparation and analysis of budgets (43 per cent), analysis of financial information (36 per cent), understanding and interpreting statistical data (26 per cent) accounting principles and methods in the health services (25 per cent) analysis of future trends (11 per cent).

The first 10 preferences listed by DONs in the Rawson study (Rawson, 1986:53–56) for continuing education were:

1.  computer applications in the health services;

2.  preparation and analysis of budgets;

3.  analysis of financial information;

4.  understanding and interpreting statistical data;

5.  operational research and systems analysis;

6.  accounting principles and methods in the health services;

7.  concepts, implications and laws of industrial relations;

8.  research methods;

9.  conflict resolution methods;

10. public speaking.

Many of these topics are just as necessary for first-line managers although their preferences may well be different.

# 7. INSERVICE EDUCATION PROGRAMMES

Stevens (1985:392) considers that inservice and continuing education programmes are closely linked to the assessment of management structures, staff activities and patient outcomes. She also maintains that 'consensus about weaknesses in staff performance can be a reasonable basis for asserting that a problem exists' and that a 'wise director' will ensure that 'projects are based on patient care deficiencies' (Stevens, 1985:384–385). The quality systems that are required for identifying performance levels are a personnel appraisal system, a system for reporting errors, incidents, patient and staff accidents, an infection control system, and a nursing dependency system. These are all components of a total quality management programme (Oakland, 1989). In addition in each ward, or unit, tools for ensuring that the competencies required for nursing the patient population are identified. Each nurse who works in the area assists in having their learning needs diagnosed in relation to the specific competencies required for the ward or unit. However O'Connor (1986:80) warns that if the learning needs are diagnosed then action needs to be taken, within a reasonable time, to remedy the deficiencies identified. Assessments are undertaken at regular intervals to ensure that skills are maintained. This process assists in meeting criteria in the Accreditation Standards.

# 7.1 DESIGNING TEACHING PROGRAMMES

There are four major theoretical perspectives of learning, the *behaviourist,* the *cognitive,* the *humanist* and the *social action* perspectives. Our methods of selecting the content to be taught and the means for teaching the content will be influenced by one or other of these perspectives.

## 7.1.1 Behaviourist

The major early researchers in this area are Pavlov, Thorndike, Skinner and Bandura and information on their methods is available in most introductory psychology texts such as Sharpe and Ross (1990:273–286).

Adherents of the behaviourist perspective believe that learning is the result of conditioning and that behaviour responds according to the type of reinforcer used. Reinforcers may be either positive, as occurs with praise, or negative as occurs with punishment. Both praise and punishment are 'extrinsic' reinforcers when given by others. 'Intrinsic' reinforcers are the feelings of achievement, pride or satisfaction we have when we have reached our goals (Sharpe and Ross, 1990:276).

A behaviourist believes that if a nurse or patient is given positive feedback, encouraged or praised as learning proceeds, then they are likely to continue with the learning process. Withdrawal of rewards or punishments can extinguish or lead to the cessation of learned behaviours. A nurse using this method of teaching is taking responsibility for changing the patient's behaviour and this implies that the change will be effective (Vargas, 1977:9). When using this method, the problem is analysed through recording behaviours, identifying the factors in the environment which are responsible for the behaviours and determining ways to change consequences in order to change the behaviour. Counter-conditioning can substitute coping responses for non-coping responses.

The behaviourist approach would be an appropriate method for the nurse manager to use with a nurse who was rejecting a difficult patient or a patient who must give up smoking.

Behaviourists also believe that behaviour can be learned from models. Nurse managers often act as role models for other members of staff through the ways they react to superiors, clients or patients and other health care personnel. The nurse managers may also have been influenced in their behaviour by their teachers and other health professionals with whom they have worked.

## 7.1.2 Cognitive

This perspective developed from the work of Piaget who believes that cognitive development occurs through people's interaction with other people, materials and technology in their environment and the information these interactions provide. Adherents of this perspective believe that intellect occurs over a number of domains (Gagne, 1974). They believe that learning occurs in an hierarchical fashion, moving from the known to the unknown and from the simple to the complex. Chaining or chunking of information occurs as new knowledge is linked to previously acquired knowledge. Information is stored first in short-term memory and then through repetition is put into long-term memory for recall later. This perspective is very closely linked to the behaviourist perspective. This method would be appropriate for teaching an asthmatic patient how to prevent and control an asthmatic attack (see *Respiratory Disorders: Asthma*, Patient Teaching Loose-Leaf Library, Springhouse Corporation).

The teacher does an assessment of learner needs based on the student's prior knowledge and identifies the skills, knowledge and attitudes required for the teaching to be effective. Evaluations are conducted to provide feedback to the teacher and enable modifications to the programme in order to maintain effectiveness of outcomes.

### 7.1.3 Humanist

In this view both the cognitive and affective areas are involved. This perspective grew from the work of Rogers (1961, 1983) and Maslow (1943, 1968) which focused on the personal needs of the learner and how these needs may be affected by early learning experiences.

When this perspective is paramount the teacher believes that the individual is self-motivated to learn and should be free to make their own choices. Each person is unique with their own self-concept and this influences the way in which each student approaches learning. Each nurse's or client's perceived needs are considered important and the learning environment is open, warm and trusting so as to facilitate the learning process. The teacher assists in clarifying values and learning is self-directed. Boud (1988, p. 226) believes the strength of this approach lies in the appreciation of students as individuals and in 'assisting them to find their own way through their learning problems'. An example of this approach is to be found in White et al. (1988) and in the case study approach used by Barclay (1989).

### 7.1.4 Social action

This is a fourth perspective of critical thinking which leads to social action for a changed society and is closely linked to the humanist tradition. Both the teacher and the learner need to be aware of the values they hold and the historical and societal influences from whence they came. Boud (1988:226–227) states that this perspective is the result of 'an ideological shift' from 'functionalism and the importance of the individual to dialectics and collective action' and is 'pursuing *freedom through learning*'.

Chief proponents of this view are Illich (1976) and Friere (1972:973, 985). Illich's thrust is that in industrialised societies those responsible for providing education have managed to convince a significant proportion of the population that they are incompetent and education must continue for life. (Illich, 1976:14).

Friere (1972:45–59), when analysing 'teacher-student relationships', found that a great deal of 'education was suffering from narration sickness'. The teacher deposits gems of knowledge into student 'receptacles'. Friere calls this the 'banking concept' of education and warns that students will never learn to think critically if this method of teaching is used. Friere proposes that problem-based education is preferable and is a joint effort. Both the teacher and the learner are participants in the learning process and each will develop as a result of the shared learning experience. This concept can be just as useful for nurse managers' teaching experiences with nurses, patients or clients. The factors that influence learning include the learner's and teacher's previous experience; perception of need of both teacher and learner; nurse-patient or staff interaction; the socio-cultural context within which learning occurs; and the stress response level of both the participants.

Learning styles vary. Some people learn best by doing, others by reading, by discussing, or by listening. Some learners prefer to use a number of senses together when learning, such as writing while they listen. Others use intuition (Denis and Richter, 1988). The method chosen by the learner to optimise learning depends on their individual strengths and weaknesses, their ability to organise information, past successes and past failures. Kolb (1984:45) sees a need to integrate both 'scholarly and practical learning styles' as information is already 'filtered' by the teacher's personal biases. For this reason Kolb (1984:45–46) strongly recommends experiential learning to counter this filtering process as both the teacher and the learner interpret the experience simultaneously according to their own learning styles. Kolb (1984:49) sees learning as equally important to the organisation as productivity and profits. Education is also seen as the key element of TQM or continuous quality improvement (Oakland, 1989:20). One of the key beliefs of TQM is that we are all both givers and receivers of services. Our patients receive our services and are entitled to receive value for money. The nurse has a responsibility to ensure that the patients and their relatives or support persons have received sufficient education to enable them to maintain or improve their health status. The nurse receives services from other staff to facilitate this teaching process. Both givers and receivers of services have a responsibility for quality service.

There is an old adage that 'more is caught than is taught'. This exemplifies the power of role models to influence attitudes and behaviour. We often model our behaviour on the behaviour of others we consider successful and our attitudes can depend on our exposure to information and experiences (Ewan, 1984:42, 56). In order to capitalise on our learning experiences, Kolb (1984: 49) recommends that time be set aside for discussion at the end of a session. This time is used to reflect on what has been learned within the session or from the project. Kolb insists that the different learning styles of

> action and reflection, concrete involvement and analytical detachment are all essential for optimal learning. When one perspective comes to dominate others learning effectiveness is reduced.

Zentner and Murray (1985:175–176) have identified a number of principles of adult learning. These include the issues of the learner's self-concept and self-esteem; respect for and value of adults' past learning experiences; the need for a non-threatening learning environment; and the ability to learn at their own pace. The principles also include recognition of the fact that adult learners are highly motivated to learn in areas which are relevant and have immediate application to their current work environment, lifestyle and interests. They get a high degree of satisfaction if they can assume control of these factors through the learning process.

An effective manager will use these principles and methods to encourage staff to assume responsibility for their own learning objectives in order to meet the performance standards documented in the job description. When the nurse learner accepts this responsibility there may be less concern about performance standards.

A crucial principle in adult learning is the necessity to provide positive reinforcement. This is provided by a preceptor, supervisor, or the nurse unit manager through feedback about accomplishments or failures, as soon as possible after the event. This guidance is given in a non-threatening manner. The person providing the feedback sees this as an educational opportunity to further develop the learner. It is an opportunity for personal growth for both the assessor and the learner.

# 8. PATIENT EDUCATION

Registered nurses have a teaching role in their daily nursing activities. This role is specified in the standards of the Australian Council of Healthcare Standards in their Accreditation Guide, Standard 3, Patient Care. This standard states that the nursing care plan should include 'details of the nursing care to be given including specific nursing care, *health teaching* and *preparation for discharge or referral*'.

This teaching role can be experienced during nurses' interactions with patients or clients, their relatives, community groups or other staff members. Recent changes in health care delivery place greater emphasis on health promotion and disease prevention. This has increased nurses' opportunities to facilitate patient learning.

Successful patient education results in a change in the patient's behaviour. The degree of change depends on a number of patient characteristics, nurse characteristics and organisational factors which affect the success of the learning process.

Patient learning is affected by the patient's readiness to learn and the nurse's readiness and ability to teach the ages of the participants and their sex which can either facilitate or hinder the learning process. Other characteristics affecting patient's learning readiness are the emotional states of both participants and their religious and cultural beliefs. Physical disabilities, language difficulties and the patient's knowledge of the disease process also affect motivation and ability to communicate.

These characteristics are also affected by a number of organisational factors. The nurse endeavours to teach within the limitations of the unique organisational setting. The setting is influenced by the philosophy of the organisation and its power structure. If there is an emphasis on patient education then opportunities for teaching will include the privacy afforded to the process, the allocation of time provided to teach and the availability of instructional materials. If patient education is encouraged then time is available for both individual as well as group classes and there is ample opportunity for patient follow-up and programme evaluation.

Nurses teach at the bedside, in the workplace, in schools and in other community agencies. In all of these different settings nurses have a teaching role. Teaching methods vary according to the setting in which teaching takes place and the needs of the learners. Their client group may vary from one-to-one encounters to any number, depending on the needs of the group and their community. Teaching is an integral part of the caring process and nurses provide specialised health care knowledge. The nursing staff, sometimes in conjunction with other health professionals, identify with patients what is to be taught. The nurses determine the standards and criteria for meeting the standards required of the learner. Methods and equipment required may need to be adapted to the patient's or client's family circumstances, lifestyles and the facilities available. Conditions may not match the expectations of the nurse for sterility, cleanliness, comfort and space. Adaptation according to the circumstances is required. As long as the principles governing actions are adhered to it is possible for the teaching and learning process to proceed to an effective outcome. Harold and Johnson (1989:10–11) suggest that teaching be fully documented for the protection of both nurse and patient. When a number of nurses are caring for a patient each needs to know the approach taken, the process used, the expected and the actual results of the teaching encounter.

These days there are a great number of aids available for teaching both adults and children, such as information leaflets, booklets, models, posters, slides, filmstrips, videos, anatomical models and charts.

For the nurse manager, the education of the staff and patients is a challenge. It will remain a challenge if we build in a mutual reflection process with our clients. Reflection on what went well and why; what went poorly and why; what was enjoyable and satisfying, what was embarrassing and why was this so? How can we as nurse managers assist and improve the teaching/learning process?

# SUMMARY

This chapter describes the different forms of education available to nurses. It also addresses the relationship between continuing professional education, nursing management and patient care within the context of health care organisations. It defines the different terms used in continuing education and their relevance for nurses. The importance of fostering an organisational culture which supports education, particularly in relation to standards set by professional bodies, and the implications of the Training Guarantee Bill are discussed. Other issues receiving attention are mandatory versus voluntary education, total quality management, and the identified needs of nurse managers for education. The design of instructional programmes is discussed from four different perspectives particularly as each relates to adult learners. The importance of patient education is emphasised and the need for reflection to assist and improve the teaching/ learning process.

# GREVILLEA CASE STUDY

Grevillea Hospital has grown from 140 beds to 220 beds in two years. The nursing staff consists of 90 RNs, 110 SNs, 30 ENAs. The length of patient stay in hospital, during this period, has decreased from 7.2 days to an average of 4.5 days. The occupancy rate is now 92 per cent. There has been a high turnover of staff in the last two years also. The hospital is located in a dormitory suburb, 25 kilometres from the centre of a major city, and has few social and cultural facilities. Despite the high turnover of staff, morale generally is as good as can be expected, and the staff of the hospital are working towards accreditation.

The Director of Nursing, Mr Frankston, has been at Grevillea for 18 months and has already made many improvements. A philosophy has been developed with, and accepted by, the nursing staff and a committee is currently developing links between philosophy, policies and practice. A Quality Assurance Committee has been formed and a Patient Classification System has been implemented for determining staffing on a daily and long-term basis.

The Charge Nurses are not yet negotiating their staff on a shift by shift basis as some nurses are reluctant to take the responsibility for staffing their wards. There has been an increasing number of complaints recently about the rosters, because, with the high turnover, there has been a tendency to move staff from ward to ward at short notice, and even from one ward to another during a shift. The nursing assignment pattern used varies, according to the ward or unit and shift, from task assignment on night duty, patient allocation in the medical wards to primary nursing in the intensive care unit. Mr Frankston feels inservice and staff-development programmes are required. However, Mr Frankston was asked to reduce staff at the last board meeting because the hospital was going to finish the year with a deficit of half a million dollars unless something was done over the next four months to reduce spending.

## QUESTIONS

1. How can Mr Frankston justify In-Service Co-ordinators when he has been asked to reduce staff?

2. Why should Mr Frankston feel he needs to consider a staff development programme?

3. What are the likely benefits to be derived from the establishment of a staff development programme?

4. What are the likely disadvantages of a staff development programme?

# REFERENCES

ANRAC (1991) *Report to the Australasian Nurse Registering Authorities Conference,* Volume 2, Assessment technology, Assessment and Evaluation Research Unit, Education Department, The University of Queensland.

Australian Council of Healthcare Standards (1990), *The accreditation guide: standards for Australian healthcare facilities,* ACHS, Zetland.

Barclay, L. (1989) 'Sexuality and the role of the nurse', in Gray, G. and Pratt, R. (eds), *Issues in Australian Nursing 2,* Churchill Livingstone, Melbourne.

Benner, P. (1984) *From novice to expert: excellence and power in clinical nursing practice.* Addison-Wesley, Menlo Park, Ca.

Betz, C. L. (1983) 'Needs assessments and evaluation: methods utilised in continuing education programs', *Journal of Continuing Education in Nursing,* 15, 2, 39-44.

Boud, D. (1988) 'A facilitator's view of adult learning', in Boud, D., and Griffin, V. (eds.) *Appreciating adults learning: from the learner's perspective.* Kogan Page, London.

Brewer, A. (1983) *Nurses, nursing and the new technology: implications of a dynamic technological environment.* School of Health Administration, University of New South Wales, Kensington.

Cooper, S. S. and Hornback, M. S. (1973) *Continuing nursing education.* McGraw-Hill, New York.

Craig, D. P. (1978) *Hip pocket guide to planning and evaluation.* Learning Concepts, San Diego.

del Bueno, D. J. (1976) Continuing education, in Marriner, A., (ed) *Volume 1: Current perspectives in nursing management,* The C. V. Mosby Company, St. Louis.

Denis, M. and Richter, I. (1988) 'Learning about intuitive learning: moose-hunting techniques', in Boud, D., and Griffin, V. (eds.) *Appreciating adults learning: from the learner's perspective.* Kogan Page, London.

Duffield, C. (1989) 'The Delphi technique', *Australian Journal of Advanced Nursing,* 6, 2, 41-45.

Ewan, C. E. (1984) *Teaching skills development manual: a guide for teachers of health workers.* School of Medical Education, University of New South Wales, Kensington.

Friere, P. (1972) *The pedagogy of the oppressed.* Penguin, Harmondsworth.

Friere, P. (1973) *Education for critical consciousness.* Sheed and Ward, London.

Friere, P. (1985) *The politics of education.* Bergin and Garvey, South Hadley, Massachusetts.

Gagne, R. M. (1974) *Essentials of learning for instruction.* Dryden Press, Hinsdale, Illinois.

Gonczi, A., Hager, P. and Oliver, L. (1990) 'Establishing competency-based standards in the professions'. National Office of Overseas Skills Recognition, Research paper No. 1, December, Australian Government Publishing Office, Canberra.

Harold, C. E., and Johnson, P. (eds.), (1989) *How to teach patients.* Springhouse Corporation, Springhouse, Pa.

Heimstra, R. (1976) *Lifelong learning.* Professional Educators Publication Inc., Lincoln, Nova Scotia.

Health Department of Victoria (1985), *Report of the Committee of Enquiry into Nursing in Victoria,* Volume 1, May; Volume 2, October (McClelland Report).

Health Department of Victoria (1988), *Report of the Study of Professional Issues in Nursing,* February (Marles Report).

Houle, C. O. (1961) *The inquiring mind.* University of Wisconsin Press, Madison.

Illich, I. and Verne, E. (1976) *Imprisoned in the global classroom.* Writers and Readers Publishing Co-operative, London.

Jarvis, P. (1983) *Adult and continuing education: theory and practice.* Croom Helm, London.

Jarvis, P. and Gibson, S. (1985) *The teacher practitioner in nursing, midwifery and health visiting.* Chapman and Hall, London.

Jones, B. (1982) *Sleepers wake! Technology and the future of work,* 2nd edition. Oxford University Press, Melbourne.

King, B. (1981), 'Learning needs of registered nurses'. *Australian Nurses Journal,* 11, 3: 42–43.

Kolb, D. A., Rubin, I. M. and McIntyre, J. M. (1984) *Organisational psychology: an experimental approach to organisational behaviour,* 4th edition. Prentice-Hall, New Jersey.

Kubat, J. (1976), 'Correlates of professional obsolete', *Journal of Continuing Education in Nursing,* 7, 2: 18–22.

Marles, F. (1988), *Report of the Study of Professional Issues in Nursing,* February, Health Department of Victoria, Melbourne.

Maslow, A. H. (1943), 'A theory of human motivation', *Psychological Review,* 50, 370–396.

Maslow, A. H. (1968) *Towards a psychology of being,* 2nd edition. Van Nostrand Reinhold Company, New York.

Mason, E. J. (1984) *How to write meaningful nursing standards,* 2nd edition. John Wiley and Sons, New York.

Masters, G. N. and McCurry, D. (1990), 'Competency-based assessment in the professions'. National Office of Overseas Skills Recognition, Research paper No. 2, December, Australian Government Publishing Office, Canberra.

McClelland, J. (1985), *Report of the Committee of Enquiry into Nursing in Victoria,* Volume 1, May; Volume 2, October, Health Department of Victoria, Melbourne.

Oakland, J. S. (1989) *Total quality management.* Heinemann, Oxford.

O'Connor, A. B. (1986) *Nursing staff development and continuing education.* Little Brown and Company, Boston.

Puetz, B. E. (1983) *Networking for nurses.* Aspen, Rockville.

Rawson, G. (1986), 'Senior health service managers: characteristics and educational needs'. No. 57 Australian studies in health service administration, School of Health Administration, University of New South Wales, Kensington.

Rogers, C. R. (1961) *On becoming a person.* Houghton Mifflin, Boston.

Rogers, C. (1983) *Freedom to learn for the '80s.* Charles E. Merrill, Columbus, Ohio.

Royal Australian Nursing Federation (1983) *Standards for nursing divisions.* RANF, Melbourne.

Sharpe, P., and Ross, S. (1990) *Living psychology,* 2nd edition. Scribe, Newham, Victoria.

Springhouse Corporation (1990) *Patient teaching loose-leaf library.* Springhouse Corporation, Springhouse, Pa.

Sprouster, J. (1987), *T.Q.C. Total quality control: the Australian experience,* 2nd revised edition. Horwitz Grahame, Cammeray.

Stevens, B. J. (1985) *Nurse as executive,* 3rd edition. Aspen, Rockville.

Styles, M. (1983), 'International nursing: the Brazilian meetings — quo vadis? Conco se vai la?' *Australian Nurses Journal,* 13,2,29–32.

Vargas, J. S. (1977) *Behavioural psychology for teachers.* Harper & Row, New York.

White, R., Ewan, C., Hatton, N., and Lovitt, L. (1988) *Critical incidents in clinical teaching: perspectives from the social and behavioural sciences: an instructional manual for nurse educators.* World Health Organisation Training Centre, School of Medical Education, University of New South Wales, Kensington.

Zentner, J., and Murray, R. (1985), 'Health teaching: a basic nursing intervention', in Murray, R. B. and Zentner, J. P. *Nursing concepts for health promotion,* 3rd edition. Prentice-Hall, New Jersey.

# CHAPTER 1.5

# Legal and professional issues

## JUDITH MAIR AND KATE BLACKMORE

After reading this chapter, you should be able to:

1. identify legal principles as they relate to the workplace;

2. apply principles of law to personnel practices;

3. apply principles of law to clinical practice in nursing.

---

An understanding of legal and professional issues in health care practice has become essential for all health care practitioners, particularly those who are involved in management. The following information should serve to identify and introduce readers to legal principles and professional issues related to nursing practice.

The Australian legal system is based upon the English common law which was introduced when the First Fleet arrived in Sydney Cove. Since that time, there has been a gradual development of the law to suit Australian conditions, and today our courts and parliaments are no longer bound by English common law precedents and legislation.

The primary source of law in Australia is a combination of common law and legislation. Common law consists of decisions made by judges which are based upon the doctrine of precedent. Judges look to past cases to determine the principle of law to be applied to the facts in the case before them. Important cases are reported in law reports relevant to particular courts. Legislation is law made by parliamentarians through the parliamentary process. Because we have a federal system of government, legislation is promulgated by the Commonwealth parliament as well as by each state parliament. However, the Commonwealth parliament's law-making powers are restricted by the Australian Constitution. In some cases it has exclusive power; in other cases there is concurrent power with state governments. Where there is an inconsistency between federal and state law on the same matter, then the Commonwealth federal law prevails. In all other matters the states retain the right to make laws.

The main federal law-making power with respect to health relates to the provision of pharmaceutical and medical benefits, quarantine and defence. State legislation is the main source of law with respect to the control and management of public and private hospitals, control and notification of disease, registration of health professionals, and other health care practices. The various states enact their own laws on these topics and the law may differ from state to state. The common law is the major source of law which covers clinical practice.

Law is not the only means by which standards in health care can be evaluated and controlled. Various government departments — for example, those which regulate work practices in health care institutions — provide policy guidelines which should be followed by those institutions. While not strictly binding in law, these policies are useful in determining whether or not a particular health care institution is meeting standards expected by law should a dispute come to court.

Law relating to employment is of particular interest to health care institutions which employ nurses, and to the nurses themselves as employees. Although part of the law of employment is to be found in the common law, much of it, such as anti-discrimination law and industrial awards, is now embodied within legislation. The law of employment also relates to discipline and dismissal. Unions have a role to play in negotiating for adequate wages and conditions for members, and in representing them in industrial disputes. As well, the right of a nurse to practise is governed by legislation in each of the states.

Career paths for nurses have been enhanced in recent times, particularly for clinical nurses. New developments in clinical career structures offer a viable alternative to entering nursing administration or education in order to progress in a nursing career. However, as clinical nurses are placed in positions where they are expected to take a greater responsibility in the delivery of health care services, there is an implication that the law will expect a higher standard of care from them. In addition, it is a general principle that higher paid positions demand greater accountability from the incumbents.

Most of the law relating to clinical nursing practice is found within the common law. For example, the law relating to assault, false imprisonment, negligence and negligent advice is found within precedents recognising the right of persons to individual autonomy and bodily integrity. The law of contract and of bailment is concerned with the rights of individuals with regard to, inter alia, health care and personal property.

Medical records are legal documents which can be readily used by a plaintiff or defendant in a court action involving health care, which means that these records must be prepared accurately and in sufficient detail to satisfy various legal requirements. Introduction of freedom of information legislation has given patients a legal right of access to their medical records. This means that nurses must ensure that report writing is carried out in the knowledge that a patient may subsequently read what has been written.

Criminal law, as well as civil law, is relevant to clinical nursing practice. Criminal law operates to protect interests which are important to society; criminal law offences relevant to health care include criminal assault and negligence. Law relating to child abuse is also relevant.

Both the common law and legislation provide for protection of workers from hazards at their place of employment, and for compensation if they suffer a work related injury. Organisations delivering health care also have a duty to avoid injury to persons, other than their employees, who enter upon their premises. The duty to others may be found in legislation, or through the law of occupier's liability.

One further issue concerns who is to be held responsible in the event that a patient successfully sues for breach of a legal right in health care. The health professional responsible for the breach bears a personal liability but the patient is most likely to sue the employer of the health professional under the doctrine of vicarious liability, provided that the health professional is an employee. In other respects, the health care institution can be held liable under its own personal duty of care to each and every patient.

Finally, the court in which it is most usual for a nurse to appear as a witness is a Coroner's court. Coroners in each state have power to investigate certain types of deaths, to establish if there has been any criminal involvement in the death. A nurse who is called as a witness may have been on duty or nursed a patient at some time while the patient was receiving health care and may not necessarily have been directly involved in the patient's death.

The following discussion will elaborate on the above points from the aspect of the patient, the professional nurse manager and the health care institution. Each of the issues will be explored more fully in the following text. Nurse managers will be directed to legal references which have been written specifically for health care practitioners in order to obtain a more detailed discussion of the various issues identified.

# 1. THE PATIENT

As well as being subject to the laws which govern the behaviour of all members of a particular society, the nurse is subject to additional legal responsibilities and obligations with respect to patient care (Mair, 1989:171). Such legal obligations may be either civil or criminal. Nurses who breach the civil rights of patients may be required to compensate them at common law. Where a nurse is in breach of the criminal law, a prosecution is brought by the state and upon conviction the nurse may be punished by a fine and/or imprisonment. This section will focus upon specific legal problems that nurses may have to face in caring for patients in health care institutions and in the community.

## 1.1 CIVIL LAW PROBLEMS

### 1.1.1 Negligence

The tort of negligence is applicable where a person suffers harm because of a breach of duty of care owed by another. Negligence is not a state of mind, but conduct that falls below the standard regarded as normal or desirable in a given community (Fleming, 1987:94). If a patient wishes to sue for harm alleged to have been caused as a result of a nurse's failure to exercise the appropriate standard of care, the patient would have to prove:

1.  that the nurse owed a duty of care to protect the patient from an unreasonable risk of harm;

2.  that the nurse failed to conform to the required standard of care in the circumstances existing at the time;

3.  that the patient suffered material injury; and

4.  that the nurse's failure to conform to the appropriate standard of care caused the injury complained of.

The duty of care question is determined by considering what the defendant ought to have foreseen. It is an objective question and the defendant's conduct is measured by the 'reasonable man' test. The mere fact of foreseeability is not sufficient; the test is *reasonable* foreseeability. Irrespective of how the test is applied in the community generally, there is little doubt that a duty of care can easily be proved when the test is applied to the practice of nursing (Mair, 1989:176). A duty of care can arise with respect to a class of persons as well as to individuals. It is not necessary for each and every plaintiff to be identified at the time an alleged act of negligence occurs. It is reasonably foreseeable that patients are likely to be affected by the acts or omissions of persons delivering their health care, therefore a duty arises to deliver that care at an appropriate standard.

To determine whether a breach of duty has occurred, the standard of care applicable in the circumstances must be considered. The standard of care is reasonable care, not perfect care. The standard expected of the health care worker is that which is attributed to the class of health care workers to which the defendant belongs. Thus the conduct of a registered nurse will be measured against that of the hypothetical reasonable registered nurse. Persons who hold themselves out as possessing special skills will be required to exhibit a higher standard of care. Thus nurses who are clinical nurse consultants and clinical nurse specialists can be expected to meet a higher standard of care than those who are working at ward level. When nurses undertake tasks which are beyond their capacity, thereby causing harm to patients, they can be held to be negligent. In an Australian case a probationary nurse was held to be negligent when she instructed a patient to self-administer ear drops which subsequently caused the patient harm. A doctor had given the nurse a verbal order to give the patient glycerine and acid carbol drops and to instruct him how to use them. The nurse thought the doctor said acid carbol drops. After checking the order with a registered nurse she went ahead and gave the drops to the patient. The nurse was held to be negligent because she undertook a task which was beyond her capacity at the time and this caused harm to the patient *(Henson and Another v Board of Management of Perth Hospital).*

In considering the standard of care required in particular circumstances, the nurse must take into account characteristics of the patient which may place that patient at additional risk. The very young, the very old, those under sedation and the mentally disturbed all call for special care (O'Sullivan, 1983:86). The circumstances in which the treatment is administered may also be relevant in determining the standard of care required. A nurse rendering assistance at the roadside to a person injured in a motor vehicle accident could not be expected to deliver care at the standard required in a fully equipped hospital with other assistance readily at hand. Provided the nurse exercised reasonable care and skill in the circumstances there would not be a breach of the duty of care (Mair, 1989:176). The same argument applies when care is administered in the home should an unanticipated emergency arise.

In order to succeed in an action of negligence, a patient must prove that damage resulted from a breach of duty. Provided the type of damage was reasonably foreseeable, the damage may be physical and/or mental. The defendant will also be liable to compensate for loss which flows reasonably and naturally upon the initial injury *(Smith v Leech Brain & Co. Ltd.)*. Loss of past wages and future income, loss of enjoyment and/ or expectation of life, loss of opportunity in life, and pain and suffering are examples of damages that may be claimed. If death occurs as a result of negligence, legislation generally provides that certain close relatives can bring an action provided they can prove pecuniary loss as a result of the death.

Finally, the plaintiff must prove that the breach of duty caused the alleged harm. To determine a direct casual connection, the 'but for' test is often applied; that is, but for the act of defendant, would the plaintiff have suffered the injury? It could be argued that a nurse who renders assistance at the roadside to a motor accident victim, and contrary to reasonable practice, decides to move the injured person, could only be successfully sued if the defendant could prove that any injury, such as paraplegia, was caused by the nurse's actions and did not arise from any other cause.

There are three main defences to an action in negligence. The first of these is the partial defence of contributory negligence: to the extent that the plaintiff was also responsible for what happened, any award of compensation will be proportionately reduced. This defence is mainly used in motor vehicle accident cases and might be applicable where a person failed to wear a seat belt or drove with an elbow protruding from a window, or where a pedestrian stepped from behind a parked bus onto a busy road (Mair, 1989:178). In health care, an argument of contributory negligence could be made when a patient does not follow advice given by the nurse to protect the patient.

The defence of *novus actus interveniens* applies when a further act of negligence by another party occurs after an initial act of negligence. If the second act of negligence causes a break in the chain of causation flowing from the first negligent act, then the first negligent person is not responsible for the further injury. However, the person responsible for the first negligent act can be held responsible for injuries resulting from the second negligent act if the second act was foreseeable. For example, if the negligence of a midwife caused brain damage to a baby during delivery and the newborn was admitted to an intensive care nursery where a second nurse caused further injury through a negligent act, the first nurse could be held responsible for the second injury as well as the first. In such a case, indemnity could be sought from the second nurse in the event of a successful claim brought on behalf of the injured newborn. In one case, a supervisory nurse was held negligent for giving a fatal dose of a drug to a child. The physician responsible for the child's care had failed to adequately note the mode of administration of the drug on the notes. An argument put by lawyers for the physician was that the nurse's negligence broke the chain of causation flowing from the physician's inadequate notation. This argument was rejected by the court; both the doctor and the nurse were negligent *(Norton v Argonaut Insurance Co)*.

A third defence of *volenti non fit injuria* means that a person cannot succeed in an action of negligence for injuries caused as a result of a normally accepted risk of an activity voluntarily entered into. This defence usually applies to sporting injuries or injuries resulting from inherently hazardous work where the injured person knew the risks and accepted them, and it is not generally applicable to the provision of health care services. However this defence, and/or the defence of contributory negligence, might be applicable in a case where a person had knowingly agreed to be a passenger in a car driven by a person affected by drink or drugs.

In all cases of alleged negligence, an injured plaintiff cannot sit tight and hope to achieve the maximum amount of compensation possible. The plaintiff is required to take reasonable steps to minimise the damage which has been caused by the breach, and this includes seeking reasonable medical care and advice. To the extent that there is a proven failure to mitigate, any compensation award will be reduced accordingly.

## 1.1.2 Negligent advice

The tort of negligent advice is a form of negligence action which can be brought for damage caused by the giving of advice rather than by some act or omission on the part of the defendant. An action for negligent advice can also be brought with respect to the giving of information, as distinct from advice, where the defendant has a sufficient interest to see that the information is correct; for example, the provision of a pro forma diet to a diabetic patient where the diet is not appropriate for the particular patient's needs.

For an action in negligent advice to be successful, the plaintiff must show that the adviser is a professional, or claims to have equivalent skills; that the adviser was willing to use those skills to advise the plaintiff in the knowledge that the plaintiff intended to rely on the advice in making a decision; and that it was reasonable for the plaintiff to do so. The mere fact that the advice was wrong does not entitle the plaintiff to succeed. The plaintiff must prove that the defendant failed to exercise reasonable care in the giving of the advice, according to the standards of a reasonably competent practitioner, and that the plaintiff suffered loss as a result of following the advice *(Hills v Potter)*.

A disclaimer of responsibility, express or implied, will protect an adviser, but any attempt to escape liability by disclaiming responsibility for advice given in the context of health care would be inappropriate and counter productive given that health care professionals are often required to advise patients (Mair, 1989:179). Nurses should ensure that they remain up-to-date with knowledge relating to their particular practice and never convey an impression that they have particular skills when they lack the capacity to give advice in that matter. When called upon to give advice on matters about which they lack knowledge, nurses should not give the advice and should refer the patient to an appropriate experienced and competent practitioner.

## 1.1.3 Assault and battery

Assault and battery are torts (civil wrongs) which serve to protect an individual's right to autonomy and self-determination. Assault consists of intentionally creating in another person an apprehension of imminent harmful or offensive contact (Fleming, 1987:24), whereas battery is committed by intentionally bringing about a harmful or offensive contact with the person of another (Fleming, 1987:23). The least touching of another in anger is a battery, and touching another without consent also constitutes a battery where the touching is not a normal incident of everyday life. Although there is a legal difference between assault and battery, the term assault is usually used to represent both.

Lack of consent to health care treatment is the basis of legal actions brought against health care workers in relation to these torts. Because an assault is complete once touching has occurred without lawful justification, a patient need not show that damage occurred as a result of the touching; the fact that treatment was carried out in good faith for the benefit of the patient is no defence where the patient is capable of giving an appropriate consent and has not done so.

Consent may be obtained verbally by asking the patient's permission before commencing treatment and receiving an affirmative response; implied by the patient's overt physical response to suggested treatments; or in writing signed by the patient and witnessed. In an emergency where a person is unable to consent, a nurse is entitled to proceed to carry out means which are aimed at saving the life of an injured person under the 'doctrine of necessity'. In such circumstances the consent of a relative or other person is not necessary. In one recent Canadian case *(Malette v Shulman* et al.) a doctor was held liable to compensate a woman for assault after he had given her a blood transfusion to save her life when she was unconscious after an accident. A nurse had previously drawn his attention to a signed and witnessed card, prohibiting blood transfusions under any circumstances, which had been found in the woman's purse.

Irrespective of the form in which it is obtained, a consent must be valid. To be valid the consent must be voluntarily given, cover the treatment to be carried out, informed to some degree, and given by a person legally competent to do so. To be voluntary the consent must be given freely by the patient in the absence of fraud or duress. A consent which is obtained while a patient is at a disadvantage — for example while under the effect of sedation — may be considered null and void *(Demers v Gerety; Beausoleil v Sisters of Charity).*

The consent must cover the treatment to be carried out and any treatment which is incidental; in the absence of an emergency any treatment carried out which has not been previously consented to is unlawful. In a Canadian case *(Murray v McMurchy)* a doctor sterilised a woman, without prior consent, whilst she was under an anaesthetic for a Caesarean section operation because he thought that fibroids in her uterus might cause a problem in future pregnancies. The court held that the operation was unlawful as the condition was not an immediate danger to the woman's life and health.

With respect to informed consent, provided the patient has a general understanding of what is to be done and has given a consent, then any issue relating to the degree of information given is a matter for the general law of negligence and is determined by what a reasonable practitioner would or would not have told a patient (Informed Decisions About Medical Procedures).

Legal capacity refers to mental capacity and children. Legislation in the various states covers consent to treatment by mental health patients. Where a person is otherwise mentally incapable, the defence of necessity is applied to permit treatment which is necessary to preserve the life of the person. In some cases a disabled person may have a court-appointed guardian to make such decisions or a guardian may be appointed under legislation.

With children, a combination of common law principles and legislation applies. At common law minors may consent to a procedure which is for their therapeutic good provided they understand the nature and consequences of the proposed treatment. The application of this principle requires a balance between the intellectual and emotional maturity of the minor and the complexity or seriousness of the proposed treatment (Mair, 1989:176). Minors of quite low ages can presumably give a valid consent to simple procedures not involving a great risk of harm (O'Sullivan, 1983:46). In New South Wales the Minors (Property and Contracts) Act provides that consent to medical treatment given by a parent or guardian of a minor aged less than 16 years is a defence to an action for assault and battery. The Act also provides for consent to be given by a child of 14 years or upwards without parental consent. Below the age of 14 years the consent of the parent or guardian is required. The definition of medical treatment includes treatment carried out by persons following the orders of a medical practitioner.

In emergencies, where a parent or guardian has not given a consent, most states have legislation which enables doctors to perform life-saving treatments on children without parental consent. Where treatment is non-urgent and parents or guardians are refusing to consent, or there is any dispute regarding consent, the matter may be referred to the Supreme Court of a state or the Family Court where a decision can be made which is in the best interests of the child. Decisions involving developmentally disabled children, especially those involving sterilisation, can be dealt with by these courts *(In re a Teenager: In re Jane)*.

There are some defences against an action in assault which are relevant to the delivery of health care. In emergency cases the doctrine of necessity justifies the application of treatment without consent provided the treatment is aimed at saving the life of a person or to prevent a serious danger to future health. Thus it is legitimate to carry out necessary treatment on a person who is unconscious without the consent of that person or any other person. Legislation in various states may authorise particular acts without consent, for example, the Motor Traffic Act 1909 (NSW) makes it mandatory for doctors to obtain blood samples for blood alcohol analysis when drivers of cars involved in motor traffic accidents require treatment in casualty. Treatment may also be administered under court authorisation.

## 1.1.4 False imprisonment

The tort of false imprisonment protects people from being subjected to an intentional and total restraint of movement without lawful justification, whether by total confinement or by being prevented from exercising the privilege of leaving the place in which they are (Fleming, 1987:26). The confinement must be total — if the person can leave by some reasonable alternative exit there is no false imprisonment. Locking patients in a room with no reasonable avenue of escape or barring patients from exercising their privilege of leaving a health care institution could amount to false imprisonment in the absence of lawful justification. Thus it has been held to be a false imprisonment when a patient was detained in a hospital for failing to pay an account *(Gadsden General Hospital v Hamilton)*.

The use of bed rails and manacles can also be a false imprisonment if used without lawful justification. In addition, a patient who reasonably believes that any attempt to leave a health care institution will be prevented by a nurse could be falsely imprisoned even if there are no physical restraints. There need not necessarily be force used in order to commit a false imprisonment. A doctor successfully sued for false imprisonment when he was escorted to a mental hospital by a police officer following the issuance of appropriate documents. The doctor was told he was to be taken to hospital. He protested but accompanied the officer to a car in which he was taken to the hospital. The High Court judge hearing the case referred to the lack of physical force used but found that the plaintiff had a justified apprehension that, if he did not submit to what was asked of him, he would be compelled by force to go to the hospital. Therefore, a restraint was imposed upon the plaintiff which amounted to an imprisonment *(Watson v Marshall)*. However, in such cases the patient would have to prove the submission to the nurse was complete and was reasonable. The tort can be committed where a client is too ill to move *(Grainger v Hill and anor)*, or is unaware of the imprisonment because he is in a state of drunkenness, asleep or insane *(Meering v Grahame-White Aviation Co. Ltd.)*.

Hospitals generally have a policy of requesting patients who wish to leave against medical advice to sign a release form and see a doctor. The policy is appropriate and hospitals are entitled to request compliance. If a patient voluntarily agrees to the request there is no problem. However, it is doubtful that hospital staff could detain a patient to enforce compliance with the hospital requirements. Should a patient leave without advising staff, or refuse to stay to sign a release form and see a doctor, the events should be clearly documented in the nursing notes.

There are some defences that can be raised against an allegation of false imprisonment and one of these is the common law defence of necessity which permits the restraint of persons who are a danger to themselves or others. For example, the restraint of an elderly patient who is suffering from Alzeimer's disease could be justified if the patient is likely to be exposed to a serious risk of harm if allowed to wander at large.

However, the necessity must be real and not merely for the convenience of staff (O'Sullivan, 1983:37). The restraint of a patient attempting to jump out of the window of a multi-storey building would be justified, as would the restraint of a psychotic patient who was threatening to harm staff and other patients. A second defence exists where an act of parliament authorises the detention of persons; for example, mental health acts and acts protecting public health.

## 1.1.5 Contract and bailment

The law of contract governs agreements made between parties which give rise to rights and obligations to those parties. A contract can be as simple as buying a newspaper or as complex as the purchase of property. Originally, contract law was a matter of private law between the parties and the courts were reluctant to intervene. However, the rise of complex business practices and the inequality of bargaining power between some of the parties has led to an increase in legislation governing contracts providing penalties for unlawful business practices, and in some cases providing remedies for persons who suffer a loss as a result of a contract. The common law courts are still involved in determining damages awards for breach of contract, misrepresentation and fraud.

Patients who enter hospitals and other health care centres enter into a contract with the institution. The relationship between a specific doctor and a patient is also one of contract. The rights and obligations of the parties are referred to as the terms and conditions of the contract. As with many contracts, these terms and conditions are not encapsulated in a single document. To the extent that they are unwritten, the common law implies certain terms and conditions. An implied term of a contract between a hospital or doctor and a patient is that treatment will be administered with reasonable care and skill (Staunton and Whyburn, 1989:100). The law requires that there be a sufficient signed memorandum for some contracts to be enforceable; contracts involving an interest in property are an example.

The parties to a contract involving health care are the patient and the health care institution when the patient enters hospital or another health care facility, and the patient and a medical practitioner when the patient is a private patient. When a nurse is employed to deliver nursing care in a health care facility, she acts as an agent or servant of the facility and is not in a direct contractual relationship with patients. Private duty nurses, who are engaged directly by patients, and private home birth midwives, contract directly with their patients (Staunton and Whyburn, 1989:102).

To be enforceable at law, a contract must exhibit the following elements:

1.  there must be an offer and acceptance of the offer;

2.  consideration must pass from all parties to the contract;

3.  the parties must intend to enter into a legally binding relationship;

4.  the parties must have legal capacity to enter into contracts;

5.  the contract must not be for the performance of an illegal act.

As in all contracts there must be an offer and an acceptance. A patient offers to pay for health care services in return for the provision of those services by a health care provider. Acceptance of the offer is made when the patient is taken on by the health care provider.

Valuable consideration is another vital element. Consideration requires that the parties to a contract must give something in return for the promise of the other. This can be a promise in exchange for a promise, a promise on one side in exchange for an act or vice versa. In the case of a contract between a patient and a health care provider, the consideration passing from the former is payment for services and the consideration passing from the latter is the provision of health care services. Payment need not be direct, and in most cases is made through Medicare or through private insurance. Where a patient receives private care and is not privately insured, payment is direct.

There must be an intent to enter into a legal relationship. This means that both parties intend that the contract between them will be enforceable at law and allow for legal actions to be taken by either party for breaches of the terms of the contract. In professional relationships such as those between health care providers and patients, the law will presume that there was an intent to create a legal relationship between the parties. Thus patients are entitled to sue for breaches of contract such as failure of a health care professional to deliver treatment with care and skill thereby causing harm to the patient. Health care providers can sue for unpaid fees where fees are to be paid directly by the patient.

A person must have legal capacity to enter into an enforceable contract. Contracts made with a minor (below the age of 18) are not usually binding upon the minor. However, a minor is bound by contracts for 'necessaries' such as accommodation and food. The provision of health care services can be considered a 'necessary' for a minor who requires treatment: therefore, the minor can be held liable to pay for those services. Special rules also apply when persons are mentally ill, developmentally disabled or drunk.

Finally, contracts will be unenforceable if they are considered to be illegal or against public policy. A contract to assist a patient to die would be illegal and unenforceable.

The law of contract is separate from an action in negligence, although one incident may give rise to an action in both breach of contract and negligence. If a person is injured as a result of the negligent act of a person with whom no contract exists, then the only cause of action would be in negligence. However, if a patient in a hospital suffers injury because of the negligence of hospital staff, the patient could bring an action both in contract and in negligence *(Thake and Anor. v Maurice)*. In reality, patients rarely resort to an action for breach of contract preferring to rely on negligence.

The law of bailment is a form of contract and applies when one person (the bailor) delivers goods to another (the bailee) so that they may be used or stored until they are to be delivered back to the bailor. When patient's goods are handed to a hospital for safekeeping the law of bailment governs the relationship. Bailment may be for reward or gratuitous: in the former case the bailee will be held liable to compensate for the loss of the goods according to the ordinary rules of negligence; in the latter case the bailee is only liable if gross negligence is shown. With regard to patients' property which has been handed over to a hospital for safekeeping, the hospital is normally considered to be a 'bailee for reward' because there is a monetary interest involved in the admission of patients. Therefore, the hospital has an obligation to exercise reasonable care in securing the safety of patients' property. Should a patient's valuables be lost or damaged through the negligence of the hospital or its staff, the hospital will be required to compensate the patient for the loss or damage.

A hospital can also become an involuntary bailee for patients' property. In a New Zealand case, a hospital was held liable to compensate the estate of a deceased woman for a ring which was on the woman's hand up to the time of her death but which subsequently disappeared *(Southland Hospital Board v Perkins Estate)*. The woman's control over her property ceased at her death and the hospital became an involuntary bailee for the ring.

If patients are admitted to hospital with valuables it would be prudent to request them to send the valuables home with a person they can trust; if the patient is incapable of nominating someone, then the valuables could be handed to a person who is legally entitled to them or who appears reasonably trustworthy. A note should be made as to the identity of the person to whom goods were entrusted, preferably signed by that person. Otherwise, the valuables should be taken in by the hospital for safekeeping. When a person is dead upon arrival in the casualty or emergency department, the property is usually dealt with by the police. If a patient dies in hospital, any valuable property should be kept safe and handed over to the legal personal representative of the deceased patient. Non-valuable items can be sent home with a relative or friend.

In order to fulfil their duty to protect a patient's valuables, hospitals have implemented policy and procedures which should be followed by nursing staff. Normally patients' goods are recorded in a document which is signed by the patient when the patient is capable of signing. When the patient is incapacitated, two nurses should be involved in recording the valuables and signing the document. The goods are then stored in a safe place which may be a locked cupboard at ward level (not the dangerous drug cupboard) if the goods are to be stored for a short period only — for example during surgery — or in a hospital safe if the goods are to be stored for a longer time. Patients are generally required to sign for the goods when they are returned to them.

If the goods are lost, the patient has the onus of proving their value. Nurses are not competent to make an evaluation of the nature and quality of particular goods such as jewellery, and therefore should not list the goods as being of any particular category and value. For example, a diamond ring in a gold setting should be described as clear stone set in a yellow coloured band even if the patient states that it is a diamond.

## 1.2 CRIMINAL LAW PROBLEMS

### 1.2.1 Assault and battery

Assault and battery can be crimes as well as torts. However, in order to constitute criminal assault there must be a forcible or hostile act of the accused without the consent of the victim. If a nurse is assaulted while on duty the matter can be reported to the police who can charge the party with criminal assault. If the person responsible for assaulting the nurse is a patient suffering from a mental condition, she might not be found guilty of assault if she lacked the required degree of *mens rea* (guilty mind) at the time of the assault. The same legal redress is available to patients assaulted by staff.

Two relevant defences to a charge of assault are misadventure and self-defence. In the former, an assault occurs by accident, whereas the latter involves the use of force by one person to repel an attack. People may use reasonable force to repel attacks upon them, but they must not use more force than is necessary to repel the attack and the right of self-defence only lasts while any danger exists. Thus a nurse would be entitled to exercise the right of self-defence if attacked by a patient or other person provided she used no more force than was necessary to repel the attack. If greater force than necessary is used to repel an attack, the person acting in self-defence can be also charged with assault. Should death result from excessive use of self-defence, a charge of manslaughter could be laid. The death of an attacker will only be considered lawful where the person attacked reasonably believes that her own life is in danger.

## 1.2.2 Criminal negligence

Criminal negligence occurs when an act which causes death goes beyond a mere matter of civil compensation to show a reckless disregard for the life and safety of another. The death of a patient resulting from treatment by a health care professional would amount to criminal negligence where that professional was grossly negligent and did something no reasonably skilled professional would have done *(R v Bateman)*.

Instances of health care workers being charged with criminal negligence are rare and are difficult to prove to the requisite standard required by the criminal law — that is, 'beyond a reasonable doubt'. Should a nurse be charged with a criminal offence in relation to the death of a patient, the charge would normally be one of manslaughter. Charges may result from a referral to the relevant Crown law authorities by a coroner investigating the death of a patient.

## 1.2.3 Child abuse

Child abuse comprises both general abuse, neglect and sexual abuse. With respect to general abuse and neglect, legislation in the various states provides for reporting and investigation of cases and for legal action to be taken against child abusers. It also provides for children to be made wards of the state for their care and protection, should this be considered to be in the child's best interests. In general, medical practitioners must report all cases of suspected child abuse and neglect and will be in breach of the law if they fail to do so. Persons who are not medical practitioners are not required to report suspected cases of child abuse unless relevant state legislation prescribes them. In some states nurses have a legal obligation to notify cases of child abuse.

Nurses in New South Wales are not prescribed persons but are required, by ministerial direction, to report suspected child sexual abuse. The New South Wales government recently introduced mandatory notification by school teachers and counsellors of suspected child sexual abuse. Persons who are not prescribed may report cases of suspected child abuse but are not obliged to do so.

Confidential reports are usually made to a government department responsible for the welfare of children, either directly or through the police. Provided that a report is made in good faith and is based upon reasonable grounds, legislation generally provides legal protection for reporters against civil actions such as as defamation and malicious prosecution which suspected child abusers may seek to bring against them. Once a report has been received an investigation is carried out. To aid in the investigation legislation usually provides for mandatory medical examinations. The authorities can then decide what action to take, if necessary, to deal with the situation. The criminal law deals with other forms of sexual assault on children such as carnal knowledge and incest.

## 1.3 MEDICAL AND NURSING RECORDS

Medical and nursing records are legal documents, therefore it is important to keep accurate and complete records of all treatment and care administered to patients. The records are reports of the progress of patients from when they are admitted to hospital, or other health care facility, until they are discharged from care or die. Accurate and complete documentation can benefit a nurse faced with an action by a patient when the record discloses that adequate and reasonable nursing care was delivered. Failure to keep adequate records can cause a nurse to be found liable even when adequate treatment was administered: failure to record the treatment which is given can be taken in law to be evidence that such treatment was in fact not given. Failure to keep complete and adequate records can be negligent since it can easily be proved that a reasonable health professional would keep patient records in order and up to date *(Whitree v State of New York)*. Failure to do so could foreseeably cause a patient to suffer harm — for example, a patient may be given two doses of a drug because a first dose was not recorded. While it is important that a patient's records be complete and up to date, a nurse should not write more than is necessary since this in itself can complicate a matter. However, it is still advisable to make a note if a patient refuses treatment or will not accept the nurse's advice (O'Sullivan, 1983:146).

Reports should be objective and those responsible for writing them should avoid making value judgements. 'Patient in pain' is a subjective statement and should be recorded as 'patient complaining of pain' together with the location of the stated pain and the nursing action taken.

Reports should be written as soon as possible after the event if they are to be accepted as reliable evidence in a court action. Errors in reporting should not be erased since this can arouse suspicion that there is something to hide. Mistakes should be ruled through neatly so that it remains possible to see what was written in error. Likewise, interlineations and notes made in margins should be avoided as they can suggest that something has been added to a report at a later date. It is for this reason that nurses are advised not to leave lines between reports. Amendments to the records should be signed and dated. For example, if a nurse recorded in a patient's notes material that was relevant to another patient, she should draw a neat line through the incorrect material, note that it was written in error, and sign and date the amendments.

Nurses should also be aware that information gained from patients in the course of administering care is confidential, and that patients are entitled to expect that nurses will maintain a high degree of confidentiality when dealing with health care records. If such confidentiality is breached, the legal rights of patients are limited, but nurses should aim to preserve confidentiality to the maximum extent possible. The right of confidentiality belongs to the patient and access to a record by others can be granted with the consent of the patient. The patient's consent to disclosure of information can be oral or written. In all other circumstances, access should be limited to other health professionals on a 'need to know' basis — that is, to those who have a genuine need for information in order to treat a patient adequately. Other justifications for breaching confidentiality include legal process, statutory authority, necessity and the criminal law.

Although patients have a right to expect that their medical records and nursing notes will be kept confidential, they have no legally enforceable right, in the absence of statutory authority, to have access to the records themselves. Examples of statutory rights are freedom of information acts. The Commonwealth government and various State governments have enacted legislation which gives persons a right to have access to various documents including personal documents. There is also a right to request that personal documents be amended if they contain false or misleading material. However, the acts only apply to government departments and agencies and are not applicable to private enterprise. Thus patients in public hospitals could seek access to their records but patients in private hospitals presumably could not.

Even when there is no legal right of access, patients should be able to see their records as a matter of policy whenever possible. Patients can have a health care practitioner with them when they are accessing their record in order to see that they understand the nature of what has been written and why it was written. Where information contained within a record could harm a patient, the patient's own practitioner could make a decision as to whether access should be granted and, if so, how. For example, the record might show that the patient has a provisional diagnosis of a terminal disease which has not been confirmed, and this could result in the patient suffering nervous shock by reading about it in the record. Access may be denied, or permitted provided provision for adequate counselling has been arranged.

## 1.4 CORONIAL LAW

Each state has its own Coroner's Court which is set up under legislation to provide the means whereby certain types of death and fires can be investigated. These courts are conducted by magistrates and usually act as courts of inquiry rather than in an adversarial manner. Coroners are interested in determining whether there are any suspicious circumstances surrounding deaths and fires. They are not primarily concerned with civil negligence, although relatives may seek to initiate a separate action in a higher court based on civil negligence causing death. If a coroner is critical of the actions of a nurse relating to the death of a patient, a report may be fowarded to a relevant nursing board which can determine whether the nurse has been guilty of professional misconduct. If a coroner suspects criminal negligence has been involved with the death, she can refer the matter to the relevant Crown Law authorities, or, where permissible, may commit the person to trial.

Generally a coroner is charged with investigating deaths where there has been a violent or unnatural death, a suspicious death, a death the cause of which is unknown, where the identity of the deceased is unknown, or where homicide is suspected. Deaths from anaesthetics and deaths in mental hospitals are specifically mentioned in some state legislation.

Not all coronial investigations become formal inquests. Those deaths which call for a mandatory inquest are outlined in the relevant legislation of each state. For example, a coroner in New South Wales must hold an inquest into deaths caused by anaesthetics and deaths of patients in mental hospitals irrespective of the cause of death. Coroners have the power to order post-mortem examinations and other examinations and tests considered necessary to facilitate an investigation. If necessary, an order of exhumation of a body may also be made.

Coronial inquiries are usually held without a jury, but a jury may be empanelled in some states where a minister directs or a relative requests one. Coroners are not required to follow the normal rules of procedure and evidence of a higher court of record; however, legislation generally provides that witnesses need not answer questions which tend to incriminate them.

Witnesses may attend voluntarily, but coroners can also require witnesses to attend and give evidence under oath or produce documents. Witnesses who fail to attend or produce documents after service of a legal process may have a warrant issued for their apprehension. Nurses will not be excused from giving evidence on the grounds of confidentiality. Refusal to take an oath or affirmation, refusal to give evidence under oath or produce documents without lawful justification, or giving false evidence are offences for which a witness can be fined and/or imprisoned.

Persons who have a sufficient interest in the proceedings may make a request to appear before the coroner, alone or with legal representation, to examine and cross-examine witnesses. These persons may apply to have a copy of the transcipt of the case upon paying a prescribed fee. When an inquest is finished the coroner reports her findings and these findings may provide the basis for relatives to decide to initiate civil proceedings, or for the relevant authorities to take further action with respect to the death. Coroners can refer concerns regarding the competence of health professionals to the relevant professional body which can then conduct an investigation into whether they have been guilty of professional misconduct.

# 2. THE PROFESSIONAL NURSE MANAGER

Professional nurse managers need to be aware of the laws relating to the registration and employment of nursing staff. They need to be aware of the rights and obligations of the staff and the institutions that employ them. This section will discuss nurses' registration, the contract of employment and anti-discrimination.

## 2.1 NURSES' REGISTRATION

The registration of nurses is a matter of state law. All states and territories in Australia have enacted legislation creating Registration Boards (known in Victoria as a Council) which are required to establish and maintain acceptable standards of nursing care. Board membership varies from state to state, but all have nursing and non-nursing representatives.

The power of the Boards is delegated by the Minister of Health in each jurisdiction and is mainly concerned with the registration and enrolment of nurses, the approval of nursing courses, investigating complaints, and imposing sanctions on nurses and others for breaches of the legislation. Although each state or territory board has similar functions, there are some differences and nurses should make themselves familiar with the legislation operating in the state or territory in which they are working. It should be noted that the power of these Boards is also to be found in various regulations, rules and by-laws as well as in the principal acts. These Boards are required to maintain rolls and registers of nurses. Registration is granted upon proof that a nurse has completed a recognised course and has reached a prescribed age. Prospective applicants must also be of good character and proficient in the English language. The Boards process applications from nurses trained in other states and overseas. Nurses trained in one state of Australia generally have little difficulty in obtaining registration in another, but could be required to undertake additional training where the educational standards differ. Nurses trained overseas might not have their qualifications recognised, or might be required to undergo a period of clinical practice, and/or undertake examinations set by the relevant Board of the state or territory in which they wish to practise as a registered nurse, before being granted registration.

Before nurses can practise in a particular state or territory, they must be registered according to its laws. All states except New South Wales maintain different registers for different disciplines of nursing. In New South Wales a composite register is maintained: both the Register (for registered nurses) and the Roll (for enrolled nurses) are divided into List A and List B. Registered nurses are able to practise generally and are not restricted to the areas in which they have previously been specifically registered. Proof of registration will normally be required by a health care employer before a person commences employment as a registered nurse. To remain on a register a nurse must pay an annual fee and remain of good character. Most health care institutions require proof of annual registration. Nurses may hold registration in a number of states provided they pay the requisite registration fees. Provision exists for temporary registration in some cases. Temporary registration may be appropriate where registration is needed for a limited time to carry out research, or in the case of nurses visiting the state or territory for a short time only. Overseas registered nurses may be required to have temporary registration as an entry requirement to undertake further studies in nursing in Australia.

The Boards have the power to carry out investigations into allegations of misconduct against registered nurses and to take disciplinary action. A complaint may be made to a Board by a person who pays a nominal sum or a Board may have a matter referred to it from a criminal court or a Coroner's court. The broadest complaint is that of professional misconduct. There are no precise guidelines as to what constitutes professional misconduct but it may include conduct that falls below the standard required by the relevant Board and/or unethical conduct. It can also include addiction to drugs or alcohol, making false and misleading statements in order to obtain registration or enrolment, or having a conviction for a serious criminal offence. Under the New South Wales Nurses Act 1991, professional misconduct '... means unsatisfactory professional conduct of a sufficiently serious nature to justify the removal of the nurse's name from the Register or roll'. Nurses suffering mental or physical incapacity may be allowed to continue practising subject to conditions imposed by a Board, or the relevant act may require a Board to cancel the registration or enrolment of an accredited nurse if the nurse becomes a mentally incapacitated person.

Whenever a complaint is received, a Board must first arrange an inquiry or investigation into the alleged conduct. The Boards have power to dismiss complaints considered frivolous or vexatious. Where an inquiry is to be held, appropriate notice must be given to the nurse in order to allow her to prepare a defence. The nurse has a right to appear before the relevant Board in person or be represented by legal counsel. Although the proceedings are informal and Boards are not required to follow the rules of evidence of a court, they can administer oaths, compel attendance of witnesses and seek evidence. Under the New South Wales Nurses Act 1991, Professional Standards Committees will hear complaints and conduct inquiries and a Tribunal is to be responsible for hearing complaints and appeals involving suspension or cancellation of a nurse's accreditation or appeals against a finding of a Committee.

The imposition of a penalty is discretionary. Penalties may be removal of a nurse's name from the register, suspension of registration for a serious offence, a caution or reprimand, and/or imposition of conditions on practice. In some states there is power to impose a fine. Where a nurse's registration is cancelled in one state or territory, most Boards are required to notify other Boards.

Depending on the jurisdiction, an appeal can be made to a court or other body. An appeal may be against a failure to register, a suspension or cancellation of registration, or a failure to re-register after a period of deregistration. Appeals against a penalty imposed after an inquiry or investigation are generally in the form of a rehearing, and the appeal body may either confirm the Board's action, or quash the conviction and, where appropriate, order that the appellant be restored to the position she would have been in prior to action taken by the Board. In New South Wales, appeals may be taken to the Nurses Tribunal and a subsequent appeal to the Supreme Court. Nurses who have their registration cancelled or suspended are usually required to surrender their certificates to practise and any badges issued by the Board.

To be more fully informed of the legal requirements regarding nursing registration, nurses should obtain a copy of the relevant legislation of the state or territory in which they are working or propose to work. The legislation is generally available from a government printing office or may be found in a hospital or law library.

## 2.2 THE CONTRACT OF EMPLOYMENT

The contract of employment is also known as a contract of service. Contracts of service must be distinguished from contracts for services. In the latter, the persons contracting to provide work are independent contractors. The distinction can make a difference in terms of liability for harm caused to others and in respect of industrial awards and statutory rights related to employment. Nurses who are employed in hospitals and community organisations will almost certainly be under a contract of services. However, nurses who enter into a contract with an agency may be independent contractors who will be solely responsible for their own actions and not entitled to statutory or award benefits such as long service leave, annual leave and workers' compensation. In the event of a dispute, a court will determine the nature of the agreement.

A proved contract of employment is necessary before the rights and duties implied by the common law will apply together with the provisions of an industrial award. If there is any inconsistency between the common law and an industrial award, the award is paramount. However, awards do not cover everything and the common law is restored to ascertain such matters as the rights and obligations of employers and employees. Statutory law will also be applicable; for example, anti-discrimination and health and safety legislation.

A contract of employment conforms to the same rules as contracts in general. Employment contracts are not always fully documented. They may be part written, part oral, and part statutory. As referred to above, the common law implies certain terms into contracts of employment where the contract is silent and there is no applicable term to be found in an award. In the case of nurses, policies laid down by their employers and relevant government departments will also apply.

As in all contracts there must be an offer and an acceptance. A job advertisement is an invitation for a person to apply for employment but is not an offer of employment. If an applicant meets the criteria for the position, an offer may be made. It should be noted that many advertisements for higher positions now contain a statement that the employer reserves the right not to fill the position. Once an offer is made it is necessary for the offeree to communicate acceptance to the offeror. An offer may specify the mode by which it is to be accepted — for example, in writing — or it may be silent in which case a oral acceptance may be enough. It is possible for an offer to be withdrawn before acceptance, but, where an acceptance is in writing, the date of posting is the relevant date of acceptance. Acceptance must correspond with the terms of the offer. If the acceptance introduces new terms such as a different wage or conditions, it is regarded as a counter offer which may be accepted or rejected by the employer. The offeree cannot then retract and accept the original offer since that offer has lapsed.

In a contract of employment valuable consideration consists of an employer's offer to pay wages in return for work performed by the employee. There must be an intent to enter into a legal relationship. When a nurse enters into an employment relationship with a health care institution, it is with the intent to be legally bound. Thus, a volunteer worker will not normally be deemed to have intended a legal relationship and therefore will not be an employee. Minors can be employed as health care workers, but state legislation may provide for minimum age and conditions upon which they can be employed. Contracts of employment to carry out unlawful acts, or ones which are against public policy, will be unenforceable at law.

An employee's duties under the contract include obeying the lawful commands of the employer. An order to do work for which the employee was not engaged is not legitimate and can be disregarded. Thus a nurse can refuse to obey an order involving a task requiring an electrician. Employees are also entitled to disregard orders which would expose them to a criminal penalty. An order requiring a nurse to do an illegal act can also be disregarded. For example, a nurse could refuse to participate in the administration of deep narcosis therapy, a treatment which is prohibited in some states.

An employee is required to act with due care and skill in the performance of tasks under the contract. A nurse who consistently fails to deliver appropriate nursing care for patients with reasonable care and skill could be dismissed. An employee also owes a duty of fidelity to the employer; a breach of this would occur if, for example, an employee disclosed a trade secret obtained during the course of employment. Nurses might be involved in a field of medical science where particular procedures are being developed. To reveal the methods used without consent of the employer would expose the nurse to legal action by the employer. Former employees can also be held to be in breach of this duty if they use data they went out of their way to acquire during employment. However, with the exception of trade secrets and matters of a confidential nature, an employee can use 'know-how' acquired during previous employment.

Employees must also account for all monies and property received during the course of employment which belong to the employer, make available to the employer inventions or processes created by the employee during the course of employment, and disclose to the employer all information received which is relevant to the employer's business.

The main duty of the employer is to pay remuneration according to the contract or a relevant award. A contract may specify the wages to be paid. Where there is an award, the wages must be the minimum specified under the award. Where a contract is silent as to the level of wages and there is no award, the common law implies that a reasonable wage will be paid, and that wage is determined by what is the normal rate of pay for the type of work performed. In any event, legislation provides generally for minimum wage rates and an employee can take action to recover unpaid wages for work done.

An employer is normally under no duty to provide actual work for an employee except where the employee is paid by commission or, in some cases, is dependent upon the work to maintain particular expertise. Under common law the employer is generally not required to provide for medical attention, to provide a character reference or to protect the employee's personal property. However, the employer is under a duty to provide a safe place and system of work, and safe entry and exit to the premises. In addition, the employer must adhere to statutory regulations requiring minimum standards of safety at the workplace. The employer is also under a duty not to discriminate against people in employment practices on grounds, inter alia, of sex, race, marital status, pregnancy, sexual preference or disability. This duty is imposed by both Commonwealth and State legislation.

The term of an employment contract may be specified; for example, a contract of five years. After that time, the contract comes to an end with no obligation on the employer to renew it unless the contract provides for the possibility of renewal. Some agreements between universities and area health services to fund clinical positions have a fixed term. If no fixed term is specified, the contract is regarded as indefinite; that is, the contract of employment continues until terminated by either side. Contracts of employment in universities can provide for tenure, which is permanent employment. Where a contract specifies a period of notice of termination then that must be followed. For example, a contract may specify that an employee must give six months' notice before leaving. If the contract is silent as to notice of termination the correct period of notice is that which is followed by custom in the trade. This is often based on the relevant pay period. If there is no such custom then a period of notice must be reasonable in the circumstances. Either party has the right to terminate upon giving the required notice.

The employer has a common law right to summarily dismiss an employee without giving notice in the event of misconduct by the employee. An employee who is summarily dismissed can then take legal action for breach of contract and, if it is proved, the employee can recover the salary that would have been payable if the correct period of notice had been given. The right to dismiss is also fettered by the right of a worker, generally through a union, to make a claim for unjust dismissal and to seek reinstatement. If an employee is suspended for misconduct the employer is obliged to continue the employee's wages for the period of suspension unless otherwise provided for. Special rules apply to the dismissal of public servants.

Contracts of employment may also be brought to an end by the death of the employee, or by the death of the employer where the employer is an individual. Where there is change of ownership of a business, employees usually continue on in the employment of the new owner and retain their leave entitlements. A contract of employment may be frustrated by the illness or incapacity of a worker when the employee is unable to perform the work. Contracts of employment may also be terminated by mutual agreement of the parties.

## 2.3 ANTIDISCRIMINATION

Antidiscrimination legislation in Australia is complex, diverse and in certain instances — notably concerning race — could be argued to be furthering the kinds of behaviour it purportedly sets out to prevent (Markus, 1988:59–9; Kalantzis, 1988). Legislation has been enacted at both Commonwealth and State levels which unevenly addresses discrimination on the ground of race, sex, marital status, physical or intellectual impairment, political or religious belief, and sexual preference. The following outline of the principles embodied in key legislation is by no means complete and it is strongly recommended that copies of the relevant Commonwealth or State legislation, or guides thereto, be obtained for more detailed information.

The key pieces of Commonwealth legislation are the following:

Racial Discrimination Act 1975
Sexual Discrimination Act 1984

Affirmative Action (Equal Employment Opportunity for Women) Act 1986

Section 9(1) of the Racial Discrimination Act makes it unlawful for someone to 'do any act involving a distinction, exclusion, restriction or preference based on race, colour, descent or national or ethnic origin which has the purpose or effect of nullifying or impairing the recognition ... of any human right or fundamental freedom in the political, economic, social, cultural or any other field of public life'.

Of relevance to nurses is its application to employment including terms of employment, conditions of work, opportunity for training and promotion and dismissal.

The Sexual Discrimination Act and the Affirmative Action Act specifically address long-standing gender inequalities in Australian society. The Sexual Discrimination Act makes it unlawful to discriminate on the basis of sex, marital status or pregnancy. Like the Racial Discrimination Act, this Act enshrines the conciliation process as the means of treating discriminatory practices. Therefore, in order for these acts to be of any significant value in combating such practices there must be a formal complaint. Since the acts were passed there have been many such complaints and there are Commonwealth and State agencies established throughout Australia for obtaining information and advice and for registering complaints. For example, in New South Wales there is the Affirmative Action Agency and the Human Rights and Equal Opportunity Commission as well as State agencies which provide similar services related to state legislation.

The Affirmative Action Act is more proactive in its objectives, requiring certain employers to develop and implement affirmative action programmes for women. The Act promotes a systematic means of overcoming the more structural aspects of discrimination in order to achieve equal employment opportunities (EEO). By nature it is not intended to achieve immediate reform but rather work as a long-term strategy, gradually breaking down prejudices and real obstacles to opportunity for women in the workplace (Ronalds, 1987).

As well as these Commonwealth enactments, most states have antidiscrimination legislation and these are quite varied. For example, the New South Wales legislation specifically includes sexual preference as a ground of unlawful discrimination but does not include religious or political conviction, whereas Western Australia includes the latter but not the former.

For the professional nurse manager, the importance of these various pieces of legislation lies in an awareness of the right to non-discriminatory practices, whether concerning herself or himself or others under her or his supervision. While the legislation does not alter any of the fundamental inequalities which exist in our society, and will not eradicate discrimination — on whatever ground — there are material gains to be had from using it for many individuals and groups.

# 3. THE ORGANISATION

This section focuses on the duties and obligations of health care organisations to patients, staff and others. The topics to be discussed include occupier's liability, workers' compensation, occupational health and safety, and vicarious liability.

## 3.1 OCCUPIER'S LIABILITY

Occupier's liability refers to the duty of care owed by occupiers of premises to persons entering therein. The duties are exclusively linked to occupation since responsibility is based on control, not ownership, as a corollary of the power to admit and exclude (Fleming, 1987:419). Possession need not be exclusive. The term 'premises' has a broad interpretation and includes ships, motor vehicles and lifts as well as land and buildings. Hospitals and private homes certainly come within the concept of premises when we consider the duty of care owed to staff, patients and visitors.

Traditionally the law has limited the duty owed according to the purpose for which entry was made. However, the common law now supports the concept that the general law of negligence is part and parcel of the law of occupier's liability, and a case is to be decided on general principles of negligence rather than the traditional categories *(Australian Safeway Stores Pty Ltd. v Zuluzna)*.

However, as the law in some places still emphasises the categories of entrants, it is necessary to review the various levels of duty owed to the different categories of entrants. The standard of care is related to the purpose of entering. Persons who enter premises under contract are generally owed the highest duty of care. The duty may be specified in the contract, but if the contract is silent on the matter the law will imply that the occupier has a duty to make the premises as safe as reasonable care and skill can make them for the purpose of the contract. The duty of care is limited to the purpose of the contract and is non-delegable. A person hiring a room in a hotel is a typical example of a contractual entrant. Here, the duty is limited to the interior of the hotel building and does not apply when the entrant is walking in the grounds, where a lower duty of care is owed *(Bell v Travco Hotels)*. Health care institutions would owe a contractual duty of care when part of the premises was let out on hire for a special purpose — for example, a conference.

The second category consists of invitees. Invitees are those who enter with the invitation of the occupier and in whom the occupier has some financial interest. Typical examples are persons entering shops. Patients in hospitals are invitees and may even be considered contractual entrants. The duty of the occupier is to exercise reasonable care to avoid harm to invitees which may be caused by unusual dangers of which the occupier is aware or ought to be aware. 'Ought to be aware' means that the occupier could have become aware of the danger if a reasonable and prudent inspection had been carried out. Invitees are expected to take reasonable care for their own safety. Unusual dangers have been held to be many and varied, from spilled yoghurt in a grocery store *(Ward v Tesco Stores)*, to an unsecured mat on the polished floor of a hospital *(Weigall v Westminster Hospital)*.

A new category of persons, known as those who enter 'as of right', has developed to cover people who enter public premises such as libraries, parks and other public buildings. However, it appears that such persons are to be considered as equal to invitees and are accordingly entitled to the same duty of care. It can be argued that visitors to hospitals are entrants as of right and entitled to the minimum standard of care with regard to the premises as that owed to patients. It is for this reason that it is important that warning signs are used to warn visitors and others when there is a potential risk of harm. For example, signs and barricades should be used when floors are being washed or polished. Community nurses visiting the homes of clients would be classed at the very least as invitees *vis-à-vis* the occupiers. If a community nurse suffered injury while entering or on the premises, he or she would have a right of action against the occupier in negligence or could resort to workers' compensation.

A third category are licensees who enter by invitation of the occupier but in whom the occupier has no fianancial interest. A typical example is a visitor to a private home. The duty of the occupier is to avoid injury from hidden dangers actually known to the occupier at the time of the incident. If a visitor were to suffer harm caused by a danger not actually known to the occupier at the time of the incident, the visitor could not succeed in an action against the occupier. It has been held that a canvasser who comes to the home by invitation is a licensee and only becomes an invitee when the occupier does business with him. Thus a canvasser was not able to recover damages for injuries suffered when he fell while leaving the occupier's premises when the occupier turned off a light before the canvasser had completely left the grounds *(Dunster v Abbott)*. A health care institution would not be liable to compensate an injured licensee who suffered harm from hidden defects not known or discoverable by the Hospital Board or its staff.

A fourth category of entrants are trespassers to whom the occupier owes a duty of humanity. An occupier is required to avoid deliberately or recklessly injuring trespassers by the occupier's own act. Thus an occupier cannot deliberately set up devices intended to cause injury to trespassers, nor be reckless as whether harm is caused to trespassers by the occupier's activities. In other respects an adult trespasser must take the static state of the premises as he or she finds them. That is, a trespasser cannot complain of harm caused by the normal use of premises. In a recent Australian case it was held that the general law of negligence is applicable to harm caused to trespassers *(Hackshaw v Shaw)*. In that case the occupier of a farm fired shots at a car which was leaving the premises after an occupant had been seen stealing petrol from a pump on the farmer's land. A young woman passenger in the car was injured and was able to recover compensation from the farmer. However, the court held that the plaintiff was guilty of contributory negligence and reduced the damages award accordingly. In another case damages awarded to a trespasser for injury caused by a dog were reduced because the trespasser ignored a warning notice *(Cummings v Grainger)*. Staff and administrative personnel of health care institutions should not attempt to deter trespassers in a way that could foreseeably cause harm to them, or without regard to whether or not the trespassers could be harmed.

The law requires a high duty of care with respect to children. Where children are likely to be attracted, the occupier must take positive steps to avoid harm. Merely issuing a warning is not enough as children may not comprehend such warnings or may forget them. The extent to which an occupier must act positively can depend upon the extent of the risk, the ease with which it can be avoided and the financial cost involved

*(Southern Portland Cement Ltd v Cooper).* Thus hospital administration and staff should be alert to those areas which may be attractive to child trespassers and which may cause harm. As well as posting warning signs it may be necessary to take active steps to keep children away from the dangerous areas. Access should be restricted to areas in health care institutions, such as intensive care units, where there may be risks to child trespassers. In addition, visitors should be advised to keep children under control while in high risk areas.

Because of the duty owed to entrants, it is necessary for nurse managers to consider risk factors to staff, visitors and patients in the working environment. Where the layout of a ward or the activities of staff pose a foreseeable risk of harm to others, there is a duty to avoid that harm. It should be noted that in three states of Australia (South Australia, Victoria and Western Australia) legislation covering occupier's liability imposes a statutory duty of care upon an occupier, thereby providing an alternative statutory remedy.

## 3.2 WORKERS' COMPENSATION

The rights and obligations of employing organisations with regard to workers' compensation legislation are of critical importance to occupational health nurses. Within the broader health services arena they are less important and the rights and obligations of the nurse as an employee become vital.

For nurses, familiarity with the chief provisions of workers' compensation legislation as they relate to an organisation in their state is imperative. The past 10 years have seen major changes in this legislation in most states. These changes have tended to reduce even further the already limited monetary liability of employers and the state and to introduce more stringent regulations governing workplace safety and rehabilitation.

Workers' compensation is essentially a form of insurance: employers pay premmiums on a compulsory policy which insures them against the costs associated with a worker suffering injury or disease associated with her or his employment which results in death, incapacity for work, permanent loss or impairment of a part of the body or faculty, or the incurring of medical or hospital expenses. Under the New South Wales Workers Compensation Act 1987, all workers employed by an organisation *must* be covered by this policy and a failure to insure places an employer in breach of the Act and therefore liable to fines and other penalties.

As employers, all organisations, no matter how small, have many other statutory obligations under the Act. However, for the occupational health nurse the most important of these concerns the keeping of records. Under section 90 of the Act, an employer is required to keep a 'Register of Injuries' in which is recorded all 'Notices of Injury' (s.99) the organisation receives from workers. These entries can be made by the worker or by someone acting on behalf of the worker such as the occupational health nurse. No compensation may be recovered under the Act unless this Notice of Injury is recorded, and it must be recorded as soon as practicable after the injury has happened and before the worker has voluntarily left that particular employment.

The entry in the Register must contain the following information:

1. name, address, age and occupation of the injured worker;

2. industry in which worker was engaged;

3. operation in which worker was engaged at time of injury;

4. date and hour of injury;

5. nature and cause of injury;

6. remarks.

Since this recorded information almost certainly would be used in the assessment of any workers' compensation claim, its importance cannot be overemphasised.

It is obvious that prevention of injury or disease or death is of immense importance. But it is equally important to understand the workings of the compensation system.

If one concentrates solely on the mechanics of occupational health and safety in prevention and education without knowledge of the legal or medico-legal system which ultimately will determine quality of life for someone damaged in the course of work, then as nurses we fail in our duty as carers and managers and place ourselves at risk as employees.

Under current legislation in New South Wales, an injured worker has a right to monetary benefits, reimbursement of health and medical expenses, vocational retraining, rehabilitation assistance and interpreter assistance in pursuing a claim. A worker also retains a right to employment.

In brief, monetary benefits consist of weekly payments for any periods following the injury during which the worker is totally or partially incapacitated for work. In the case of partial incapacity, frequently a medical practitioner will specify the person fit for light duties. In this case a worker has the right to request an employer to provide suitable employment. This is important for occupational health nurses and nurse managers in recognition of their own rights but also for the welfare of fellow workers. For example, many nursing positions necessitate lifting. If a nurse or other health worker in the organisation is injured at work while lifting and because of that injury is certified fit only for light duties, she has the right to ask her employer for work which requires no lifting or other activity likely to impede recovery.

Sometimes an employee will know that there is no such position available within an organisation but again it is essential that she presents the medical certificate to the employer and requests light duties. If, after this request, the employer does not provide suitable employment the worker may be entitled to additional benefits under the Act. In this regard, it is also important for nurses to know that under the amended Industrial Arbitration Act 1940, it is an offence to dismiss an employee within six months of incapacitation solely because the employee is not fit for employment as a result of the injury, unless the person is medically certified as permanently unfit.

With regard to rehabilitation, all employers are obliged under the Act to have in place a rehabilitation programme developed with workers and any industrial union representing those workers. Employers are also obliged to ensure the worker is offered the help of an accredited rehabilitation provider. This programme, as well as information on other rights — such as choice of medical practitioner — must be made to all workers. 'Rehabilitation training' may be vocational re-education, rehabilitation treatment or medical training or a combination of these. Where such training is approved by the State Compensation Board, the expense of this retraining may be met by the Board. If, on the other hand, rehabilitation training is simply a change in duties at the workplace then the organisation has the obligation to initiate these changes but only after consultation with the designated Rehabilitation Co-ordinator, the worker, the union, the rehabilitation provider and/or the treating medical practitioner.

Obligations of employees under this Act are particularly important to the success or otherwise of a worker's compensation claim. Principal of these is the obligation to notify the employer as soon as possible. Failure to do so may prejudice any claim. An injured worker should immediately see a medical practitioner — even if there is no immediate need for time away from work — and obtain a certificate which contains an opinion on whether the injury is consistent with the stated cause, the time away from work required and any restriction on the worker's ability to work. This certificate must then be forwarded with a claim and any receipts for medical expenses to the employer.

Nurses frequently resort to self-treatment of seemingly minor ailments, notably back pain, and while their competence to treat such notoriously unmanageable ailments may be as good as that available from other health care providers, if the injury was sustained at work there is a straightforward obligation under this Act to see a medical practitioner as soon as possible in order to establish a record of the injury. It is also of critical importance that copies of all these documents are made and kept by the employer.

In brief, other obligations under the Act consist of permitting the worker to attend medical examinations arranged by the employer, the State Compensation Board or other relevant authority; co-operation in any rehabilitation programme affecting the worker; and, if the worker is in receipt of workers' compensation payments, then she or he must notify the organisation making the payments if there is any change in her or his employment status.

## 3.3 OCCUPATIONAL HEALTH AND SAFETY

Like workers' compensation legislation, occupational health and safety legislation with regard to the organisation's rights and responsibilities, is of particular significance to occupational health nurses but has relevance to all nurses since they will often be involved in implementing, on behalf of the employing organisation, the regulations and statutory requirements of the relevant act.

Also like worker's compensation legislation, occupational health and safety legislation has undergone a significant transformation in the last 10 years at both the commonwealth and state level. While the responsibility for occupational health matters in Australia has traditionally rested within the states and territories, since 1983 the Commonwealth government has taken on a leadership role by using Commonwealth powers to foster occupational health and safety in the workplace. In 1985, the *National Occupational Health and Safety Act* was passed establishing the National Occupational Health and Safety Commission as a statutory corporation. The four principles which inform the objectives and functions of this body are:

1. **Prevention** — by minimising the causes of hazards inherent in the working environment;

2. **Equity** — that is, protection for everyone, from all hazards;

3. **Participation** — of workers and employers as well as experts in assessment and decision making; and

4. **Responsibility** — one that continues to be largely with employers and with the state with regard to the introduction and enforcement of legislation (Brooks, 1988: 702-708).

The practical outcome of the application of these principles has been the emergence of Worksafe Australia as a primary source of research, education, information gathering and co-ordination in occupational health and safety. For nurses, the value of Worksafe Australia lies in its educational resources, which are considerable and growing rapidly, and in its overall objective of achieving uniform standards.

The legislation of most importance to nurses, however, is at a state or territory level and currently this legislation is fairly similar among the states. For example, under the New South Wales Occupational Health and Safety Act 1983 employers must ensure the health, safety and welfare of their employees and people visiting their places of work who are not their employees. An employer must:

☐ provide or maintain plant and systems of work that are safe and without risks to health;

☐ make safe arrangement with regard to the use, handling, storage or transport of plant or substances;

☐ provide information, instruction, training and supervision as may be necessary to ensure the safety and health of employees; and

☐ maintain the condition of the place of work as well as its means of access and egress in order that it is safe and without risk.

A further requirement of the Act is that in workplaces of 20 or more, where the majority of employees request it, an Occupational Health and Safety Committee must be established.

A nurse can assist the organisation in fulfilling these obligations by calling on the range of services available through the Workcover Authority — the administrative amalgamation of the Division of Occupational Health and Safety within the Department of

Industrial Relations and Employment and the Workers' Compensation and Rehabilitation authority — for advice on training, technical assistance and for educational information. However, the primary role of the nurse is in establishing and maintaining worker safety and here the interests of the professional nurse manager as an employer or worker within an organisation and that of the occupational health nurse coincide.

Nurse managers can make significant contributions to the health, safety and welfare of fellow workers through skilful and informed management practices. However, they must also be aware of the rights and responsibilities of nurses as employees within an organisation.

Management of health and safety in the workplace has traditionally been regarded as the domain of the specialist — the occupational health nurse or officer or other nominated person. Current practice, however, encourages all managers to see health and safety as an integral part of the management role. In essence, the nurse manager's goal should be the control of hazards through identification of hazards or potential hazards in the workplace, the evaluation of those hazards, and their control. In large organisations, these same tasks will be also addressed by the Occupational Health and Safety Committee. There is often a statutory requirement for establishing these committees and they provide the best available forum for productive consultation between workers, managers and employing organisations. In New South Wales, the Workcover Authority has published guidelines for managing health and safety at work (Workcover Authority of New South Wales 1989).

But it should be remembered that the nurse manager is also an employee and as such has rights and obligations under this legislation. With respect to obligations under the Occupational Health and Safety Act 1983 of New South Wales, every employee while at work must 'take reasonable care for the health and safety of persons who are at his [sic] place of work and who may be affected by his acts or omissions at work' (s.19/[a]). At first glance this section appears to place enormous responsibility on an employee. However, the important word is 'reasonable'. As Marks and Churchill point out, a judge or magistrate in assessing a 'reasonable' standard of care under the Act would be 'entitled to take into account the fact that the person was an employee, the nature and extent of his [sic] experience, qualifications, expertise and knowledge, the totality of the circumstances involved and the nature of any relevant situation with which he [sic] was confronted' (Marks & Churchill, 1988:51). In other words, this section is directed to circumstances where a particular act or omission would harm others at the workplace.

Under section 19(b), employees are compelled to co-operate with employers in their efforts to comply with the legislation. The general import of this obligation, which carries a penalty of $2000 for breach, is that an employee must not place the employer in breach of the Act. So, for example, refusal to wear gloves provided by a hospital for the handling of infectious material would place a nurse's health at risk and therefore place her in a situation whereby the organisation would be in breach of the Act.

With regard to rights under this legislation, the rights of the nurse manager are those of any employee; that is, the right to work in a safe and healthy environment. However, the Act provides no easy mechanism for individual employees to do anything about an employer who is in breach of the Act. There is no right under the Act which allows an employee to cease work even if there is an apparent safety or health risk. Rather, this Act relies on employee participation (Health and Safety Committees) in the regulation of health and safety at work, on statutory requirement for the notification of accidents and injuries, and on the fact that under common law an employee is not under any obligation to work in circumstances perceived to be dangerous.

For the nurse manager, it is essential to know who the Committee members are and if she or he perceives a health or safety risk in the workplace to bring this matter to the attention of the Committee.

## 3.4 VICARIOUS LIABILITY

Nurse managers should be aware that under the law of vicarious liability an employer can be held responsible for the acts of its employees carried out in the course of their employment. Although responsibility for an employee's acts is limited to the course of employment, this term is fairly broad and encompasses all acts which are reasonably within the scope of the employee's duties, authorised or not. This means that a health care employer can be held legally responsible to compensate an injured patient whose injuries resulted from an employee's negligence, even when the employee was doing an act in an unauthorised manner. For example, most hospitals have procedure manuals which detail the manner in which various procedures are to be carried out. If a nurse ignores the instructions in the procedure manual and causes harm to a patient, the hospital cannot escape liability on the basis that the nurse was not following laid down procedures. Vicarious liability does not negate the nurse's personal liability, it just means that the health care employer will generally be the party which is sued since it will carry insurance to cover its liability. The employing body will only escape vicarious liability where it can be proved that the employee was so far removed from the course of employment as to be 'on a frolic of his own'.

Notwithstanding the doctrine of vicarious liability, the courts have been prepared to find that an employing body such as a hospital has a personal duty of care towards patients and others *(Albrighton v Royal Prince Alfred Hospital and Ors)*. Thus a hospital can be found negligent for harm caused to a patient even in those cases where it could not be vicariously liable, for example, when the alleged harm was caused by the act or omission of a visiting medical officer. Where the policies and procedures adopted by a hospital could expose patients to an unreasonable risk of harm, a duty arises to avoid that harm.

Vicarious liability applies with respect to civil wrongs but does not generally apply to criminal acts. Nurses who are private practitioners are solely responsible for their own acts and will be vicariously liable for the acts of persons employed by them. Thus, nurses who become independent practitioners should consider taking out insurance to cover them in the event they are successfully sued by an injured patient. If an employer is successfully sued for an act of an employee, the common law provides that an action may be taken for indemnity from the employee; however, most jurisdictions now prohibit such action.

# CONCLUSION

The purpose of this chapter has been to introduce nurse managers to the application of legal and professional principles to nursing practice. Nurse managers should use the chapter as a guide to current areas of law and professional practice which are an essential part of the knowledge of a practising nurse manager.

Concepts of accountability and responsibility, together with legal obligations and rights of all parties from the point of view of the patient, the professional nurse manager and the organisation, have been identified and discussed. Nurse managers should use this knowledge to formulate suitable policies and safe practices in the workplace.

In these days of increasing litigation against health professionals, failure to observe appropriate legal and professional standards in the delivery of nursing care could find the nurse manager involved in a legal case.

Nurse managers should see part of their role as maintaining an up-to-date knowledge of law and professional accountability, and to that end should pursue further readings in the given areas. References have been included at the end of this chapter to enable readers to become more fully conversant with each of the topics discussed therein.

# REFERENCES AND BIBLIOGRAPHY

Affirmative Action (Equal Employment Opportunity for Women) Act 1986 (Eth.)

*Albrighton v Royal Prince Alfred Hospital and Ord.* (1979) 2 NSWLR 165; (1980) 2 NSWLR 542.

*Australian Safeway Stores Pty. Ltd. v Zuluzna* (1987) 61 AL JR 180.

*Bell v Travco Hotels* (1953) 1 Q.B. 473.

*Beausoleil v Sisters of Charity* (1966) 53 DLR. 2d. 65.

Brooks, A. (1988), *Guide book to Australian occupational health and safety laws,* (3rd edition), CCH Australia, Sydney.

*Cummings v Grainger* (1975) 1 WLR. 1330.

CCH Australia (1987), *Occupational health & safety committees manual,* (2nd edition), CCH Australia, Sydney.

Coulton, R., McCulloch, A., Noble, G. (1990), *The social dimensions of occupational health and safety,* Social Science Press, Wentworth Falls.

*Demers v Gerety* (1973) 515 P2d. 645.

Dix, A. et al. (1988), *Law for the medical profession,* Butterworths, Sydney.

*Dunster v Abbott* (1953) 2 All ER 1572.

Fleming, J. G. (1987), *The law of torts,* (7th edition), Law Book Company, Sydney.

*Gadsden General Hospital v Hamilton* (1925) 103 So. 553.

*Grainger v Hill and anor.* (1838) 4 Bing NC 212.

*Hackshaw v Shaw* (1984) 11 CLR 614.

*Henson and Another v Board of Management of Perth Hospital* (1939) 41 WALR 15.

*Hills v Potter* (1983) 3 All ER 716.

*Industrial Arbitration Act* 1940 (NSW).

*In re a Teenager* FCA at Sydney, No. S 5619 of 1987; *In re Jane* FCA at Melbourne, No. NM 6654 of 1988).

Informed Decisions About Medical Procedures. Law Reform Commission of Victoria (Report 24); Australian Law Reform Commission (Report 50); New South Wales Law Reform Commission (Report 61. June), 1989.

Kalantzis, M. (1988) 'The cultural deconstruction of racism: education and multiculturalism' in Marie de Lepervanche and Gillian Bottomley (eds), *The cultural construction of race.* Sydney Studies in Society and Culture, No. 4, Sydney.

Laufer, S. (1990), *Law for the nursing profession,* CCH Australia, Sydney.

Mair, J. (1989), *'The community nurse and the law'.* in Rice, V. (ed.), *Community nursing practice* (2nd edition), MacLennan & Petty, Sydney.

*Malette v Shulman* et al (1991) 2 Med LR 162.

Marks, F. (1987), *Workers compensation law and practice in New South Wales* (2nd edition), CCH Australia, Sydney.

Marks, F., and Churchill, J. (1988), *Understanding New South Wales occupational health & safety legislation.* CCH Australia, Sydney.

Markus, A. (1988) 'Australian Governments and the concept of race: an historical perspective', in Marie de Lepervanche and Gillian Bottomley (eds), *The cultural construction of race.* Sydney Studies in Society and Culture, No.4, Sydney.

*Meering v Grahame-White Aviation Co. Ltd* (1919) 122 LT 44.

*Minors (Property and Contracts) Act* 1970 (NSW).

*Motor Traffic Act* 1909 (NSW).

*Murray v McMurchy* (1949) 2 DLR. 422.

*Norton v Argonaut Insurance Co.* 144 So. 2d 249.

*Nurses' Act* 1991 (NSW).

O'Sullivan, J. (1983), *Law for nurses* (3rd edition), Law Book Company, Sydney.

*R v Bateman* 19 Cr. App. Rep. 8.

*Racial Discrimination Act* 1975 (CTH).

Ronalds, C. (1987), *Affirmative action and sex discrimination: a handbook on legal rights for women,* Pluto Press, Sydney.

*Sexual Discrimination Act* 1984 (CTH).

*Smith v Leech Brain & Co. Ltd.* (1962) 2 QB 405.

*Southland Hospital Board v Perkins Estate* (1986) 1 N.Z.L.R. 373.

*Southern Portland Cement Ltd v Cooper* (1974) AC 623.

Staunton, P. and Whyburn, B. (1989), *Nursing and the Law* (2nd edition.), W. B. Saunders/ Baillière Tindall, Sydney.

Swerissen, H., Thyer, E., and Doran, J. (1989), 'Workers' compensation in transition', in H. Gardner (ed.), *The politics of health: the Australian experience,* Churchill Livingstone, Melbourne.

*Thake and Anor. v Maurice* (1981) WLR 337.

Wallace, M. (1991), *Health care and the law,* Law Book Company, Sydney.

*Ward v Tesco Stores* (1968) 1 All ER 232.

*Watson v Marshall* (1971) 124 CLR 621.

*Weigall v Westminster Hospital* (1936) 1 All ER 232.

*Whitree v State of New York* 290 NYS 2d 486.

WorkCover (NSW) (1987), *Guidelines for workplace based occupational rehabilitation programmes.*

WorkCover (NSW) (1987), *Protection for workers and employers.*

WorkCover (NSW) (1989), *Managing Health and Safety at Work.*

*Workers' Compensation Act* 1987 (NSW).

*Occupational Health and Safety Act* 1983 (NSW).

# PART TWO

# Processes:
# The Functions of
# Management

# CHAPTER 2.1

# Communication

## RITA AXFORD

After reading this chapter, you should be able to:

1. describe the communication process in terms of the basic elements of communication and sources of misinterpretation;

2. apply basic principles of active listening and assertive communication to general and stressful management situations;

3. identify communication skills effective in promoting positive and extinguishing negative employee behaviours;

4. analyse communication activities for first-line managers in health care settings;

5. analyse common communication processes in organisations, including meetings, interviews and written reports;

6. explore communication processes useful for professional development, including public speaking and professional networking.

---

This chapter will introduce the nurse manager to fundamental research about the nature of communication and to principles of effective communication derived from this knowledge. The primary focus will be on skill development, followed by examples from a number of applications common in first-line management in health care settings. This should provide you with strong underpinnings for your own communication skill development.

Managers of all types spend a major part of their work day communicating in one form or another. Research confirms this. Davis (1967:326) reports that first-line managers spend 74 per cent of their time in communication activities.

Classically, management has been defined as working with and through others to meet the goals of both the individual and the organisation (Stoner, Collins and Yetton, 1985:7). The functions of leadership, decision-making, evaluation, selection, training, motivation, coaching and discipline can only be achieved through skilled communication. Understanding common goals and the means to achieve them is, therefore, fundamental to effective management.

The first-line manager occupies a pivotal role in the organisation as she is positioned between upper management, service providers and clients. The charge nurse regularly interacts with individual employees, patients, families, groups of staff, administrative personnel, other professional care givers, union and medical products representatives, and with the general public. She must skilfully communicate with this host of individuals in a variety of circumstances. She must be able to express ideas and plans orally and in writing and to listen attentively and accurately.

Since the success of the manager depends heavily upon this fundamental set of skills, it is useful to explore briefly how such skills are learned. Skill learning of any kind, whether it be effective communication or aseptic technique, is dependent upon first, an understanding of the basic principles underpinning the skill; second, applying the principles in various situations; and finally, practice (DeTornyay and Thompson, 1987:61). This chapter will introduce you to theories and principles of communication and describe a number of applications common in first-line management. Practising these skills, the vital third step in skill learning, is up to you.

# 1. THE NATURE OF COMMUNICATION

Stoner et al (1985:599) define communication as the process by which people attempt to share meaning via the transmission of symbolic messages. Let's examine the fundamental elements of this definition. First, communication involves people. Understanding communication therefore means trying to understand how people relate to each other. Communication involves shared meaning. This suggests that in order for people to communicate, they must agree upon definitions of the terms they use. Communication is symbolic. The gestures, sounds, letters, numbers and words we use to communicate only represent or approximate the ideas they are meant to share.

The simplest model depicting the process of communication consists of a system of three elements: the sender, the message, and the receiver (Figure 2.1.1a). The message is initiated by the sender and is simply transmitted to the receiver. This model is easy to follow and readily comes to mind when we first think about communication. It is not complete enough, however, to help us accurately understand how communication does and does not happen. For this, we need a more complex model (Figure 2.1.1b).

In this model the sender initiates the communication, encoding the information to be transmitted by translating it into a series of symbols or gestures. Media are the physical forms into which the sender encodes the message. Speech may be heard, written words are read, and gestures are seen or felt. Transmission can be conceptualised as both an act (speaking, writing, gesturing) and a physical property (paper, ink, air). Decoding is the process by which the receiver interprets the message and translates it into meaningful information. Decoding is affected by the receiver's past experiences, cultural heritage, personal expectations, physical wellbeing, etc.

'Noise' is any factor that disturbs, confuses or otherwise interferes with or distorts the communication. Feedback is the reversal of the process initiated by the receiver and contains similar barriers to accurate message transmission.

This model, although more complex, is also limited. It depicts the communication process as a single, one dimensional phenomenon. We can readily demonstrate that 'noise' has a cumulative effect in repetitions of the communication process. Meaning is distorted with each iteration, with an increasing loss of accuracy.

**FIGURE 2.1.1:** A — simplest communications model. B — communications model. (Source: George, C. S., Collins, D., Gill, B., Cole, K., 1987.)

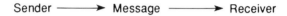

(a) **Simplest communication model**

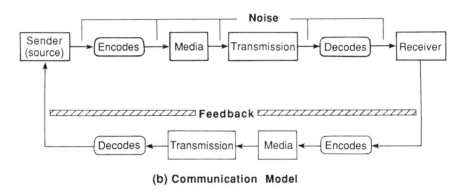

(b) **Communication Model**

As language is the dominant form of human communication, it is important to understand how we attach meaning to verbal utterances. Miller (1967:76–77) presents an explanation for this process. He explains that the simplest thing one can do in the presence of a spoken utterance is to hear it. Even if the language is incomprehensible, one can still listen to an utterance as an auditory stimulus and respond to it in terms of how loud, how fast, how long, from which direction, and so forth. Once an utterance is heard, one can accept it as meaningful. Next is interpretation, a two-step process. The first step is assigning meaning to individual words, and the second interpreting how these meanings combine in sentences. Compare the sentences: 'Healthy young babies sleep soundly' and 'Colourless green ideas sleep furiously'. Although each word is meaningful and the sentences are quite similar in terms of their syntax, the second cannot be interpreted using the usual semantic rules for English. Meaningful interpretation of individual words is affected by the company they keep.

The next level, understanding, frequently goes beyond the utterance itself and involves the context in which the words are spoken. A nurse hearing her colleague state, 'Mr Jones has just suffered a cardiac arrest' must do more than interpret the literal reference; she must understand that she should go immediately to the patient's room and assist in the resuscitation effort. Understanding the function of an utterance in terms of diverse and complex contexts involves high level understanding of shared meaning.

Theoretical explanations of communication also examine the contribution of non-verbal messages to shared meaning. Non-verbal elements include not only the overt expressions and gestures of the speaker, but also the environmental context within which the communication is occurring, as well as the roles, relationships and experiences of the participants.

Communication can also be described in terms of the dimensions of the exchange: one-way and two-way communication. In one-way communication, the sender is neither expecting nor responding to feedback from the receiver. A common example of one-way communication in organisations is the delivery of a policy statement from upper management. In two-way communication, the receiver provides acknowledged feedback to the sender. This can be observed when a manager makes a suggestion to a subordinate and receives a question or counter-suggestion.

Leavitt and Mueller (1951:401–410) explored outcomes of one- and two-way communication through a series of scientific experiments. Individuals were asked to describe an arrangement of geometric shapes to a group of listeners using words alone. The listeners were to reproduce the diagrams under conditions of one-way and two-way communication. Their findings indicate that while one-way communication takes considerably less time than two-way communication, two-way communication is more accurate. Further, receivers are more sure of themselves and of their judgements when two-way communication is used. Senders can easily feel attacked when two-way communication is used as receivers may call attention to a sender's ambiguities and mistakes. Although less accurate, one-way communication appears much more orderly than two-way communication, which was often described as noisy and chaotic.

From this, we see that managers need to evaluate their message in order to determine which mode of communication is most suitable for a given situation. If communication must be fast and if accuracy is easy to achieve, one-way communication is both economical and efficient. If orderliness is considered vital, as in a large public meeting, one-way communication might also be more appropriate. One-way communication can be politically expedient as it reduces the chance that the sender's mistakes will be publicly revealed and challenged.

When accuracy of communication is important and involvement of the participants is desired, two-way communication is needed. Instructions for carrying out a complex task, such as the operation of a new piece of nursing technology, need to allow for dialogue and questions. Two-way communication can serve to inform staff of operating procedures, enhance their confidence when using it, and improve the life expectancy of the equipment. In this case, a team conference is more economical and effective than a memorandum or directive.

Managers do well who create an efficient mix of one- and two-way communication patterns. In addition, when the need for accuracy is great, communication is enhanced by simultaneously employing multiple communication media. In this case, the nurse manager might draft a written report, follow it by a verbal exchange and repeat the message with a follow-up memorandum.

Channels of organisational communication are traditionally characterised in terms of direction: vertical and horizontal. The first-line manager is central in organisation communication flow, as Figure 2.1.2 illustrates. Formal downward communication starts with top management and flows down through management levels to line workers and non-supervisory personnel. The major purposes of downward communication are to advise, inform, direct and instruct subordinates and to provide members with information about organisational goals and policies. Upward communication also follows this hierarchy, but in the reverse order. The main function of upward communication is to supply information to the upper levels about what is happening at the lower levels. This type of communication includes progress reports, suggestions, explanations and requests for resources or decisions.

FIGURE 2.1.2: Traditional channels of communication in organisations

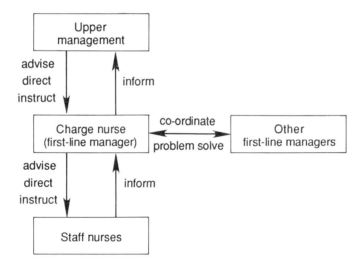

Problems common to vertical communication often relate to the varying positions of people in the organisation, their power bases, and their perceived needs to protect them. Downward communication is vulnerable to filtering, modification, or being stopped completely at each of the various levels as managers decide what should be passed on to their subordinates. Upward communication is likely to be filtered, condensed or altered by middle managers who see it as part of their job to protect upper management from non-essential data originating at the lower levels. Middle managers may keep information that would reflect unfavourably upon them from reaching superiors. Thus, vertical communication is often inaccurate or incomplete.

Horizontal communication usually follows patterns of workflow in an organisation and occurs between members of work groups, between one work group and another, between members of different departments and between line and staff. The main purpose of lateral communication is to provide a direct channel for organisational co-ordination and problem-solving (Hodgett, 1982:295).

This classification scheme describes in a simplistic way the formal communication channels within organisations. It bears noting that health care organisations are highly complex and utilise many formal and informal communication networks involving a multi-directional flow of information. A nurse manager regularly interacts not only with her immediate boss, nursing employees and peer managers within the institution, she formally communicates with consumers of care (patients) and their families, peer nurse managers from other institutions, community groups, employee physicians, private practitioners, other health team members, members from professional nursing organisations, the institution's trustees, union officials, the press, and representatives from sales and equipment companies.

A significant amount of communication occurs outside these acknowledged formal channels and flows through sanctioned and unsanctioned informal networks. Such communication often relieves the organisation's communication burden, reduces inaccuracy by putting relevant people in direct contact with each other, and improves employee satisfaction through the development of peer relationships (Hodgett, 1982:296).

Informal communication networks, called the 'grapevine', may be recognised by the organisation, but not officially sanctioned. The grapevine may be made up of several information networks which overlap and intersect at a number of points. It may serve social and informal communication functions as well as work-related ones. Although the grapevine is hard to control with any precision, it is often much faster in operation than formal communication channels and may be used to distribute information through planned 'leaks' or judiciously placed 'just between you and me' remarks. Some useful characteristics of grapevines are listed below:

1. people talk most when the news is recent;

2. people talk about things that affect their work;

3. people talk to people they know;

4. people working near each other or in the same chain of procedure are likely to be on the same grapevine.

Leavitt (1951:72) conducted research which examined various communication network configurations (meaning who talks directly with whom) and the accuracy of communication, the group's performance and member satisfaction. Centrality was found to be the critical feature in predicting simple problem solving effectiveness and satisfaction. For complex tasks, decentralised configurations were comparatively quicker and more accurate. Some of the patterns examined are shown in Figure 2.1.3. The 'Y' and 'wheel' formations are central, while the 'star', the 'chain' and the 'circle' patterns are decentralised configurations.

The centrality of the pattern also affects leader emergence and group member satisfaction. For both simple and complex tasks, centralised groups tended to agree that the person occupying the central position was group leader. In decentralised configurations, no one position in the network emerged as the leadership position. Group member satisfaction tended to be higher in decentralised networks for all types of tasks and were ranked from highest to lowest, circle, chain and star. The central person in the Y and wheel configuration preferred the centralised to the decentralised networks. These findings have implications for the nurse manager as she uses alternative communication networks. Rapid and accurate communication of management decisions may be made through her associates, while complex decisions which affect staff overall may best be referred to representative work groups.

**FIGURE 2.1.3:**   Communication network configurations (source: Leavitt, H. J., 1951)

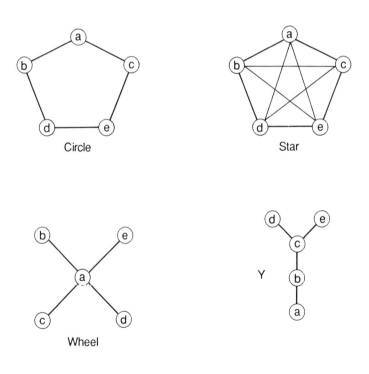

Barriers to communication, described in the communication model as 'noise', have also been studied empirically. Sayles and Strauss (1980:166–170) identified a number of commonly occurring factors which disturb, confuse or otherwise interfere with or distort the intended meaning of a message.

First, we often hear what we expect to hear. A subordinate who has been habitually criticised may misinterpret a compliment from her manager as being a sarcastic remark. A second barrier is ignoring information that conflicts with what we 'know'. A manager may ignore subordinates' complaints because she 'knows' working conditions are good. Not only are the words interpreted differently depending upon who says them, but words themselves may have substantially different meanings to different people and in different circumstances. 'A few minutes' to a nurse preparing an injection means quite a different thing to a patient in pain, or to a manager waiting to start a disciplinary interview.

The non-verbal component of communication can interfere with intended meaning in a number of ways. We regularly evaluate the source of the information; the same verbal message delivered by one's mother is interpreted differently from one delivered by a physician or one's boss. This interpretation of the non-verbal message may contribute to or detract from the accuracy of the overall communication. Non-verbal signals inconsistent with the verbal message lead to a range of interpretations of the message. Emotions and physical discomforts on the part of the sender or the receiver can cause major interference in communication. It is easy to recollect instances in which strong feelings such as pain, anger, fear or love have distorted the message intended. Past experiences with an individual can serve to create an effective filter or 'noise' from a given sender. The fable of the little boy who 'cried wolf' exemplifies this barrier to shared understanding.

## 2. COMMUNICATION SKILLS

Sending and receiving messages accurately will be addressed in the following examination of two vital communication skills, **active listening** and **assertion.** These skills provide the foundation of effective communication, mastery of which helps managers at all levels succeed.

Active listening describes communication behaviours focused on overcoming barriers to shared understanding (Sullivan and Decker, 1988:162). Active listening occurs in a climate which is supportive and includes verbal messages which describe rather than criticise and which assume a problem-solving orientation rather than one which tries to control. Spontaneity and an attitude of empathy and equality in the relationship are equally important.

The steps in active listening are few, but involve full participation by the message receiver. First, attend to your non-verbal listening behaviours. That is, use appropriate body language which clearly demonstrates that you are attending to the message. Second, use 'door-openers' and questions which encourage the speaker to elaborate on the meaning of the message. Clarify vague or uncertain words. Next, paraphrase the message, both its feeling and its content. And finally, obtain confirmation of your paraphrase. Table 2.1.1 provides verbal examples of these behaviours. Active listening, like all other skills, requires practice, the results of which are well worth the effort.

TABLE 2.1.1: Active listening behaviour

| COMPONENT | DESCRIPTION | EXAMPLE |
|---|---|---|
| Door-openers | A description of the speaker's body language or an invitation to talk. | 'You're beaming today'<br>'Tell me more'<br>'Go on ...' |
| Open question | General questions which provide space to answer | 'What's on your mind?'<br>'What are your thoughts on this proposal?' |
| Paraphrase of message | Concise summary of speaker's feelings | 'Seems like you're feeling pretty angry at Jo right now.' |
| Paraphrase of content message | Concise summary of speaker's words | 'You're working on making a decision about this?' |
| Clarification | Questioning vague or uncertain statements | 'I don't understand what you mean by "working on it".' |
| Confirmation | Questioning the speaker about the accuracy of your paraphrases | 'Was I on target?'<br>'Correct me if I'm wrong about this.' |

Assertiveness is a term used to describe behaviours that a person can use to deliver clear messages and stand up for herself in difficult situations without violating the rights of others (Morton, Richey and Kellett, 1981:18). It is especially appropriate for nurse managers to develop assertion skills as they are members of a traditionally female profession within an environment which historically has encouraged subservient behaviour. As women managers develop in new roles of authority and responsibility, they risk exchanging passive behaviours for aggressive ones. Aggression, like passivity, tends to foster misunderstanding, to decrease effectiveness, and to increase levels of stress.

The three basic steps to assertiveness are listed below (Morton et al, 1981):

Step 1. actively listen to what is being said then show the other person that you both hear and understand them;

Step 2. separate ideas from feelings by saying what you think or what you feel;

Step 3. say what you want to happen.

Assertive skills build upon what you have learned about active listening. They too, require practice. The first step, active listening, forces you to focus fully on the other person. Do not use the time they are talking to build up your defence or counter-attack. By really listening, you can demonstrate understanding and empathy for their situation or viewpoint even if you do not wholly agree with it. Step two, separating ideas from feelings, enables you to reduce the tension in the situation. You can then directly state your thoughts or feelings without insistence or apology. The word 'however' is a good linking word between step 1 and step 2. The word 'but' is usually not helpful as it tends to contradict your first statement. 'However' can become overused and routine, so it is useful to practise reasonable alternatives such as 'on the other hand', 'nonetheless', 'in addition', 'even so', 'nevertheless', 'alternatively', etc. Step three, saying what you want to happen, is essential to indicate in a clear and straightforward way what action or outcome you want. This not only serves to clarify your own thinking, it lays the foundation for future negotiations.

Once you have mastered these basics, there are additional assertive behaviours which can enhance your competence and confidence as an assertive communicator. Using assertive body language is one of these techniques. Body language is not new; we practise it in our day-to-day lives. Assertive body language means developing an awareness of our bodily expression of meaning and assuring a 'good fit' in the verbal and non-verbal messages we are sending. Assertive, congruent body language is especially helpful in stressful situations. Table 2.1.2 explores some detectable differences between assertive, aggressive and passive body language.

TABLE 2.1.2: Assertive body language (source: Morton et al, 1981)

| | ASSERTIVE | AGGRESSIVE | PASSIVE |
|---|---|---|---|
| Posture | Upright/straight | Leaning forward | Shrinking |
| Head | Firm not rigid | Chin jutting out | Head down |
| Eyes | Direct, no staring, good and regular eye contact | Strongly focused staring, often piercing or glaring eye contact | Glancing away Little eye contact |
| Face | Expression fits the words | Set/firm | Smiling even when upset |
| Voice | Well modulated to fit content | Loud/emphatic | Hesitant/soft, trailing off at ends of words/sentences |
| Arms/hands | Relaxed/moving easily | Controlled Extreme/sharp gestures/ fingers pointing, jabbing | Aimless/still |
| Movement/walking | Measured pace suitable to action | Slow and heavy or fast, deliberate, hard | Slow and hesitant or fast and jerky |

The 'broken record technique' is another useful assertion technique. It can be helpful when you find the receiver paying little attention to what you have to say or to your situation. This approach makes sure that your message gets through without nagging, whingeing, or whining and is achieved by delivering the message clearly, consistently and repeatedly. An example might be: 'Lateness is a behaviour that is unacceptable on this ward. I understand that you have a childcare problem, but the hard facts are that it is not acceptable to be late for work. However, we can give you an ADO tomorrow to give you time to look into alternative arrangements for Mary. What I can't do is accept your being late for work.'

An important assertive communication technique for first-line managers, that of saying 'no', is stressful for many people. There are a number of different reasons why people find it difficult to say 'no'. Some people like to please others and feel that 'no' is an unwelcome response. Others are afraid of an aggressive reaction. Some people are unthinking or unrealistic about what they are able to deliver. If your first reaction is to say 'no', then it is important for you to stop and think about your response. If you believe 'no' to be the right response, then you want to find a way to say it as directly as possible without making excuses, apologising, or giving long-winded explanations. A firm belief that you have the right to say 'no' without feeling guilty is the key to an assertive 'no'. Saying 'no' firmly and reasonably may require practice. Anticipate situations in which you are likely to have to say 'no' and practise the words you will use beforehand. 'No, Dr Grant, copying "obs" onto a worksheet for you is not a priority for the nurses on this ward.'

A person who is behaving aggressively tends to expect disagreement, and so proceeds without listening. 'Fogging' is a strategy useful in slowing them down and means giving an unexpected response — a way of side-stepping the attack for the moment while retaining your point of view and your integrity. It is accomplished by agreeing with some part of what they say. It is called 'fogging' because the effect is like suddenly being faced with a fog-bank. Fog is not hard, concrete or solid, but because it is difficult to see through, it becomes necessary for the aggressor to hold back a bit and pay attention to what is being encountered. 'Yes' takes an aggressor by surprise and helps to put the brakes on. If someone said, 'Well, that was a pretty stupid way to behave in a meeting,' and you want to fog you might say, 'Yes I can see that you think it was a pretty stupid way to behave.' You are not agreeing that you behaved stupidly, only that you can see this is what they believe. Fogging gives you time to get things on a more even keel and can reduce the heat in a potentially explosive situation.

Problems can be confronted and your needs made known without attacking the other person or burying your true feelings about a difficult matter. Through 'ownership of feelings' in an assertive message, the sender accepts responsibility for her own feelings and describes behaviours. Messages that own the sender's feelings usually begin with or contain the word 'I'. Messages which describe behaviour concentrate on what one person sees, hears and feels about another person's behaviour as it affects the observer. The focus is on the specific situation as it affects the sender. 'Stop being such a motor-mouth. Can't you see I'm trying to finish the roster' is an example of an aggressive response to a situation. Conversely, 'I am feeling anxious because you're continuing to talk to me. I need to finish the roster now,' expresses and 'owns' the sender's feeling and acts to defuse the tension in the situation.

Consistent body language, employing the broken record technique, saying 'no' without guilt, fogging, and owning one's feelings are assertion behaviours which enhance the basic steps of assertive communication: (1) active listening; (2) separating ideas from feelings; and (3) saying what you want to happen. Practice can make you skilful in delivering clear messages and standing up for yourself in difficult situations without violating the rights of others.

In work-related situations it may be difficult to know what the 'rights of others' are exactly. Chenevert (1985:109) identifies 10 basic rights for women in the health professions:

1.  you have the right to be treated with respect;

2.  you have the right to a reasonable work load;

3.  you have the right to an equitable wage;

4.  you have the right to determine your own priorities;

5.  you have the right to ask for what you want;

6.  you have the right to refuse without making excuses or feeling guilty;

7.  you have the right to make mistakes and be responsible for them;

8.  you have the right to give and receive information as a professional;

9.  you have the right to act in the best interest of the patient;

10. you have the right to be human.

She states that nurses have these basic rights and that each individual is responsible for acquiring these rights for herself. No-one is responsible for 'giving' them to her. As first-line managers, awareness of nurses' rights is vital and demonstrating assertive communication can empower staff to assume accountability for their own rights.

Now that we have explored basic strategies for active listening and assertive communication, our next task is to examine common situations and settings in which first-line managers use these and other specialised communication skills.

# 3. COMMUNICATION ACTIVITIES FOR FIRST-LINE MANAGERS

In the preceeding pages, management was defined as working through others to meet the goals of the organisation and the individual. It follows, therefore, that the first-line manager's role involves communicating these goals and providing the means, the opportunity and the will to achieve them. These are achieved, in part, through the management activities of motivation, discipline, delegation and conflict resolution.

## 3.1 MOTIVATION

Managers need to understand motivation in order to assist employees to reach their full potential. Motivation is defined as that which arouses, channels and sustains people's behaviour (Stoner et al, 1985:531). The principles of motivation include clear communication as well as strategies for helping people to achieve both the organisation's set goals and their own, as set out below.

| | |
|---|---|
| *Design* | Clear concise message |
| *Look* | For non-verbal clues |
| *Listen* | Actively |
| *Own* | Your own feelings |
| *Describe* | Behaviours |

Motivation is puzzling to study because motives cannot be directly observed or measured; they must be inferred from people's behaviour. Theories have been developed in attempts to explain and predict behaviour, and to link behaviour to consequences. This action-consequences relationship is a fundamental principle underlying a manager's ability to motivate employees to work towards goal achievement.

Early motivation theorists, such as Taylor and Gilbreth in the 1930s and 1940s, believed that peak performance was achieved by finding the most efficient way of doing a job and then training employees in the method. The Australian-born Elton Mayo, a human relations scholar, asserted that social contact was equally important. Managers motivate employees by acknowledging their social needs, making them feel useful and important, and managing the social forces in the organisation. In the 1960s, behavioural theorists such as Maslow and McGregor claimed that motivation was much more complex and that employees were motivated by many factors — not only money and the social rewards of the workplace, but the need for a sense of accomplishment and involvement in meaningful work (Stoner et al, 1985:534). From this perspective, managers and employees share responsibility for achieving organisational and individual objectives.

The manager's role in the process of motivation consists of two key elements: communicating the goals and providing the feedback. Communicating the goals is information giving and involves the basic steps of active listening and assertion. Feedback about employees' behaviour as it relates to these goals involves the following: (1) stating clearly what the employee did that deserves recognition; (2) expressing sincere personal satisfaction with the employee and the performance; (3) explaining why it is important to continue in this manner; and (4) asking what you can do to help her continue with these behaviours.

Blanchard and Johnson (1982) wrote a popular booklet which briefly encapsulates the fundamentals of motivation. They assert that a manager's time is best spend investing in people. They are quite clear that people who feel good about themselves produce good results and that the best way to achieve this is to 'catch them doing something right'. The behaviour we want to foster, while initiated by a clear understanding of goals, is maintained by the consequences (feedback) of such behaviour.

Motivation is not the only influence on a person's performance level. There may be circumstances in which an employee's motivation has little impact on their performance. Campbell and Pritchard (1976) argue that performance is a function of a group of factors including aptitude level, skill level, understanding of the task, choice to expand effort and to persist, and a host of other facilitating and inhibiting conditions. This topic is also discussed in the chapter on human resource management.

# 4. DISCIPLINE

When employees are unsuccessful in meeting organisational goals, the manager must attempt to identify reasons for this failure and counsel the employees accordingly. Some problems which arise concern professional competence or job performance, while others involve work habits. The latter are by far the more common employee problem and include, among other things, tardiness, taking excessively long tea breaks, untidiness and shirking.

Like motivation and rewards for desirable behaviour in the workplace, elimination of poor habits involves explicit information about consequences, plus consistent negative reinforcement. While an intermittent positive reinforcement schedule is most effective in rewarding constructive behaviours, consistency is the key for extinguishing poor work habits. The following list describes the fundamentals of positive discipline and is based upon the underlying assumptions of Skinnerian reinforcement theory (DeTornyay et al, 1987):

1.  reward individuals fairly, not equally;

2.  reward publicly, discipline privately;

3.  positive reinforcement involves explicit information about what will get rewarded and intermittent reward;

4.  extinction involves explicit information about consequences and consistent negative reinforcement;

5.  failure to respond modifies behaviour.

One can also view the manager-employee counselling process in terms of a set of progressive steps leading up to more and more serious disciplinary action. This process has been developed and formalised for the protection of all involved: the employer, the employee, and clients and patients, and involves a participative approach to problem resolution. The first step in the process is that of a verbal warning or admonition. It should be done in a private interview; active listening skills are required, and a clear format should be followed. The manager states the problem clearly and specifically. Then she asks for the employee's view of the situation. When clear about this, the manager asks the employee for alternative solutions. It may take some clarifying and assertion on the manager's part to communicate what is and what is not an acceptable plan for resolving the problem. Next, both agree on the plan, and finally get commitment and set up a review date. It is essential that the plan is clear and acceptable, that the review date is firm, and that the commitment to both are kept. It is useful to state explicitly 'this is a verbal warning'.

If the undesirable behaviour recurs, a written warning or admonition is the next step. The same procedures are followed as with the verbal warning, but there must also be careful, objective written documentation of the interview. It is essential that the manager is familiar with the organisation's written policies on disciplinary proceedings. Persistent behaviour which requires suspension or dismissal is usually referred by the first-line manager to her immediate superior or above. Care and attention to the fundamental steps and appropriate documentation help the organisation protect workers' rights and patients' safety.

Problems which involve dealing with an impaired employee often appear first as poor work habits. Differentiating chemical dependence problems from poor work habits is the first order of responsibility for the first-line manager. Table 2.1.3 describes characteristic drinking and work behaviours of the impaired employee. Intervention is considered to be beyond the scope of the manager. The manager's responsibility is for detection and referral of the employee to counselling services. This is usually accomplished through organisational supports such as the human resources or personnel department.

# 5. DELEGATION

Managers' communication activities frequently involve instructing and directing employees. In addition to giving information, instructing and directing involve the fundamental management activity of delegating. Delegating is more than just getting someone else to do the work for you. If done well and wisely, it is an important staff development activity. The benefits of effective delegation include achieving better use of special skills and scarce human resources, reducing job pressure and related stress, keeping the organisation running smoothly while you are away, spreading the workload more evenly, improving the morale of subordinates, identifying potential managers, and getting new ideas and fresh viewpoints into the workplace.

The principles of clear communication underpin effective delegation. In addition, the manager must be clear on the level of independence and responsibility which is being shared (Engel, 1983:226). Communication allows the manager to use delegation to motivate and develop her employees, and is also essential for enabling employees to

TABLE 2.1.3: Characteristic drinking and work behaviours of the impaired employee (source: Charter Medical Corporation)

|  | BEHAVIOUR | VISIBLE SIGNS |
|---|---|---|
| Early phase | Drinks to relieve tension | Late (after meal break) |
|  |  | Leaves job early |
|  |  | Absent from office |
|  | Alcohol tolerance increases | Fellow workers complain |
|  |  | Overreacts to real or imagined criticism |
|  |  | Complains about not feeling well |
|  | Blackouts (Memory lapses) | Lies |
|  |  | Misses deadlines |
|  |  | Mistakes through inattention or poor judgement |
| Middle phase | Lies about drinking habits | Decreased efficiency |
|  | Surreptitious drinks | Frequent days off for vague ailments or implausible reasons |
|  | Guilt about drinking | Statements about undependable |
|  |  | Begins to avoid associates |
|  | Tremors during hangover | Borrows money from co-workers |
|  |  | Exaggerates work accomplishments |
|  |  | Hospitalised more than average |
|  | Loss of interest | Repeated minor injuries on and off the job |
|  |  | Unreasonable resentment |
|  |  | General deterioration |
|  |  | Spasmodic work pace |
|  |  | Attention wanders; lack of concentration |
| Late middle phase | Avoids discussion of problems | Frequent time off, sometimes for several days |
|  |  | Fails to return from meal breaks |
|  |  | Grandiose, aggressive or belligerent |
|  | Fails in efforts at control | Domestic problems interfere with work |
|  |  | Apparent loss of ethical values |
|  |  | Money problems |
|  | Neglects food | Hospitalisations increase |
|  |  | Refuses to discuss problems |
|  | Prefers to drink alone | Trouble with the law |
|  |  | Performance far below expected level |
| Late phase | Believes that other activities interfere with drinking | Prolonged unpredictable absences |
|  |  | Drinking on the job |
|  |  | Totally undependable |
|  |  | Repeated hospitalisations |
|  |  | Visible physical deterioration |
|  |  | Money problems worsen |
|  |  | Serious family problems and/or divorce |
|  |  | Uneven and generally incompetent |

successfully carry out the activities being assigned to them. The process outlined below will:

1.  explain the need for delegation;

2.  explain the task and ask the employee's view;

3.  specify the amount of responsibility and authority being assigned with the task;

4.  confirm the employee's understanding;

5.  set up and keep the review date.

# **6.** CONFLICT RESOLUTION

Many communication situations encountered by the first-line manager involve conflict. This is only natural when dealing with people with different goals and backgrounds, often under stressful circumstances. It has been demonstrated that in some cases a certain level of conflict will produce better performance and serve as a motivator. Conflict management is based on this premise. Managers need to assess the importance and impact of the conflict before deciding whether to intervene to help resolve it (Huseman, Lahiff and Hatfield, 1982:65).

Principled negotiation is a strategy for resolving conflicting interests. The first principle in resolving conflict, according to Fisher and Ury (1985) is to separate the people from the problem. Every participant is a person, first and foremost. Second, they recommend separating the problem to be negotiated from the process of negotiation. This requires that participants not argue over positions: an inefficient strategy which may endanger personal relationships. Bargaining over positions often produces unwise compromise agreements.

Separating the people from the problem from the process allows one to focus on interests. Behind opposing positions lie shared, compatible interests, as well as the conflicting ones. Wise solutions reconcile interests rather than focusing on compromise positions. How does one identify interests? Ask why. Ask why not. Make a list. Recognise that each side has multiple interests and that the most powerful interests are basic human needs. Don't defend your ideas, invite criticism and advice. If you are attacked, recast it as an attack on the problem. Ask questions. Pause and reflect. The ability to talk about interests is the key to finding 'winning solutions'.

Now, invent options for mutual gain. By identifying what participants share and do not share, new ways to view the alternative outcomes can be created. Look forward, not backward. Explore a broad scope of options, not a narrow, single-minded outcome. Finally, develop and use objective criteria to evaluate the relative merit of the alternatives being explored.

What if the participants in the conflict do not play with the same rules? The best strategy in this case has already been described: separate the people from the problem; focus on interests, not positions; invent options for mutual gain; and insist on using objective critiera. Awareness of some common tricky tactics can be helpful in anticipatting and not being caught by these strategies. Participants may deliberately deceive by providing phony facts, ambiguous authority, or less than full disclosure. They may use psychological warfare such as personal attacks and threats to add to the stress in the situation. Pressure tactics such as refusal to negotiate, extreme demands and ultimatums can be difficult to deal with. Don't be a victim, deploy the principles you have just learned, as outlined below (Fisher et al, 1985):

1.  separate the people from the problem;

2.  focus on interests, not position;

3.  invent options for mutual gain;

4.  insist on using objective criteria.

# 7. COMMUNICATION PROCESSES WITHIN ORGANISATIONS

Communication skills have been applied in a variety of management activities. In this next section, we will examine in some detail commonly occurring organisational processes which also necessitate well developed communication skills.

## 7.1 COMMUNICATION IN GROUPS

In exploring organisational communication in groups, we will first examine how group communication differs from individual communication, and will describe commonly identified roles group members play and how they facilitate or retard group effort. Following this, we will examine meetings, an important, often misused process for group communication and decision making in organisations.

Group communication differs from individual communication in terms of a phenomenon known as group syntality (Gillies, 1982:152). This term describes how a group demonstrates collective behaviours which become increasingly integrated over time. A group's response to a planned course of action is similar to that of a single entity. A group experiences moods such as hostility, depression and elation which alter its characteristic behaviours and its energy output. A group demonstrates that it has a memory for group experiences. And finally, a group can preserve its own characteristic habits and flavour despite ongoing replacement of a proportion of its members.

Bales and Slater (1955) describe a number of different roles individuals may play and their effect on communication within the group. The active supporter demonstrates solidarity, raises other members' status and gives help. This role opens communication by rewarding constructive behaviours of others. The passive supporter agrees, shows passive acceptance, understands, concurs and complies. This role, while less influential in group decision-making, contributes positively to group integration. The morale booster relieves tension, jokes, laughs and shows satisfaction. Communication blocked by group tension can be opened by input from this player. The idea generator offers and asks for suggestions and direction. The role fosters autonomy of others. The evaluator/ problem solver readily gives opinions, evaluates ideas, offers analyses and expresses feeling. In asking for suggestions, direction and possible ways of acting, this role fosters task-oriented communication. The gatekeeper will give and ask for information, repetition and confirmation. This role keeps the rules of the meeting in force. These six roles all open communication whether about the task at hand or in support of the people or processes which accomplish it.

Non-supporter roles disagree, show rejection and withhold help. While these roles can serve to refocus the group if it is moving towards unreasonable decisions, they often stifle communication if their interactions are overly passive or aggressive. The morale deflator shows antagonism, devalues others and is defensive. While generally detracting from group morale, cohesion can result from a united front against these behaviours.

These roles enacted by different members at different times serve a constructive function in the group's development. Consistent non-supportive behaviours can be a cue for the manager or group leader to intervene with an individual member in order to maintain the group's integrity and effectiveness.

## 7.2 MEETINGS

Within all organisations there are meetings. These vary in number and type across and within each organisation. Health care organisations, being complex and service-oriented, are no exception. Beaumont (1987) describes meeting in organisations in terms of the organisational hierarchy and their formality. The highest level meeting in an organisation is the board of executives (also called board of trustees or board of directors). It may operate with an informal structure, but generally the decisions are recorded formally as it is ultimately accountable to stockholders or to the public. Other groupings of top level executives may meet regularly or irregularly and generally maintain informal processes.

Meetings internal to the organisation generally reflect the manager's leadership style and, to a lesser degree, the organisational culture. Interdepartmental staff meetings within large organisations are usually conducted exclusively at the managerial level. While it might be desirable to include staff, often politically sensitive information is discussed which precludes wide representation. Mostly these are formal proceedings with 'visiting expertise' provided when required. Departmental staff meetings vary in formality depending, among other things, on size. These meetings may have informational, decision-making, goal-setting, and/or team-building functions. The broadest base of participation by staff is often the most useful and satisfying.

External to the organisation are other meetings vital to its functioning. Union meetings are usually formal and highly structured as these meetings deal with sensitive issues such as wages and working conditions, grievance procedures and discipline problems. Outside contractors including suppliers, buyers and technical informants may meet using informal processes, but with agreements formally recorded.

Organisations vary considerably in their use of committees as decision-making bodies or vehicles for communication. Committees may be described as 'standing', meaning they are a formal part of the organisation's hierarchy with written terms of reference to guide them. Ad hoc committee, sub-committee, task force and working group are terms used to describe committees which may or may not appear on an organisational chart. They may have a short or permanent tenure and can function as a significant part of the organisation's decision-making processes.

Meetings serve a variety of communication functions in organisations. They may be used to give directions and job assignments, to specify areas of responsibility, and to give procedural information. Meetings can be production/service oriented if their purpose is to analyse a production or client problem, to discuss alternatives or to plan for implementation of solutions. This is the category for the traditional nursing 'handover' between shifts. Meetings can also be content oriented and serve to share new information relating to the 'business we are in'. In health care organisations, 'ward rounds' fit into this category. Other common functions of meetings include information dissemination and team building.

Two important questions face the first-line manager when considering committee functions. First, how to decide when to initiate an ad hoc committee and use group process for decision making rather than make individual task assignments? And second, when to join a committee (given the myriad of demands placed upon her time)?

Forming a committee and using groups for decision making is a wise strategy if it can utilise a diversity of member resources and opinions and increase members' motivation to participate. Often groups recognise and correct errors sooner than individual decision-makers. When planning change, it is worth noting that group decisions are more readily accepted, especially by those who helped make the decisions. Conversely, using individuals as decision-makers reduces pressure towards conformity, encourages individual initiative, centralises responsibility and authority, and facilitates more rapid problem solving.

Given that time is a valuable and scarce resource for all managers, critical questions about the usefulness of committee membership need to be asked before deciding whether or not to join a committee. It is useful to ascertain to whom the committee reports, its parameters (general or specific, advisory or decision making), and its support systems (clerical, fiscal, etc.). Additionally, you should want to know what power or influence the committee has to implement and evaluate its decisions. While you may not be able to ask directly, try to determine why were you selected for membership. Was it for a specific skill or knowledge that you possess, or was it as a scapegoat for the group? Finally, ask yourself if you are prepared to be a member. A half-hearted commitment is often worse than useless and may be damaging to your future.

First-line managers need to have a clear understanding of the roles and rules which govern effective meetings. Keenan (1990) affirms that meetings should be held only when the agenda justifies the cost of the meeting and only with the necessary people. It is important to distribute background information on meeting topics in advance of the meeting with sufficient time to allow members to familiarise themselves with the agenda and topics under consideration. An agenda written in terms of expected outcomes with time allotments helps keep the discussion focused. While the leader must be familiar with 'rules of order', leading meetings with 'rules of trust' fosters a much more effective and less competitive environment. Finally, record, distribute and follow up on all decisions and commitments.

A typical agenda order for formal meetings is outlined in the following list (Renton, 1979):

1. chair's address;

2. apologies;

3. confirmation of previous meeting's minutes;

4. business arising from minutes;

5. correspondence;

6. business arising from correspondence;

7. treasurer's report (and approval);

8. reports from sub-committees;

9. old business;

10. new business;

11. next meeting;

12. adjournment.

A well set agenda is the blue-print for a good meeting. Remember to separate the transmission of information from problem-solving time, and refer topics that are better handled by smaller groups or by individuals to sub-committees or working parties. Start and finish on time. Fatigue reduces group productivity and a maximum of 90 minutes is a useful guideline. Therefore, keep the number of topics reasonable in order to complete them in the alloted time. Careful sequencing of your topics is important. Place major decisions at the top of the agenda so that fatigue and time shortage do not adversely effect the outcomes. Ask yourself if topics build on one another and if several items could be dealt with more effectively if grouped together.

Minutes, while generally written by the group's secretary, are ultimately the chairperson's responsibility. Minutes should clearly report each item, relevant discussion, action taken, and person responsible. Many secretaries use these four categories as headings and record minutes in a column format. Minutes should report the name of the committee or group, the date of the meeting and all who were in attendance. According to accepted rules of order, this record of the group's activity should be reviewed and approved by the membership at the next meeting.

As groups make collective decisions, the leader needs to be familiar with accepted procedure and protocol. The organisation may have terms of reference which spell these out. If not, a number of handbooks exist which provide the rules regarding recognition of speakers, motions, seconds, discussion, amendments, voting and points of order.

Beside preparing the agenda and the meeting room environment, the chairperson is also responsible for providing leadership. The following questions can be used for self-assessment in evaluating leader effectiveness:

☐ could the members see and hear each other clearly?;

☐ did every member genuinely have an opportunity to participate?;

☐ were the objectives (stated in the agenda) achieved?;

☐ was there a general feeling of satisfaction from the members?.

Members also have a responsibility. They are obliged to come on time and be prepared, having read the agenda and any other background information circulated. Apologies should be conveyed if members are unable to attend and courtesy should govern activities and communication.

# 7.3 INTERVIEWING

A second organisational process in which managers often engage is the selection interview (a matter also discussed in Chapter 2.2). The interview is the single most common technique used in the hiring process (Huston and Marquis, 1989:171–172). The selection interview is an information-seeking meeting between an individual applying for a position and a member or members of an organisation doing the hiring. In the interview, the interviewer is trying to evaluate information from sources including the application form, other interviews, and sometimes test scores. The applicant is trying to gather information about the job and the organisation. Selection interviewing of nursing staff may be conducted by the personnel department staff, by the nurse manager with or without representation from her staff, or by both. They may be one-to-one interviews or interview panels. It is important to realise that both parties are interviewing and evaluating each other. Keen interviewing skills assist in obtaining the best, most complete data in the short time allotted.

Effective interviewing practices incorporate the principles of equal opportunity employment. Familiarity with the official guidelines will assist managers in fair employment practices at this most fundamental level. Effective interviewing also involves planning the interview, presenting oneself, responding to the applicant, getting information, giving information and processing the information obtained.

The first step in planning the interview is to become familiar with the application form, the job requirements and job description, and areas to be covered in the interview. Plan and organise questions pertinent to the job and the applicant. Prepare for the interview in an environment free from interruptions. Presenting oneself is the next key step. The interviewer makes an impression on the applicant, both as an individual and as a representative of the organisation. The interviewer's tone of voice, eye contact, gestures, posture and personal grooming all make an impression on the applicant. The manager's response to the applicant is also important. Reacting appropriately to the applicant's comments, questions and non-verbal cues, conveying interest in the applicant, and encouraging an atmosphere of warmth and trust, all demonstrate concern for the applicant's feelings while still maintaining control of the interview.

Interviewers are ultimately seeking reliable information to help in employment decision-making. Therefore, in addition to preparing well-thought-out and appropriate questions, the interviewer should probe incomplete answers and problem areas during the interview itself. A number of probes which can help you get the information you want and need without seeming to interrogate the applicant are listed below (Huston et al, 1989):

1.  in what way?;

2.  how did that come about?;

3.  what would be an example of that?;

4.  how do you feel about ...?;

5.  tell me more about ...;

6.  what was it about that particular (job, school, etc.) that you liked?;

7.  ... found particularly challenging?;

8.  how did you happen to ...?;

9.  to what do you attribute that?;

10. what prompted your decision to ...?;

11. what else comes to mind?;

12. what was your reaction?

Giving information is another key element of the selection interview. The applicant is interviewing and selecting the organisation as much as the manager is interviewing and selecting the potential employee. Come prepared to communicate appropriate and accurate information about the organisation and available jobs for which the applicant would qualify. Ask for and answer any questions from the applicant.

Although selection interviews are widely used, research evidence suggests that they can easily become subjective and ineffective in the decision-making process (Huston et al, 1989). Selection errors in interviewing can be reduced by choosing the best of several applicants rather than making a 'yes/no' decision on each applicant alone. Planning and structuring the interview increase its effectiveness and reduce bias by providing the interviewer with similar information relevant for all candidates. Personal characteristics may be identified, but should be evaluated only in the context of job requirements.

Information processing and decision-making are the last steps in this process. Taking notes is encouraged as this increases the accuracy of interviewers' recall of information about each applicant, and notes can be retained to justify a selection decision should this be required later. Interviewers need practice in assimilating, remembering and integrating information relevant to selection decisions. Opportunities to participate in this process should be made available to staff as a developmental activity. Debriefing afterwards is an important instructional tool.

## 7.4 WRITTEN COMMUNICATION

A third communication process that managers must master is that of writing a coherent document. Report writing is more structured and less elaborate than other forms of prose. Memoranda are less formal and follow a tight format. All writing, whether for a project proposal or a public speaking engagement, is achieved in much the same way. We will focus on the writing process itself and then overview the format and syntax of management reports.

Writing is a cognitive function with a psycho-motor component. While few of us are troubled by the motor skills needed for writing, many of us are afflicted with 'writer's 'block'. We will therefore explore the cognitive aspects of writing in light of effective strategies for overcoming such blocks (Flower, 1985).

We know that the brain has both short-term and long-term memory. Also, there is evidence that our creative and analytical functions are quite different and probably occur in different locations of the brain. We have all used 'stream of consciousness', a form of daydreaming strategy, and can recall that ideas float easily and fancifully, rather than diligently towards a goal or task completion. The number of ideas and the creativity that can be generated by this process is impressive. We are capable of processing information on several tracks at once, and we know that we learn by practice. With this in mind, it may be useful to observe someone who is in the process of writing and troubled by it. Please review the following paragraph.

> My name is Rhonda Riter. I am trying to write about writer's block. In today's world ... writers today face writer's block for a number of reasons ... writer's block is of universal concern ... In today's environment, writer's block is a question that plagues many beginning writers ... In the current environment, writer's block is a problem of great ... of universal concern that plagues ... Writer's block is a matter of almost universal concern ... In the high-pres-

sure, information -intensive environment of today, one problem that plagues many beginning writers is ... This is a problem because ...

(Flower, 1985)

This is an example of a 'trial and error' approach to producing sentences and is one of three commonly employed ineffective writing strategies. The writer is trying to combine words and phrases until one version sounds acceptable. In her first major thought, she has tried out at least six alternative phrasings: 'in today's world', 'writers today', 'in today's environment', and 'a matter of', 'a question of', 'one problem that ...'. These trial and error stabs at producing sentences often yield a 'writer's confusion' as juggling so many alternative wordings overloads the short-term memory. The trial and error strategy is not only confusing, it is slow. Our writer could have continued to hammer away at this one sentence and tried more than a hundred possible combinations and grammatical transformations with this phrase alone. A writer needs to develop strategies to narrow this enormous field of options down to a set of things one wants to say, rather than testing all possible ways of saying it.

Read the next paragraph, Rhonda's struggle with a second ineffective writing strategy.

Writer's block is a problem because ... Due to the phenomenon of writer's block ... Because of its omnipresence, many writers fail to complete their articles ... thereby forfeiting their ideas ... thereby letting their ideas fall by the wayside ... Because of the omnipresence of writer's block ... Persistent writer's block affects many of us ... Writer's block persists even when good ideas ... Writer's block, an omnipresent fear for writers with valuable ideas ... For many writers, having their ideas blocked is a persistent fear because of the loss of valuable ideas ...

(Flower, 1985)

The writer who uses this 'perfect-draft' strategy is attempting, at the beginning, to write the perfect final copy. This is slow, laborious, costly and inefficient. Looking at this paragraph as a whole, we see that instead of planning ideas, jotting down constructive notes, or defining her writing goals, Rhonda has started out by trying to produce a perfect set of sentences. She is trying to generate her ideas and structure the language in the flowing sequence of a finished text. The creative brain and the analytical brain are having to fight it out for her attention throughout this process. In addition to the difficulty and cost in terms of time and paper, many creative thoughts are lost.

Look now at the following paragraph as Rhonda struggles on.

OK, writer's block ... Writer's block ... maybe something will come. I'll just think about it for a while ... Although many people fail to recognise it ... Although ... Although what!? I don't know! Oh well ... Although many people fail to ... don't recognise it, a most important determinant of writing success

is ... is ... is what? Try again ...
Not only is writer's block one of the most important, but ... but ... but. This is maddening. I'm getting nowhere writing sentences. Writer's block ... oh, what in tarnation do I know about writer's block. I think I'm having it! How can I write about writer's block when I'm in the middle of it!! What an awful paper to be writing. Wonder what I'll fix for dinner tonight. My, that window sure is dirty.

(Flower, 1985)

Some writers wait until they see the whole piece clearly in their mind or until words and sentences start 'flowing' and they know just what they want to say. This is a well-known but chancy strategy. The problem here is that the mind rarely sticks to the task at hand. At first, the writer is focusing her attention on producing sentences. Expressions which sound promising are giving her needed momentum, but don't provide needed direction. The mind, as it is wont to do, flits on to the next thing that pops in to it ... dinner tonight, the dirty window pane. Rhonda's gone off the track, but she is really close to a powerful and effective writing strategy. It takes only a little direction to move from 'inspiration seeking' to 'brainstorming'. Read the following text:

All right, writer's block is a universal ... universal problem for writers when under conditions of pressure ... a universal situation in which writers placed under pressure of today's environment ... oh, here I go again what are the key ideas about writers block?
— it's due to the environment
— lack of time is a 'biggie' too
— our self-image is not as a writer
— is this unique to nursing?
— how can we get writing experience?
— critique networks can help
That's not perfect, but it captures the important ideas. It'll be easier to make sentences out of those ideas later when I'm out of the idea-generating mode. OK, now for more brainstorming.
What is it about the environment?

(Flower, 1985)

Now we see something different happening. With 'brainstorming', instead of producing perfect sentences the writer concentrates on the generation and flow of ideas. Note also that instead of letting the mind 'free associate', the writer concentrates on her ideas. The ideas are not criticised. Their order and construction do not matter. That comes later. Congruence and flow of ideas are analytical processes and, while necessary, they do hinder the creative processes if they compete for attention now. The next strategy can be employed at any time but is particularly useful after a few minutes of brainstorming. Notation techniques can help connect ideas and tell us which are subordinate thoughts and which super-ordinate, as can be seen in the following text:

> What is writer's block ... it's like ... A roadblock ... Stops traffic ... Stops flow of ideas ...
> Query: Do my thoughts actually flow?
> Response: If writer's block actually stops something from moving, this assumes that 'something' is already there. That's a distinction I might play with. How about writer's blank?
> Writer's Blank versus Writer's Block
> No thoughts
> Thoughts come from:
>     Reading
>     Listening and talking
>     Seeing problems
> Obstructed thoughts
>     How to get thoughts moving:
>     Reduce distractions
>
> (Flower, 1985)

Rhonda has now started to structure the relationship between her ideas. She has made notes to reflect big ideas versus little ideas. While ideas are still being created, this is more of a clarification process accomplished by working with phrases visually in order to organise ideas, relationships and concepts. It helps to write subordinate phrases together. Some writers find it useful to use more exotic displays of relationships such as flow charts, decision trees, brackets, boxes and arrows. The key is to write down fragments and phrases as they come to you in order to visualise relationships and to leave room to rewrite and make changes on your draft. This eases the load on your limited short-term memory by creating meaningful groupings and maximises your brain's creative and analytical abilities.

What about when you are stuck, when you are going around and around in circles? In this case, 'satisficing' is a very useful strategy and puts your mind at ease by noting a problem area. Satisficing means being satisfied with a less than satisfactory wording — one you can live with for the moment. Later you can rework the phrasing, check a thesaurus or dictionary, or just sleep on it. The mind is amazing in that it will help you out when you least expect it. That 'perfect' phrase may come to you with no effort when you re-read your draft tomorrow, or it may pop into your thoughts in the shower, in the car, or as you drift off to sleep. No worries, you have marked these trouble spots on your draft so they won't slip by when you edit.

Finally, we know we learn from practice. We learn from simple concepts to complex ones and likewise from the familiar to the unfamiliar. A final look at Rhonda shows her using a well-practised strategy to get over a block.

Writer's block is not only one of the most dreaded, it is one of the most important … Oh rats!! I'm getting nowhere again. Let's see, what do I really know about this. Sometimes I get it when I don't know what I'm talking about, and sometimes it's when I don't really have anything to say. But, honestly sometimes I do have something to say, and this is really the most frustrating … what I mean is … when I have good ideas, but too many pressures, whether work deadlines or family concerns, that's when writer's block is most common. So, I have good ideas, but competing demands … hmmm. Let's re-work this. Maybe the strategy is to get something, just something of the ideas or thoughts down on paper RIGHT NOW.

(Flower, 1985)

This is really two strategies in one. The first is 'what I mean is'. This is a strategy for when you get bogged down. Start by saying to yourself 'What I mean is …' and switch from writing prose to talking to yourself. We have lots of practice talking and less practice writing. So, let's use our practised skills here — self-talk. Do it quickly, do it on paper, and do it now. Just say what you think. Some people find an alternative strategy useful. They write the ideas in a letter to a close friend or someone interested in the project. You don't have to send it. The intent is to get your ideas unblocked and down on paper — right now!

Now, and only now, are you ready to begin the editing process. Editing has its own set of problems largely related to the fact that it is often uncomfortable. No-one likes to be criticised. This perception of the editing process as criticism is a harmful one. Editing and critiquing are not criticism. They are the next logical step in the writing process.

There are four steps to this process and it begins only after you have your creative ideas on paper. Read through your rough draft of ideas and make logical connections. One idea should flow to the next. Big ideas should become your topic sentences and littler supporting ideas the subordinate sentences within the paragraph.

Next, edit your work for coherence, conciseness, and force. What you say should be easily understood by your readers, should be said in few, rather than many words, and should use an appropriate variety of emphasis techniques. You can check your effectiveness by reading your work aloud. Compare it to listening to a dynamic speaker: you want it to be short, to the point, and delivered with enough variety to keep a reader interested.

In summary, writing is most effective if one can separate idea generating from the editing process. Brainstorming, notation and satisficing strategies are more efficient than trying to set down a perfect first draft. Ideas that are not written down are soon lost, so write right now. Short bursts of writing time can be as effective as long ones. Editing should be a separate activity done with the intent to strengthen and polish the ideas. Connection, coherence, conciseness and force are the key ingredients to the editing process.

# 7.5 MEMOS AND REPORTS

Memos and reports are the most commonly used written communication format within organisations (Davies, 1981). They differ from each other in their length, format and degree of formality. Memoranda are the least formal and are a means of ensuring that what might otherwise be communicated orally is committed to writing, thus creating a 'paper trail' of an organisation's activity.

Memos have a standard heading. This device encapsulates the basic data in the briefest form possible. A memo generally consists of a few sentences, cut to the very essence of the communication. Figure 2.1.4 provides an example.

A report is a longer communication which often includes a statement for a proposed action, supporting rationale, data and/or a budget. Reports need to be organised to deliver the most important information first and to provide a clear statement of intent. It is important to write for the specific reader audience. Well-written reports generally avoid verbose statements, flowery prose or high-powered multi-syllable terminology. While it would seem that the strategies proposed for facilitating effective writing may be limited only to lengthy documents, writing for publication or public speaking, the converse is true. Clear, 'punchy' reports and memos are rare as most written communications in organisations are 'first draft' endeavours. It takes very little longer to jot down a few notes about what you want to say, and then edit for coherence, conciseness and force. Such a strategy makes for effective written communication and a successful manager.

FIGURE 2.1.4: Sample memorandum

**Central Hospital**
**Department of Nursing**
**Memorandum**

**To:**       Ms. A. Sherman, D.O.N.
**From:**    Mandy Nelson, Charge Nurse 4-west
**Date:**    6 . 1 . 92
**Subject:**  Charge Nurse Meetings

We need your presence at our next meeting as we are finalising our presentation to Mr Baird regarding our request for budget software on ward computers. The meeting is scheduled for 2.00 pm on Thursday the 12th in the west-wing conference room.

## 7.6 ORAL PRESENTATIONS AND PUBLIC SPEAKING

In addition to communicating ideas to larger audiences in writing, managers are often called upon to make oral presentations. Such opportunities are often a bit daunting, but should be readily accepted and even sought after, as they provide an opportunity for the manager to develop herself professionally.

The first step in preparing for an oral presentation is to ask questions about the forum itself. Who is it for? What is the purpose? When and where it will be held? Next, clear objectives and an outline for the talk are most helpful. The preceeding strategies for writing apply equally here. Some additional elements vital to a successful public talk include a clear introduction, the body of your talk, and a summary. Written documents can be re-read for key points; oral presentation cannot. The adage 'tell them what you plan to tell them, tell them, then tell them what you told them' is very apt.

The introduction should include a clear beginning. The use of an appropriate audio-visual theme or logo is called 'set' and can be very effective in focusing your audience's attention on the topic (DeTornyay et al, 1987). The presentation objectives need to be stated clearly. It is useful to verify the baseline knowledge of the audience. Besides previewing the content areas to be covered, motivating the audience's interest and establishing their 'need to know' are also functions of a good introduction.

The body of the talk needs to be logically organised. It must be relevant to the purpose, and at an appropriate level of depth and complexity. Technical vocabulary needs to be clear and resources used cited in a non-intrusive manner.

The summary should introduce no new material. Its purpose is to review the major points, provide a feeling of achievement and establish a clear sense of closure. Returning to the theme used in the 'set' is an effective means of doing this.

The non-verbal elements of a talk are also vital to its success. Be sure everything is ready on time; a written timetable can be helpful. Check that all charts, diagrams, graphs, posters, films and slides are clear, simple and visible to all participants. Make sure that you are familiar with the room and with any pieces of presentation technology you will be using (slide or overhead projector, tape recorder, microphone, etc.). Have a back-up plan in case the technologies fail you. Handouts and an additional light globe have been known to save many a presentation.

Preparation of the physical environment may not be your responsibility as a presentor. If it is, make sure chairs and tables are arranged so that the audience can see and hear comfortably. Ensure there is adequate light and heat, freedom from noise and smoke, and knowledge about where toilet facilities are located. Materials for note taking should be available.

Preparation for delivering your talk includes transferring your talk onto cards or sheets of paper which can be handled and read easily and unobtrusively. Have them numbered in case of disaster. Always practise your talk. Practise it aloud. Practise in front of a mirror and to a friend or colleague. You should know exactly how long it will take to deliver, where the 'trouble spots' are, and what you can delete or add if timing becomes a problem.

When the time comes to deliver your presentation, rise from your chair with ease and tend to your body language. Position yourself vis-a-vis your audience. Move to a better location if necessary. Despite 'nerves', convey to the audience that you are confident. Offer no apologies — after all that preparation and practice you have nothing to apologise for. Eye contact with your audience is essential. Maintain your enthusiasm for the topic, and vary your voice volume and speed appropriately. Maintain good posture as you move easily, with a relaxed, composed 'stage presence'. Avoid mannerisms such as pacing, fiddling with spectacles, microphone or notes, folding your arms, slouching, or driving your hands deep into your pockets. It is a good idea to have a glass of water and a tissue nearby. Aim to look neat and professional rather than dazzling or spectacular. If you are on the platform when other speakers are presenting, attend to their talks rigorously.

## 7.7 NETWORKING

Networking is another professional process useful to managers at all levels, and especially to the first-line manager. While networking is not new, female socialisation patterns are different from male-oriented norms where networking is viewed as natural in establishing a set of contacts, mentors and informants. As members of a female dominated profession we have to ensure these skills and support our 'tall poppies' even though this is sometimes perceived as antithetical to nurturing, caring, passive, dependent, egalitarian behavioural norms.

The *Concise Macquarie Dictionary* defines 'network' as any netlike combination of filaments, lines, passages or the like. The notion of a human or professional network is likewise a system of interconnected or co-operating individuals. Networks may be formal or informal and may be personal or group contacts.

Puetz (1983) asserts that professional networks have an expressed purpose and are different from social networks. Professional networks are a process in which managers use contacts for information, advice and moral support for the development of their careers. Research shows that effective networking also increases feelings of accomplishment, self-worth and self-esteem.

Currently, nurse networks are largely informal, and limited to nurse-to-nurse communication. However, more and more nursing managers are taking advantage of the cross-fertilisation of networking activities within and outside of their organisation and across disciplines and levels in the organisation hierarchy.

Gibb and Gibb (1967) describe four dominant factors which differentiate successful from unsuccessful networks: trust among participants; communication feedback; movement towards set goals; and genuine interdependence in the system. This means that successful networking involves asking advice and also giving information both voluntarily and when it is sought. If you hear about a job opening and know individuals who would be good, volunteer the information to them; promote and support their development. Follow up on contacts that are given you, keep in touch with them and report back to the referee. Be businesslike in your networking. Don't be afraid to ask for what you need, but be specific in your request and do your 'homework' before asking someone to give of their time. Listen actively.

Networking largely involves the development of 'people skills'. If you are uncomfortable meeting people, set specific goals for yourself such as 'I will meet three new people at this activity or function'. Learn conversational 'ice breakers'. People like to talk about themselves, so plan questions accordingly. Be positive about yourself and about others of whom you speak. Learn names and use them. Finally, don't tell everything to everybody. Ask if information is confidential and, if so, never betray the confidence.

Networking involves investing time. As time is a limited resource, developing a systematic approach pays off. Preparing for networking activities means first clarifying your career goals. The 'tools of the trade' include a curriculum vitae and resume which is current and readily updated. Using business cards is also effective. Upon receipt of someone's card, note on the back where you met them, what the content of the conversation was, and any relevant follow-up information. Your professional appearance and demeanour are also at the crux of successful networking.

To realise the benefits of a networking system, your participation needs to be two-sided. Honest and supportive feedback is both positive and negative. Evaluate ideas critically in a supportive environment. This means separating the person and his or her self-esteem from the ideas themselves.

The benefits of networking are growing in contemporary organisations. In today's world, access to information is the most powerful predictor of success. Where previously money and rank were equated with success, today it is just as often a case of being in the right place at the right time. This is often a direct result of access to information, effective communication skills, and professional networking.

## SUMMARY

In this chapter, fundamental principles and research underpinning effective communication have been explored. Communication skill development focused on active listening and assertiveness. Practising these behaviours in addition to congruent body language, the broken record technique, saying 'no', fogging, and owning feelings in a message were recommended to the first-line nursing manager as strategies with widespread application. The managerial processes of motivation, discipline and conflict resolution were explored in light of the elements of communication contained within them. Finally, a number of management activities were reviewed. This included information about conducting meetings, selection interviewing, writing reports, oral presentations and professional networking. Success in these activities by the first-line manager was shown to be highly dependent upon the development of effective communication skills.

# DRYANDRA CASE STUDY 2

On Tuesday night there had been a bomb scare in the Accident and Emergency Ward of Dryandra Base Hospital which had meant the immediate evacuation of the area for five hours while the A&E ward was searched and the time of the announced explosion expired. It had also caused the transfer of some emergency cases to the Hakea Private Hospital. While the staff had coped with the bomb scare fairly well some deficiencies had been exposed and one of these had been reported unfavourably in the Dryandra Times. As a result of this report two further bomb scares had occurred on Wednesday and Thursday. Consequently the Board had demanded an immediate report from Radna Razneuth the Chief Executive Officer. Radna had delegated the report to Lesley Linum, the Director of Nursing and Tsui Lei, the Director of Medical Services, because the lack of readily available portable oxygen cylinders for two patients who required them during the first evacuation was seen as their responsibility.

1. Write the memo from the CEO to the DON and DMS delegating the preparation of the report.

2. Prepare the report from the DON and DMS on the incidents. The report should include policies and procedures for dealing with such emergencies. It should also include recommendations for prevention of similar occurrences in future.

3. Prepare a letter of reply from the CEO to the Editor on the unfavourable report in the Dryandra Times.

# REFERENCES

Bales, R. and Slater, P. (1955), 'Role differentiation in small decision making groups', in Parsons, T. (Ed) *Family, socialisation, and the interaction process,* Free Press, Illinois.
Beaumont, J. (1987), *Mastering the meeting,* Information Australia, Melbourne.
Blanchard, K. and Johnson, S. (1982), *The one minute manager,* Berkely Books, New York.
Campbell, J. P. and Pritchard, R. D. (1976), in Dunnette, M. D. (Ed) *Handbook of industrial and organisational psychology,* 62-130 Rand McNally, Chicago.
Chenevert, M. (1985), *Pro-nurse handbook,* The C.V. Mosby Company, St Louis.
Davies, K. (1981), 'Communication within management', *Personnel,* Vol 11, 217.
Davis, K. (1967), *Human relations at work: the dynamics of organisational behaviour,* (3rd edition), McGraw-Hill, New York.
DeTornyay, R. and Thompson, M. A. (1987), *Strategies for teaching nursing,* (3rd edition), John Wiley & Sons, Brisbane.
Engel, H. M. (1983), *How to delegate: a guide to getting things done,* Gulf Publishing Co, Texas.

Fisher, R. and Ury, W. (1985), *Getting to yes: negotiating agreement without giving in,* Penguin, Ringwood.

Flower, Linda (1985), *Problem-solving strategies for writing,* (2nd edition), Harcourt Brace Jovanovich, New York.

George, C. S., Collins, D., Gill, B. and Cole, K. (1987), *Supervision in action: the art of managing others,* (2nd edition), Prentice-Hall, Sydney.

Gibb, J. R. and Gibb, L. M. (1967), 'Humanistic elements in group growth', *Challenges of humanistic psychology,* McGraw-Hill, New York.

Gillies, D. A. (1982), *Nursing management: a systems approach,* W. B. Saunders Company, Sydney.

Hodgett, R. M. (1982), *Management: theory, process and practice,* (3rd edition), Holt, Rinehart and Winston, New York.

Huseman, R. C., Lahiff, J. M. and Hatfield, J. D. (1982), *Business communications strategies and skills (Australian edition),* Holt, Rinehart and Winston, Sydney.

Huston, C. J. and Marquis, B. L. (1989), *Retention and productivity strategies for nurse managers,* J. B. Lippincott, Sydney.

Keenan, M. (1990), 'Making your meetings pay off', *Nursing Management,* 21, 58-60.

Leavitt, H. J. (1951), 'Some effects of certain communication patterns of group performance', *Journal of Abnormal and Social Psychology,* 46, 38-50.

Leavitt, H. J. and Mueller, A. H. (1951), 'Some effects of feedback on communicating', *Human Relations,* 4, 401-410.

Miller, G. A. (1967), *The psychology of communication,* Penguin Books, Ringwood.

Morton, J. C., Richey, C. A. and Kellett, M. (1981), *Building assertive skills,* The C.V. Mosby Company, St. Louis.

Puetz, Belinda (1983), *Networking for nurses,* Aspen, Rockville.

Renton, N. E. (1979), *Guide for meetings and organisations,* (3rd edition), Law Book Company Ltd, Melbourne.

Sayles, L. and Strauss, G. (1980), *Personnel: the human problems of management,* (4th edition), Prentice-Hall, London.

Stoner, J. A. F., Collins, R. R. and Yetton, P. W. (1985), *Management in Australia,* Prentice-Hall, Sydney.

Sullivan, E. J. and Decker, P. J. (1988), *Effective management in nursing,* (2nd edition), Addison-Wesley Co, Menlo Park, California.

# CHAPTER 2.2

# The nurse as a resource manager

MARY COURTNEY AND KRISTINA MALKO

After reading this chapter you should be able to:

1. identify the major obstacles to effective time management;

2. understand the frequently utilised time management strategies;

3. understand the importance of human resource management;

4. discuss the significance of planning for, recruiting and selecting staff;

5. recognise the importance of developing human resources;

6. identify the underlying principles and applications of EEO legislation;

7. describe principles of effective performance appraisal;

8. understand the relationships between job satisfaction, job performance, motivation and a supportive working environment;

9. discuss the factors influencing health care costs;

10. define basic cost-accounting and productivity terminology;

11. identify the five basic steps in the standard costing process;

12. understand the process of break-even analysis and variance analysis.

This chapter addresses the role of a manager in relation to resources. It begins with a discussion of time management and analyses the various activities which are undertaken by individuals at various levels of management. It then proceeds to discuss important aspects of management of human resources and indicates how activities should be undertaken efficiently and effectively. Finally, money resources are addressed. Factors which influence health care costs are outlined and calculations which are required by managers are provided. The conclusion is reached that only through the appropriate development and use of resources can quality care be provided and hence, achievement of organisational goals.

An organisation's resources allow the organisation to determine the goals it is capable of achieving. Before any specific goals or objectives can be identified, it is necessary to undertake a comprehensive analysis of the resources available. The quantity of resources available to the individual nurse manager depend on a number of different factors such as the bed-size and geographical location of the hospital concerned. With this in mind, the major resources for analysis will be as follows:

1. Time
   Activities managers undertake
   Major obstacles to effective time management
   Frequently utilised time management strategies

2. People
   Meeting human resource requirements
   Staffing the needs of the organisation
   Developing human resources
   Optimising working conditions

3. Money
   Factors influencing health care costs
   Productivity conscious environment
   Cost terminology
   Calculating standard costs
   Budget allocation
   Break-even analysis
   Variance analysis

# 1. TIME MANAGEMENT

Recent changes in the nursing profession have emphasised the critical nature of time management. The trend towards an increased level of registered nursing staff, the increasing patient workloads from shorter length of stay and increased acuity of patients, and the ever-increasing push from governments for cost-effectiveness, make it essential that all levels of the nursing profession manage their time more efficiently.

Time management continues to be an extremely popular topic in nursing with numerous books and articles written on the subject. Some of the more frequently cited sources are as follows: Applebaum and Rohrs (1981), Norville (1984), Morano (1984), Ashkenas and Schaffer (1982), Lucas and Austin (1984).

## 1.1 ACTIVITIES MANAGERS UNDERTAKE

Managers in general spend considerable time, effort and energy interacting with other people, both inside and outside the organisation. A study by Mintzberg of chief executives found 78 per cent of their time was spent in oral communication activities such as attending meetings, talking on the telephone, and touring their organisations (Mintzberg, 1973:38). In another study, a group of middle managers devoted 80 per cent of their time to oral communication (Lawler et al, 1968:432–439).

Figure 2.2.1 displays the time required for some of management's activities. It is interesting to note that meetings occupy 38 per cent of all activities, but require 69 per cent of all the time available.

FIGURE 2.2.1:   Time and activities spent by managers (source: Megginson (1989) adapted from Henry Mintzberg 1973:39)

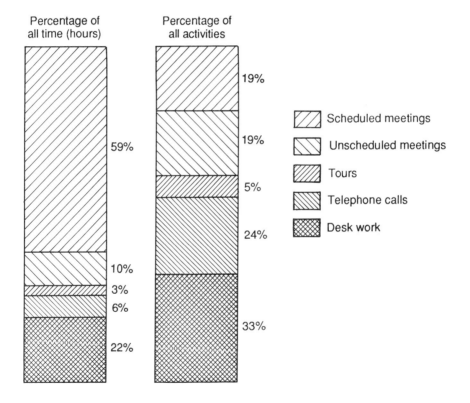

A further study by Mahoney (1965) showed how managers from low, medium and high levels in their organisations allocated their available time in undertaking several management activities. (See Figure 2.2.2)

FIGURE 2.2.2: Time spent at managerial levels (source: Megginson et al, (1989) adapted from Mahoney et al. (1965:103))

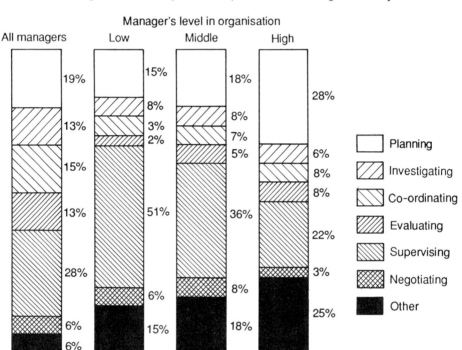

Percentage of total managerial time spent on each managerial activity

## 1.2 MAJOR OBSTACLES TO EFFECTIVE TIME MANAGEMENT

Inevitable obstacles will present themselves for the best laid plans. The following list provides some of the most common. Managers with chronic time management problems generally experience a number of these:

1.   lack of priority setting;

2.   indecisiveness/procrastination;

3.   inability to delegate;

4.   perfectionism and excessive attention to detail;

5.   inefficient meetings;

6.  telephone meetings;

7.  drop-in visitors and non-job related conversation;

8.  smoking/coffee ritual;

9.  inability to say 'no'.

## 1.3 FREQUENTLY UTILISED TIME MANAGEMENT STRATEGIES

Time management strategies are varied and not all will work for everyone. Blaney and Hobson (1988:279–287) highlight the following which may be useful in your own situation:

1.  assertiveness and politeness;

2.  list making;

3.  knowledge of yourself;

4.  uninterrupted quiet time;

5.  orderly work area;

6.  personal filing system;

7.  processing of paperwork;

8.  concentration on one task at a time;

9.  grouping of similar tasks;

10. intermediate goals for long projects;

11. starting difficult tasks;

12. standardisation of routine reports and correspondence;

13. selective reading;

14. management of telephone calls;

15. restriction of personal visits;

16. decisiveness;

17. effective operation of meetings;

18. commitments to others and co-operation;

19. development and familiarity with standard procedures;

20. delegation of work to subordinates;

21. unit or group meetings;

22. effective use of slack, idle or waiting time.

## 1.4 MANAGERIAL SKILLS

To find out what managerial skills are most likely to be used by effective managers, a study of 2000 executives was conducted. It found that 'superior managers' have 64 basic skills. Katz (1974:90–102) grouped these further into four major categories as follows:

☐ conceptual skills;

☐ human-relations skills;

☐ administrative skills;

☐ technical skills;

Figure 2.2.3 displays the relative importance of managerial skills at different managerial levels in an organisation. Interestingly, results of this study showed the importance of human relations skills across the three levels of management to be very similar, with first-line, middle and top management being 43 per cent, 38 per cent and 40 per cent respectively. This indicates that an essential component of a first-line manager's role is the maintenance of a network of contacts and human relationships to achieve organisational goals.

# 2. HUMAN RESOURCE MANAGEMENT

The most important assets an organisation has are its employees or human resources, and they should not be taken for granted. Saul (1987) indicates that in service industries, and these include health care organisations, people are the product, in contrast to manufacturing industries where people make the product. As most health care organisations are today recognising the importance of human resources, they are placing increasing emphasis on human resource management in order to meet organisational goals designed to provide a high quality of care. There is also an increased recognition that effective human resource management can make a difference to an organisation's success or failure. This is especially true in health care organisations where labour costs make up the majority of recurrent expenses. These occurrences have followed a long history in all areas of industry, where employees and their current and potential contributions to an organisation have been overlooked.

Employees and the public are demanding that employers demonstrate greater social responsibility in managing their human resources. Employers are being forced to face staff shortages, demands for working environments which are safe and which do not contribute to ill health, and legislation about discrimination and equal employment access. Other issues which need to be faced include demands made by union bodies and government agencies regarding conditions provided for employees.

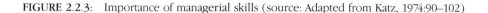

**FIGURE 2.2.3:**  Importance of managerial skills (source: Adapted from Katz, 1974:90–102)

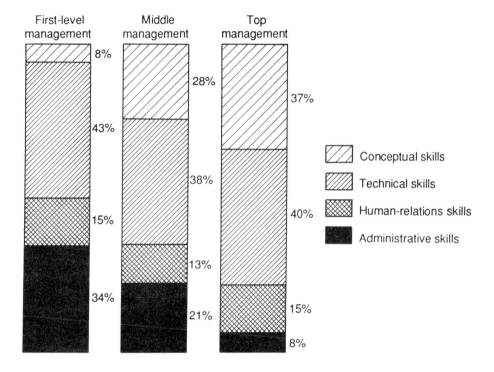

As a result of all of the demands, most large organisations have expanded the activities previously performed by personnel or staffing departments. These new departments of 'human resource management' usually have the responsibility of co-ordinating and enforcing policies relating to the human resources of the organisation. However, all supervisors and managers within an organisation are responsible for performing human resource management practices in their relations with individuals who work in their areas. This is of particular importance in organisations which, because of size or financial constraints, do not have formal human resource management departments.

According to Clark (1988:11) human resource management is the management of the formal relationship between an employer and employees in order to facilitate the achievement of organisational goals. Schuler et al (1988:9) go further and state that human resource management involves the 'utilisation of several functions and activities to ensure that they are used effectively and fairly for the benefit of the individual, the organisation, and society'. Therefore, human resource management is an integral factor which must be considered in strategic planning. Its aim is to assist the achievement of an organisation's goals by planning for, attracting, selecting, developing and compensating people who are willing and capable of contributing to the attainment of these goals. The attainment of organisational goals necessitates the presence of organisational fit, where the mission and objectives, policies and practices, structure and culture, and workforce characteristics of an organisation and each of the departments within it are internally congruent. Associated with this is a need for managers to have an understanding of human behaviour and motivation, and the skills to use this understanding.

There is no position more frustrating than that of the first-line manager, who must represent top management to the employees and the employees to top management. No-one is in a more difficult position. Yet, no-one is more potentially influential in attaining organisational goals through the drive to build morale and promote and provide quality care without increasing costs. Therefore, first-line managers need to be involved in each of the following phases of human resource management practice for their departments.

## 2.1 MEETING HUMAN RESOURCE REQUIREMENTS

### 2.1.1 Planning

This involves forecasting short and long term human resource requirements. 'More specifically, human resource planning involves forecasting human resource needs for the organisation and planning the steps necessary to meet these needs' (Schuler et al 1988:43). You need to have access to information regarding any potential changes of function for your area so that you can develop staffing strategies which will support these changes if required. If there are no potential changes you still need to have an accurate idea of the staffing requirements for your area. The most efficient way of doing this is through the design and analysis of job requirements.

### 2.1.2 Job requirements

Activities undertaken by personnel in an organisation are referred to as jobs. Descriptions and specifications of all jobs need to be determined in such a fashion that they contribute to the attainment of organisational goals by assisting with recruitment, selection, orientation and development of staff, while satisfying the employment related needs of the individuals who undertake or perform them.

> If the design of a job does not facilitate the achievement of ... (organisational goals), ... that job should be either redesigned or eliminated ... If the duties

of each job are made clear and distinct from those of other jobs, it is less likely that any activity required to be performed within the organisation will be neglected or duplicated (McCarthy and Stone, 1986:78).

In order to design jobs appropriately, a job analysis needs to be undertaken. This is a process where data is gathered which provides information on the duties of a job and the required qualifications or characteristics an employee must possess to perform it. The information is contained in job descriptions and job specifications. A job description is a statement describing the duties, responsibilities and tasks of a particular job which is to be performed. Out of this a job specification is developed. This states the knowledge, skills and abilities required of a person to adequately perform a particular job. The information on descriptions and specifications may be prepared and presented separately or in the one document.

McCarthy and Stone (1986:84) and Schuler et al (1988:84) recommend that the primary sources of data when analysing jobs should be the employees who are undertaking these jobs and their immediate supervisors, with the assistance of an analyst if one is available. The information can be collected in interviews and questionnaires, in workshops of groups of individuals with similar roles or who work in a similar area, by observing performance, and by the keeping of diaries or logs by employees. Bassett and Metzger (1986:112) advise that job analyses which are based upon performance standards which have been developed through a co-operative effort between employees and managers are more meaningful than those produced by managers alone, and are thus more likely to be effective.

If a job description and a job specification are required where a position does not exist or if they have never existed in a formal way, they can be obtained from other areas or similar organisations and modified to suit your specific needs. You should never merely copy job analyses which have been produced for another purpose, as in order for them to be useful they should take into consideration the specific needs, aims and culture of your department or organisation, and the purpose for which they will be used. Because of this, there is no one best way to write job descriptions and specifications. However, there are a variety of recommended ways from which you can select, depending on need. We shall not address these here, but in most human resource management texts, a few general guidelines are provided.

Job descriptions should be concise and worded as simply and as clearly as possible. According to Smith and Elbert (1986:120) poorly written job descriptions 'lead to unclear job duties, ambiguous standards of performance, and overly subjective performance feedback' in appraisals. They should begin with a title. This is followed by the departmental location of the job, the person to whom the job holder is responsible and the date of the latest revision of the description. Next should be a job duties section which specifies in precise detail what is to be undertaken. Ignatavicius and Griffith (1982:38) advise that all duties, tasks and responsibilities should be stated in behaviourally based terms with the use of action verbs followed by direct objects. They indicate that you may also find it helpful to categorise and prioritise duties according to purpose, for example, direct care, supervision, management, communication and professional development. Although other authors do not recommend generalities, Rowland and Rowland (1985:295) suggest that a job description should include a statement such as 'and other related duties as required' to provide the flexibility needed from time to time as circumstances change. The job specification, which outlines the knowledge, skills, abilities and special expertise required for the job, can then be developed. It must match the job description and be derived from it. Written specifications play an essential role in recruitment in that by establishing the qualifications required of applicants they provide a basis for attracting and selecting appropriate people, and discouraging or eliminating unsuitable applicants.

Once job descriptions and specifications have been written, piloted and refined they should be referred to regularly for accurate training, development and appraisals. Some organisations make the mistake of writing them, possibly using them in recruiting, and then filing them away for posterity. Periodic checks are required to ensure that descriptions and specifications are not out of date and that they continue to be accurate statements of what is needed for good performance. It is recommended that they be at least referred to, and amended as required at the time of each performance appraisal, and whenever staff are recruited for positions.

## 2.2 STAFFING THE NEEDS OF THE ORGANISATION

### 2.2.1 Recruitment

'Recruitment is the process of searching for and identifying job candidates in sufficient quantity and of sufficient quality to meet organisational human resource needs' (Clark, 1988:167). Therefore, it involves attracting the right people, in the right numbers, with the required abilities to fill identified vacancies. These vacancies can be created because staff leave or because of a restructuring process requiring the creation of new jobs. Vacancies may be filled in a number of ways. You may appoint someone from within the organisation, make an external appointment, or restructure the service so that the need for that position no longer exists.

The first decision which needs to be made is whether recruitment will be internal or external. Some organisations believe that it is a good staff development practice to recruit and promote from within the organisation wherever possible, and only recruit externally at the entry level or if there is no-one within the organisation with the requisite skills and knowledge (Clark, 1988:169). The advantages of recruiting internally are that people see that they have a chance of promotion and thus morale and motivation can be improved, and you know what you are getting. On the other hand, the advantages of recruiting externally include the addition of individuals with fresh new ideas, knowledge and experience, and they may not require specialised training which the internal applicant may need. Some organisations allow for this need for training and development of their own personnel, but others believe that it is preferable to get the people who are already experienced in the specified areas. A major problem associated with internal recruitment is that the position of the successful applicant may subsequently need to be filled, unless it is eliminated as part of a planned restructuring process. You also may be developing an atmosphere of 'inbreeding', with minimal innovation, unless potentially costly developmental education is undertaken. You need to compare these disadvantages with those associated with external recruitment, which include possible hostility and lowering of morale of present staff, and costs of orientation. If you do decide to proceed with external recruitment, you will need to be aware that current staff may apply if they see the position as being a desirable transfer or a promotion, and they cannot be excluded from consideration if they meet stated requirements.

Many mechanisms are available for recruiting personnel. The nursing profession has adopted the passive traditional approach for many years. This entailed waiting for applicants seeking employment to approach individual organisations. However, when there are staff shortages and demands for staff in specialised areas, most health care agencies adopt a more aggressive approach. The most common form of recruitment is through advertising in circulars, on billboards (for internal recruits), and in newspapers and professional or trade journals (for external recruits). Beginning nurses are increasingly being recruited through attendance at open days at universities and colleges, or at career markets. In some instances, where there is an extensive shortage, organisations undertake large scale public relations activities, such as that commenced by the New South Wales Department of Health in 1989 to attract people to nursing.

Once you have decided on how you will advertise and what mechanisms you will use, you need to develop a strategy which will make the position attractive. Nurses are now much more selective about their choice of employment than ever before. Therefore, your recruitment mechanisms must incorporate a successful marketing strategy which incorporates developing and maintaining a positive public profile. In a research study reported by Rowland and Rowland (1985:395) it was found that the top three factors which attracted nurses were flexible shift and scheduling policies, high nurse/patient ratios and positive reputations of hospitals. Therefore, particularly if you are having trouble recruiting sufficient staff with required qualifications and experience, you should consider adopting innovative management practices in your area which are seen to be desirable by potential employees.

## 2.2.2 Selection

Several different methods are used to obtain information about applicants. They include the use of application forms, interviews, tests and references. 'Regardless of the methods used, it is essential that the information obtained be clearly job-related or predictive of success in that job' (McCarthy and Stone, 1986:124). Application forms are a quick systematic means of obtaining a broad range of information about an applicant. They should be used as a basis for further exploration of the applicant's background and suitability. Increasingly in nursing we are required to provide a curriculum vitae which is a good source of information; however, McCarthy and Stone (1986:127), warn of the problems inherent in these. Applicants may overstate their virtues and minimise any deficiencies. Employment consultancy firms do a roaring trade in providing well written, if not always accurate, outlines. However, written applications can be used to undertake a short-listing process, to reduce the number of applicants who are to be sub-sequently interviewed. This process facilitates the elimination of people who do not meet essential critieria for the job. If none of the candidates meet these criteria, it may be better not to proceed. Appointment of a weak or unsuitable person could result in endless problems in the future. When short-listing, you may consider that some candidates could perform the job if provided with education and guidance. If this is the case, the job description may need to be altered. However, caution is necessary if major deficiencies exist as it is unrealistic to expect miracles from staff development. If there are insufficient applicants with suitable qualifications, the position may need to be reclassified to a higher level, in order to attract more suitable candidates. If there are several people who meet the essential criteria, then the committee can then look at desirable criteria, in order to produce an appropriate short list before proceeding to an interview.

While the validity of conducting interviews is questionable, and despite the fact that they may contribute very little information beyond what is provided in written applications, they are widely used and need to be considered. The job interview has three prime purposes: to gather specific information in order to find the right person for the position; to establish a relationship that will allow assessment of the applicant's obvious qualities; and to foster in the applicant a favourable view of the position, the service and the people who are in the organisation. Most interviews are conducted by a panel. This is done in an attempt to prevent unfairness in selection such as nepotism, and to ensure that the decision-making is shared by several people. However, you are advised to keep this panel as small as possible. The choice of who sits on the panel is based on organisational policies, but should include the person who will be the successful applicant's immediate superior. Panel interviews have several disadvantages and these need to be considered. Applicants may become nervous when faced with a number of people; panel members may be inadequately prepared or excessively aggressive; accord may not be reached; and if a majority rule is invoked, a person may be appointed against the wishes of the applicant's future immediate supervisor, which may cause problems.

Whoever chairs the session should ensure that job descriptions and specifications are circulated as soon as possible before the interview, along with the applications. These papers should be kept confidential. The panelists should meet sometime before the interviews commence. Each member of the panel should concentrate on a specific area, and the same questions should be addressed to each applicant, albeit varied somewhat to suit the specific circumstances of individuals.

Equal Employment Opportunity (EEO) legislation is designed to prevent job discrimination, and employers are obliged to develop policies which ensure that staff selection and promotion are based on merit, and that an applicant's qualifications and ability to perform the job are assessed in a fair manner. Discrimination can be defined as 'any practice that makes distinctions between individuals or groups so as to advantage some or advantage others' (Department of Employment and Industrial Relations,

1982:1). A variety of discriminatory issues have been identified, and you are cautioned not to address any of these in the interview process unless they are specifically related to ability to competently perform the job in question. McCarthy and Stone (1986:163) identify these topics as: race, colour, sex, religion, political opinion, national extraction, social origin, age, marital status, criminal record, medical record, sexual preference, trade union activities, nationality, personality attributes and disabilities. Some organisations have an EEO policy which requires that panelists provide a list of non-discriminatory criteria upon which selection decisions have been based, and some further require that an EEO representative is present on all panels. You should be aware of the policies of your organisation and comply with these.

The interview room must be supportive with privacy and comfort, so as not to disadvantage any applicants. The sitting arrangement needs to be considered as this will convey certain messages, and may influence the behaviour of applicants. The applicant should be welcomed, introduced to members of the interview panel and made to feel as much at ease as possible. A confronting, challenging style of interview is likely to create problems. The purpose of the interview is not only to seek more information about the applicant, but also for the applicant to get information upon which to base a decision about staying or not. If an interview panel appears hostile it may deter a potential employee from taking up a position.

Once the process of how the interview will progress is outlined, the panel can proceed to inquire about an applicant's strengths, weaknesses, aspirations and specific areas of concern which have been predetermined. Information should then be provided by members of the panel about the organisation and the particular position. Each applicant should be provided with an opportunity to visit the work environment either before or after the interview, and to ask questions.

According to Pincus (1982:44), one of the most common problems with selection interviews is the tendency for interviewers to make up their minds too early and thereafter filter out any information which is not in accord with their views. Other problems include gathering information which is not job related or predictive of success in a position, allowing one attribute such as confidence in the interview to influence evaluation, and not obtaining information about past behaviour in the form of references (Schuler et al 1988:154).

References are a great problem. Although they can offer a wealth of information not supplied by the candidate, many are of little help. Applicants will rarely ask someone for a reference if they are not sure of getting a positive report. On occasions a referee may be dishonest. An individual may be wanting to either get rid of someone or retain a person for their own service and may write a reference accordingly. In the health care system, telephone referrals are frequently preferred. A short conversation is often more honest and more revealing than a written reference and is usually less of a burden on the referee. You must be careful not to invade the privacy rights of an applicant by making enquiries of the current employer if they are not cited as a referee. One way of overcoming this problem is to specifically state in the advertisement that at least one reference must be from a senior colleague.

The final selection process to be referred to here, which is used minimally in health care settings, is testing. Over many years a wide range of general ability, specific aptitude and personality tests have regularly come into vogue only to be discredited. Rowland and Rowland (1985:302) indicate that where hospitals can afford to be selective 'nurses are not hired unless they can demonstrate ability to perform certain major functions such as the proper calculation and administration of medications'. However, most modern organisations use orientation and staff development for such testing and remedial activities. Finally, because of the disrepute associated with the use of many unvalidated and unreliable tests and the expense involved in their production, caution with their use is advised.

## 2.3 DEVELOPING HUMAN RESOURCES

'The functions of recruiting and selecting human resources are only the initial stages in building an effective workforce. Managers, supervisors and employees also require training and continual development if their potential is to be utilised effectively' (McCarthy and Stone, 1986:175). Recognition of this has been recently endorsed by the Federal Government which has legislated for a mandatory budget allocation to staff development. Staff or human resource development should be designed either to improve an individual's performance in their present job, or to prepare the individual for a different job within an organisation. Its aim is to provide experiences that enhance the attainment of both organisational and personal goals while maximising the growth of the individual (Smith and Elbert, 1986:46). This can be achieved because staff development contributes to removing performance deficiencies, providing staff with the skills to be more flexible, innovative and adaptable, and increasing the level of commitment of employees to the organisation. Those aspects of human resource development which will be addressed here include orientation, inservice and continuing education, and performance appraisal. Their relationships to career development, job satisfaction, motivation and a harmonious working environment will also be explored (see also Chapter 1.4).

Although most institutions have personnel who are responsible for overseeing and conducting staff development programmes, it is the responsibility of the area manager to ensure that deficiencies and needs are identified and communicated to these personnel. Your responsibility also extends beyond this level. If you have staff who are demonstrating initiative and are undertaking educational programmes away from your organisation, you will demonstrate a commitment to staff development if you support them, as long as this support does not compromise the attainment of organisational goals. For example, you are compromising nursing care if so many staff are released from work to attend lectures at any one time that staff shortages result.

If the manager does not have a commitment to staff development then all the programmes in the world will not assist the staff. Likewise, staff development will only remedy a situation in which the employee wants to and is capable of benefiting. It will not rectify selection errors. If the wrong person is employed, or if the person is hostile towards development, then again it is not likely to achieve the stated aims. You need to determine whether or not staff development will make a real difference and finally accept that it is not a universal panacea and will not cure all of an organisation's ills.

Schuler et al (1988:305–327) identify three major phases of any staff development programme. First you must determine needs. Ascertain organisational or departmental needs by examining short- and long-term objectives, and by studying information available from the central administration department. In your own area, you have to know about specific job-related needs and the needs of individual staff members. You can find relevant information in documents about future projects, job descriptions, performance standards, performance appraisals, and by asking staff what they consider to be necessary or desirable. Once you have identified needs, the next step is developing and implementing a programme. The third phase is evaluation of the programme: needs should be reassessed, and the entire process continued. Although, as previously stated, there are usually personnel specifically responsible for all these activities, input from staff and management will contribute to greater efficiency and effectiveness.

## 2.3.1 Orientation

This is the process of inducting a new employee into an organisation. Because most nurses already have some experience, the major purpose of an orientation is not to review basic skills but to help participants build upon past nursing experiences and adapt to the new working environment and its philosophy, policies and practices. Smith and Elbert (1986:26) indicate that because this is the first extensive contact between the staff member and the culture of the organisation it 'may establish predispositions that are indelible. Hence, every effort should be made to ensure that the impressions and attitudes that evolve are compatible with hospital goals and intentions'. Furthermore, if an appropriate and supportive orientation is not conducted, potentially good employees may become disgruntled, perform badly, lack job satisfaction and ultimately leave.

McCarthy and Stone (1986:178) advocate the use of a checklist to avoid overlooking items that are important to employees, and the use of orientation packages which the new employees can read at their leisure or when needed, and when they are less stressed and more able to absorb information. Because of the problems encountered in many traditional forms of orientation where new employees are provided with rules and regulations in lectures and then abandoned to their areas of employment, a number of institutions are undertaking contract orientations. This involves an agreement between the new employee and an educator on behalf of the employer. It is designed to encourage new staff to learn at their own pace, on their own. According to Huang and Schoenkneckt (1984:53) it is a system based on adult learning theories. They outline these theories:

1.  adults learn when they feel a need to learn;

2.  adults build their present learning based on their past experience;

3.  adults are usually self-directed;

4.  adults can usually define their learning needs and help plan their learning programmes.

Following the provision of initial general information of an essential nature such as safety and security policies and practices and employment conditions, each person undertaking the orientation is provided with a booklet outlining the orientation requirements and is assigned a preceptor. The preceptors are role models in providing patient care. They act more as resource persons than as active instructors. The orientees seek and plan their own learning experiences with guidance from these preceptors and area managers. This type of programme is especially beneficial with new graduates who may be undertaking an extended orientation/education programme.

## 2.3.2 Education

Because organisations must assure the clinical competency of staff and the achievement of nursing practice standards, education is a critical staff development responsibility, warranting a substantial allotment of available resources. Employees' skills have to be updated. If not, they become less and less capable. Therefore, the organisation and area managers have to take on a nurturing role in providing opportunities for employees' professional and personal growth. Lifelong learning is a major management responsibility that will help maintain the high contribution of employees. Staff education is categorised in a number of ways. Smith and Elbert (1986:25–27) refer to inservice and continuing education as the two major categories. Inservice education usually refers to on-the-job training, learning from experience, and short specific-purpose courses conducted on-site, for example, 'to update nurses on new techniques, methods or findings' (25). On the other hand, continuing education usually refers to courses which run over an extended period, either within the organisation or at another venue. It may also involve extended periods of study at a tertiary institution.

You may choose to adopt a contract learning programme similar to that outlined for orientation for the staff in your area. Whichever system you adopt it is essential that you demonstrate a commitment to the educational needs of your staff and that you recognise the importance of education to them as individuals and to the organisation. One of the trends to gain recent popularity in human resource management is job enrichment or career development. By assisting staff with their career development, through the identification of educational needs and career counselling, you will not only be assisting with the development of individuals, but also contributing to the production of a pool of promotable professional people. Clark (1988:269) says that this tends to increase staff loyalty to the organisation and decreases labour turnover. Sovie (1981:30–35) supports this view and states that we must pay more attention to professional maturation through development if we are to be successful in promoting professional careers in nursing.

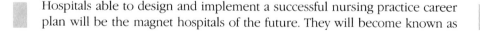

Hospitals able to design and implement a successful nursing practice career plan will be the magnet hospitals of the future. They will become known as institutions where professional nurses are recognised and valued for their contribution to patient care, where professional nursing is practised, and finally, where nurses advance in career patterns that are personally and professionally satisfying (Sovie, 1981:31).

## 2.3.3 Performance appraisal

Performance appraisals are undertaken for a variety of reasons. Clark (1988:233) identifies five administrative reasons for conducting appraisals:

1.  to mould employee behaviour according to organisational norms;

2.  to enhance the consistency between employee actions and organisational goals;

3.  to improve the quality of human resources planning in relation to training, development and promotion;

4.  to improve the quality of salary reviews and other rewards;

5.  to provide a record in cases of dismissal, demotion, grievance or appeal.

Another and no less important reason for conducting appraisals is staff development. Employees want to know how they are doing, they want feedback regarding educational needs and they want rewards for achieving performance goals. Appraisals have gained much notoriety because this has not been recognised, and accordingly they have been used as a punitive measure to censure staff who are not complying with what is seen to be desirable behaviour. In fact there have been so many problems with performance appraisal over the years that the development of a successful system has been likened to achieving peace in the world (del Bueno, 1977:21–23). However, a great deal of work has been done to refine appraisal systems, and you are encouraged to develop a system which most closely meets your needs.

The most important use of performance appraisal data is improvement of employee motivation. Increased motivation leads to increased effort, which, if applied in the right direction by a competent employee, will increase performance levels. Two components of the employee's motivation are the links the employee sees between the level of effort and the outcome, that is, between the performance and the attainment of valued rewards. An employee who does not see improved performance as a means of earning a pay rise, being promoted, getting recognition, or receiving any other form of organisational reward will not feel compelled to seek higher levels of performance. You also need to be aware that some people may try hard to do a good job, but still fail. This may occur because individuals direct energies into inappropriate activities or where, regardless of intentions, the employee does not have the skills and abilities to get the job done. These problems reveal the need for counselling and education.

Equal Employment Opportunity legislation, as well as other forms of governmental legislation, has been designed to prevent employee discrimination. For this reason alone, it makes good managerial sense to ensure that the appraisal system in use is technically sound and well accepted by employees. It is clear that an effective performance appraisal system provides managers with valuable information for helping employees improve their performance. Appraisals should be constructed and managed in such a way that supervisors and employees believe that they provide a realistic picture of job performance. They should see that the information collected is used to either help correct problems or reward desirable performance. The way to ensure acceptance, understanding and comprehension of the system is to involve in its development phase representatives from all levels of staff who will use it.

Brief (1979:8) identifies four basic steps in the development of an appraisal instrument:

1. you need to determine what behaviours are to be assessed. The behaviour should be important in terms of overall contribution to effectiveness of patient care and it must be observable and measurable;

2. you need to ensure that the instrument you are using is valid. That is, it needs to provide an accurate measure of actual behaviour;

3. you need to determine how the appraisal will be done, by whom and how frequently;

4. you need to ensure that there is periodic evaluation of the system.

There are various methodologies for rating performance. Some of the commonest approaches are briefly outlined here:

1. **the essay method.** This is one of the most frequently used methods. Here the evaluator is required to write a statement which best describes the individual being evaluated. The statement usually should include identifying strengths, weaknesses and recommendations for future development (McCarthy and Stone, 1986:236). The major problem with this approach is that it can be very subjective.

2. **rating scales.** Here each behaviour to be rated is represented by a line or scale on which the rater indicates the degree to which the individual demonstrates the behaviour. There have been many variations of these rating scales produced over the years. One of the most recent is the behaviourally anchored rating scale which is advocated by Smith and Elbert (1986). This system is seen to minimise subjectivity and increase reliability and validity because descriptions and scales are specifically reduced. Their major problem is that they are difficult, and hence time-consuming and expensive to develop.

3. **management by objectives.** This approach seeks to judge the performance of individuals on the basis of the attainment of predetermined objectives, which have been set in conjunction with supervisors. The objectives are based on organisational goals and the job description, and are accompanied by details of how they can be achieved. Agreement is reached between the subordinate and supervisor.

At the end of a predetermined period of time the subordinate makes an appraisal of her attainment of the set objectives, then an interview is conducted with the superior, and new ones are set for the next period. Desirable behaviour is reinforced, rewarded and recognised (Clark, 1988:242). The major advantage of this system is that appraisees can get a good idea of where they are at because self-appraisal is involved. It also helps career development, and allows for greater autonomy than that provided with other methods.

It can be seen that there are many systems in use, but those which appear to work most effectively include self-appraisal (in which the employee measures his or her own performance against pre-established measures) and management by objectives. These methods provide performance appraisals that measure where the person is now and provide for a future plan, which is far better than an approach that only looks back over the past year, particularly when focused on failings. They measure performance and not personality traits and have an inherent reward system. In their book *In Search of Excellence,* Peters and Waterman (1983) found that in all exceptional companies there was a rich, varied, attractive reward system for staff. Although you may be unable to have a major immediate influence on monetary rewards, you can provide rewards in the form of positive reinforcement through recognition of desirable performance.

Regardless of what form of appraisal system is used, it will not be useful unless the information generated is effectively utilised in the appraisal interview.

> The evaluation interview provides the superior with an opportunity to discuss the subordinate's performance record and to explore areas of possible improvement and growth. It also provides an opportunity to identify the subordinate's attitudes and feelings more thoroughly, and thus improve communication between the parties that may lead to a feeling of harmony and co-operation (McCarthy and Stone, 1986:241).

Interviews should be planned sufficiently in advance to allow both parties an opportunity to prepare for the discussion. At least a week should be provided. As previously stated, the focus should be on the future rather than the past. Strengths rather than weaknesses should be stressed. There should be a concentration on opportunities for growth and development within the appraisee's current job and if management by objectives is used, you should ensure that the objectives are feasible. If the appraisal indicates deficiencies in performance, the problem should be identified and a course of action planned. You may find this to be a difficult task, but it should be done with objectivity, fairness and a recognition of the feelings of the individual who is being appraised. The appraisal interview also needs to be accurately documented, as if ineffective performance persists it may be necessary for the organisation to take disciplinary action, or to demote or ultimately discharge the employee. Accurate documentation is also required in cases of positive performance for future rewards such as promotion.

## 2.3.4 Motivation

Hospitals are plagued by high rates of turnover and absenteeism among their nursing staff. These behaviours are symptomatic of boredom, disillusionment, lack of involvement and apathy. These are attributed to lack of job satisfaction and motivation, both of which are significant in self development. Because of the nature of the manager's role, employee motivation is a major responsibility. Possibly the most important function performed is motivating and controlling employee performance while developing trust and confidence, and thus having productive, motivated employees. Because motivation is a complex process it can be difficult to understand the motivational forces operating within an individual.

Many theories have been put forward to explain motivation (and some are discussed further in Chapter 2.1), and many studies have been conducted into job satisfaction and motivation in nursing (Rowland and Rowland, 1985; McConnell, 1986). Overall, they show that while extrinsic rewards such as salaries, hours and fringe benefits may draw someone to a job, it is the intrinsic rewards which contribute to raising self-esteem through recognition, achievement, responsibility, autonomy, potential for growth and the ability to make decisions which maintain motivation and satisfaction and result in a productive worker. Therefore an open climate should be developed where there is high morale and supportive relationships between members of staff. If this is achieved the staff should be highly motivated towards achievement of organisational goals and their own professional development.

According to McCarthy and Stone (1986:266) the 'satisfaction that individuals receive from their employment is largely dependent upon the extent to which the job and everything associated with it meets their needs and wants'. McCarthy and Stone (1986:267) indicate that job performance leads to job satisfaction. This is because people derive rewards from the performance which are a source of satisfaction. The reward can be extrinsic, such as a reward or promotion, or intrinsic, the feeling one has contributed in a meaningful way. Participation in decision-making has many positive attributes. McCarthy and Stone (1986:313) further indicate that groups that participate in setting goals often place higher demands upon themselves than do their managers. We have already discussed management by objectives in appraisal. It can also be used as a general way of organising participation by staff in decision-making and the determining of objectives for your area or for the whole organisation.

Another form of staff participation which is becoming increasingly popular is the use of quality circles (Bassett and Metzger, 1986:87–89). Here, small groups of employees meet together regularly to identify, analyse and suggest solutions to problems. It is also known as industrial democracy. Clark (1988:157) defines this as referring to 'significant involvement of staff in decision-making, through structures and processes which involve the sharing of authority and responsibility in the workplace'. Therefore, it goes beyond mere representation of staff on boards or other decision-making bodies. It pervades the whole decision-making process. In this case the role of a supervisor is more one of a resource person or facilitator in the quality circles. Although there has been no legislation in Australia for industrial democracy it has been implemented in a variety of forms, and you are advised to consider the use of one of these forms of participative management in your area of responsibility.

## 2.3.5 Industrial relations

A brief discussion of industrial relations is provided because you need to have an understanding of the relationships between unions and the personnel working in your department. In Australia, governments have intervened in industrial relations, forming tribunals which are designed to regulate industrial relations by determining wages and conditions of employees and to resolve disputes if they arise. The Australian Council of Trade Unions (ACTU) operates at a national level and determines general policies on industrial and social issues and presents these to governments and industrial tribunals. There are also various federal and state bodies, and small enterprise bargaining units are being used with increasing frequency. However, on the whole, you are concerned primarily with decisions which are made by tribunals. These decisions are outlined in various awards which prescribe wages and conditions. We advise you to refer to the specific information for your state.

Clearly a union has a responsibility to bargain and negotiate for certain essential features of the employment contract. These include policies and procedures related to salaries; benefits, including pensions; working conditions of all types, including hours of duty and holidays; a grievance mechanism; promotion/seniority procedures; and perhaps, finally, job security. As these are obviously the concern of an area manager, a wide spectrum of mutual expectations provides a milieu in which employee and employer can work together towards shared goals. Therefore, managers need to understand how unions operate and be skilful in their negotiations with them. According to McCarthy and Stone (1986:343) in most work places there are

> delegates who work full-time for their employer in their chosen occupation, but who will represent the union in a particular workplace on a day-to-day basis. This usually means acting as an intermediary between the rank-and-file members and the union (particularly by way of promulgating information to members), and representing members in minor grievances with the employer.

Therefore it is necessary for you to have a detailed understanding of the awards and associated conditions under which staff in your area work and relevant grievance procedures, and develop a working relationship with the delegates. Clark (1988:97) indicates that 'one of the key elements of effective industrial relations management is the existence of an adequate and accommodating grievance procedure'. When discontent in the workforce arises because of one or more problems and the union is involved, it becomes an industrial issue. The objective of grievance procedures is to provide a forum for managers, union representatives and employees to discuss the problem and negotiate a resolution. The development of sound grievance procedures may assist in preventing minor problems escalating into a major industrial fiasco, with involvement of industrial tribunals, and will certainly contribute to maintaining a harmonious working environment.

# 3. MONEY

## 3.1 FACTORS INFLUENCING HEALTH CARE COSTS

Nurse managers should be aware of the numerous factors influencing the cost of health care and cost per unit of service. Strasen (1987:102) notes the following:

1.  physician practice patterns will affect the cost per patient. If a patient is ordered an expensive dressing in preference to the routine dressing or if intensive care is required, the average cost per patient day for the hospital will increase;

2.  patient census, occupancy rates and the volume of services produced impact on costs. The cost per unit of service will generally decrease when patient census and services are above the break-even point and alternatively when the patient census and services provision are below the break-even point, the cost per unit of service will generally increase;

3.  hospital supplies, contract rates and purchasing policies will affect the cost per patient day. Items may be purchased at lower prices by utilising group-purchasing practices which will reduce the average cost per patient day;

4.  workers' compensation claims and utilisation of sick leave significantly increase hospital cost. Hospitals can decrease hospital costs if outlays in these areas can be decreased;

5.  increases in salaries will significantly impact on costs per patient because of the labour-intensive nature of patient care. When utilising predetermined standards for all categories of hospital staff, eg nurses, pharmacists social workers etc., an increase in salaries will severely affect costs;

6.  over-utilisation of supplies increases costs per patient day — supply use must be monitored to avoid this.

## 3.2 MOVES TO A PRODUCTIVITY CONSCIOUS ENVIRONMENT

Until recent times, there have been few incentives for health care providers to assess the productivity of their organisations. With deficit funding, hospitals were reimbursed for monies used in the previous year. The incentives in fact were to do more and more for patients, with little regard for cost.

   With recent moves to a more cost conscious environment, a measure is required to quantify accurately and quickly the cost of nursing care. Patient classification systems provide methods in which patients can be classified into groups that consume similar amounts of resources.

The following formula is used to define productivity:

$$\text{PRODUCTIVITY} \quad = \quad \frac{\text{RESOURCES}}{\text{UNITS OF PRODUCTION}}$$

Implicit in the definition of productivity is the notion of maintaining some set standard at the same time as maintaining effectiveness in the results obtained.

Effectiveness, in terms of productivity, implies the capability of producing desired results — doing the right things at the right times (Mannisto, 1980:18).

So far, the assumption is made that all outputs and inputs can be measured and quantified. Several authors question this because of the problems of uncertainty in the health care environment.

Nursing service outputs are intermediate: since what nursing does is based on what the patient 'needs', it is not measurably related to the final output (Herzog, 1985:26).

It is difficult to measure a product in a department where not only the needs of the client are changing, but where the nature of the client is changing also (Margulies and Duval, 1984).

Effectiveness is a function of healing, or improving the overall wellbeing of the patient; in contrast, effectiveness has been measured in terms of treatment, or the ability to deliver services (Silvers, Zelman and Kahn, 1983:110).

Thus, productivity is basically the relationship between resources and outputs. Hoffman (1988:18) states:

Measurement and analysis of productivity assume that

1. there is one best way of creating outputs using usually limited resources; and

2. all inputs and outputs can be observed and measured to determine if the one best way is being strictly followed.

## 3.3 COST TERMINOLOGY

Nurse managers must be able to understand the terminology and speak the language of costs if they intend to communicate effectively with other members of management teams.

The following costs terms require distinction:

☐ indirect and direct costs;

☐ fixed and variable costs.


## 3.3.1 Direct and indirect costs

Cleverly (1986:202) notes that cost can be classified according to departments or responsibility centres or by the object of expenditure. In the health care setting, departments are usually classified according to the direct or indirect nature of the activity. The terms revenue or non-revenue may also be used in association with direct and indirect respectively.

That is:

        direct   —  revenue
        indirect  —  non-revenue

In the hospital environment, **direct costs** are costs that are directly connected with the delivery of patient care services. Examples of direct costs may include the following:

a.   cost of nursing services;

b.   cost of medical supplies.

**Indirect costs** however, are not directly associated with the delivery of specific patient care services. Examples of indirect costs may include the following:

a.   cost of administrative departments;

b.   professional services;

c.   medical records department;

d.   billing department;

e.   engineering department.

Whether a cost is designated as direct or indirect has little bearing on whether the cost is seen as fixed, variable or semi-variable. Such terms are used to describe the fluctuation of costs over a particular period of time or at a specific level of performance; whereas direct or indirect costs look to specific cost objectives. It is important to remember this to avoid confusion as a specific cost may bear different labels.

### 3.3.2 Fixed costs and variable costs

**Fixed costs** are incurred by the hospital regardless of changes in volume or patient days. For example, directors of nursing salaries remain the same regardless of fluctuations in census. Figure 2.2.4 below gives an example of such a relationship between cost and volume.

**FIGURE 2.2.4:**   Fixed costs

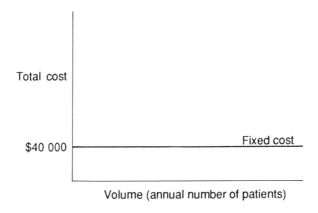

The fixed costs appear as a horizontal line because regardless of volume the costs remain the same. Examples of fixed costs which may normally occur in a nursing unit include:

a) nurse unit manager's salary;

b) director of nursing's salary;

c) infection control salary;

d) quality assurance salary.

Examples of fixed costs which may normally occur in the hospital organisation may include:

a) depreciation;

b) administration;

c) insurance;

d) capital financing.

**Variable costs** however vary with the volume of output. They are costs over and above the fixed costs. The exact amount of variation is dependent upon policy decisions. That is, they may vary directly or proportionally.

Suppose the number of supplies for each patient treated on an intensive care unit is calculated. If the throughput of patients increases by 5 per cent, then the expenditure on supplies will also increase.

Variable costs behaviour may be viewed as follows in Figure 2.2.5:

FIGURE 2.2.5:   Variable costs

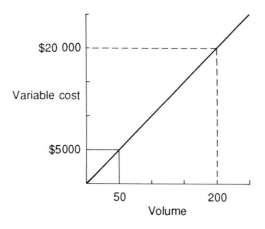

Further examples of variable costs may include:

a) linen costs;

b) food costs;

c) supplies for a specific type of patient (eg. dialysis, ICU, cardiac surgery).

The following Figure 2.2.6 shows how variable costs are incurred over and above fixed costs.

**Total costs** are the sum of fixed and variable costs.

**Cost per unit of service** or unit cost is another term that requires explanation. The unit of service in the health care setting for patient care is the patient day. Some examples of units of service for health care are shown in the following table:

| Department | Unit of Service |
|---|---|
| Dietary | Meals |
| Repairs/Maintenance | Job order |
| Theatre | Surgery minutes<br>Anaesthesia minutes |
| Recovery Room | Number of patients<br>– inpatient<br>– outpatient |
| District Nursing | Home vists |

**FIGURE 2.2.6**:  Total costs

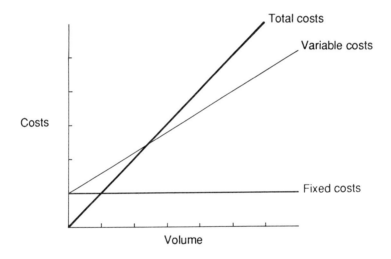

The foregoing has set a foundation for the understanding of cost behaviour. The problems of calculating costs and predicting how they will behave over time will now be discussed.

## 3.4 CALCULATING STANDARD COSTS

Since nursing programmes are often the first to be targeted for reductions, it is imperative that nurse administrators be capable of documenting the need for resources (whether nursing hours, supplies, facilities, equipment or support help) and justifying their arguments

(Marks and Smith, 1987:192)

In order to undertake such an activity, a base line of costs and their behaviour needs to be established. Valid cost profiles are required as it is difficult to create a realistic budget unless a rational basis for calculating the cost of resource inputs is defined.

Cleverly (1986:227) explains this when he says

a budget or set of resource expectations can be thought of as a standard costing system. The budget represents management's expectations of how costs should behave, given a certain set of volume assumptions.

How then does a nurse manager establish how much it will cost for a particular service and how that specific cost will behave?

Cleverly (1986:228) explains the five basic steps in the standard costing process as follows:

1. define the volume of patients by case type to be treated in the budget period;

2. define the standard treatment protocol by case type;

3. define the required departmental volumes;

4. define the standard cost profiles for departmental outputs;

5. define the prices to be paid for resources.

This increased interest in cost accounting in health care organisations has come about because of the need for management to maintain control of total expenses. Direct costs, as discussed earlier in this chapter, are easily identified and controlled by management; indirect costs are not however, as easily identifiable and are not really under the control of the manager.

Indirect costs have to be allocated to various departments or cost centres so that the manager may have a complete and accurate picture of the true expenses of each department or cost centre. By transferring indirect costs to departments or cost centres, managers can participate more fully in decision-making for overhead expenses, and they are more likely to take responsibility for the costs when they are fiscally accountable.

If a department or cost centre does not have both direct and indirect expenses allocated by the hospital, then the department could overestimate its financial contribution margin.

Various methods for allocating indirect expenses to patient care areas are shown in the following table.

Examples of Indirect Costs Allocation Criteria

| Department | Criteria |
|---|---|
| Repairs and Maintenance | • Square metres of department |
| Medical Records | • Cost per patient chart per department |
| Housekeeping | • By square metres of department<br>• By hours in department<br>• By number of services to department |
| Dietary | • Cost per meals per patient in department |
| Administration | • By number of staff hours for department<br>• By amount of expenses generated<br>• By dividing administrators' salaries by the number of departments |

A simplified example of the standard cost system for a diabetes education clinic is illustrated below:

### 3.4.1 Standard hourly cost in a diabetes education clinic

Standard cost per patient:

| | |
|---|---|
| Supplies cost | $5.00 |
| Nursing staff cost* | $8.33 |
| Overhead cost* | $3.12 |
| Total Cost per Patient | $16.45 |

Standard hourly cost for running the clinic:

| | |
|---|---|
| 3 Nurses × 3 patients × $16.45 = | $148.05 |

Underlying assumptions:

| | |
|---|---|
| Annual number of nurse practitioners | 3 |
| Number of patients per hour | 3 |
| Nursing costs per hour | $25.00 |
| Supplies cost per patient | $5.00 |
| Overhead costs per day | $75.00 |

\* $25.00 divide by 3 = $8.33
\*\* $75.00 divide by (3 patients times 8 hours/day) = $3.12

### 3.4.2 Break-even analysis

Break-even analysis can be applied to analyse the cost, volume and profit of a certain product or service in order to facilitate decision making by management.

Strasen (1987:96) identified a number of assumptions about break-even analysis that nurse managers should understand:

1. costs can be broken down into fixed and variable costs;

2. fixed costs remain essentially constant despite changes in volume or patient census;

3. variable costs fluctuate with volume or patient census;

4. charges for patient care services are considered a constant over the period of time being considered;

5. the cost of expense factors such as salaries is held constant over the predetermined time period;

6. efficiency and productivity standards are held constant over the time in question;

7. revenue and expense behaviour can be considered linear with changes in volume.

The following example will demonstrate how to calculate the least number of patients required on a ward in order to cover the direct costs of minimum staffing.

Utilising      –      a productivity standard      =      4.5 HPPD
                –      average cost of staff      =      $14/hr

**Minimum Level of Staffing**

| Shift | No. of staff | Hours |
|---|---|---|
| Morning | 3 | 24 |
| Evening | 2 | 16 |
| Night | 2 | 16 |
| Nursing Unit Manager | 1 | 5.7* |
| Total | | 61.7 |

* (40 hours divided by 7 days) = 5.7

Minimum Hours
Productivity standard = Break-even point

$$\frac{61.7 \text{ hrs}}{4.5 \text{ HPPD}} = 13.7 \text{ patients}$$

Therefore this unit would always require 13.7 patients in order to pay for the minimum staffing direct costs of the unit. Figure 2.2.7 shows a diagrammatic representation of these calculations.

Break-even analysis may also be used when an organisation is concerned with answering the following types of questions:

a. what number of bed days are required for the hospital to break even?;

b. what profit will be earned if 1650 beds are obtained?;

c. to generate $17 000 profit, how many bed days are required?;

d. when variable costs rise to $21/bed day and the hospital's capacity is limited to 1200 bed days, what charge per bed is required to return $17 000 profit?.

**FIGURE 2.2.7:** Least number of patients required

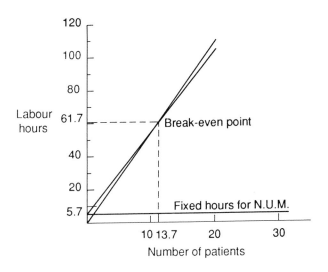

The following example will demonstrate how these questions may be answered utilising data as follows:

| | |
|---|---|
| Fixed costs | $25 000 per annum |
| Variable costs | $18 per bed day |
| Revenue | $40 per day |

We can use an algebraic manipulation on the unknown X to answer all the above questions using the equation S = FC +VC + P.

Key to symbols
S       = Selling price (ie, revenue or rate × no. of beds or cases)
FC      = Fixed cost per period
VC      = Variable cost (ie, variable cost + no. of beds or cases)
P       = Profit (this always equals 0 if finding break-even point)

Solutions
a. If S     = FC + VC + P
   40 (x)   = 25 000 + 18(x) + 0
        x   = 1136.3
            = 1137 beds are required for the hospital to break even.

b. P
= S - FC - VC
= (40)(1650) - 25 000 - (18)(1650)
= 66 000 - 25 000 - 29 700
= $11 300 profit will be earned if 1650 beds are obtained.

c. If S
40 (x)
22 (x)
x
= FC + VC + P
= 25 000 + 18(x) + 17 000
= $42 000
= 1909.09 beds
= 1910 beds days are required to generate $17 000 profit.

d. S
R(1200)
R
= FC + VC + P
= 25 000 + (1200)(21) + 17 000
= 67 200
= $56 charge per bed is required to return $17 000 profit when variable costs rise to $21/bed day and the hospital's capacity is limited to 1200 bed days.

Figure 2.2.8 provides a diagrammatic representation of these calculations.

**FIGURE 2.2.8:** Break-even point

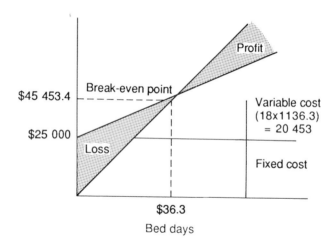

3.4.3 Variance analysis

Many health care institutions are turning to flexible budgeting to address variances in monthly volume and utilisation. Nurse administrators therefore will encounter this form of budgeting, which is becoming increasingly prevalent because of the availability of computer systems.

Three factors which cause variances are as follows:

1.  changes in volume;

2.  changes from planned efficiency;

3.  changes in the rate of wages/salaries.

From these three factors it is possible to calculate corresponding variances:

1.  volume variance;

2.  efficiency variance;

3.  rate variance.

**A volume variance** presents when the actual volume is found to be greater or less than the budgeted volume. The actual measure of volume may be for example:

☐ patient day count; or

☐ patient classification points system.

Volume variance may be calculated as follows:

Volume variance = (earned hours - budgeted hours) × budgeted hourly rate

Note: earned hours = actual activity (days) × budgeted activity ratio

**Efficiency variance.** The actual productivity of staff may be compared to the budgeted plan for staff. By dividing planned/budgeted activity into planned/budgeted hours, it is possible to obtain an efficiency standard.

$$\text{Thus budgeted activity ration} = \frac{\text{budgeted hours [payroll hours]}}{\text{budgeted activity [patient days]}}$$

Once the efficiency standard is calculated, it is possible for the nurse administrator/manager confronted with either greater or less performance than the standard to calculate an efficiency variance.

The formula for calculation of efficiency variance is as follows:

| efficiency variance | = | (actual - earned)<br>hours    hours | × | budgeted hourly rate |
|---|---|---|---|---|
| (where earned hours | = | actual activity<br>[patient days] | × | budgeted activity ratio) |

The formula for calculation of the rate variance is as follows:

| rate variance | = | (actual rate - budgeted rate) | × | actual hours |
|---|---|---|---|---|

### 3.4.4 City Hospital: case study of variance analysis

The following practical example will now be examined in order to understand the use of variance analysis. Consider the data in Table 2.2.1.

TABLE 2.2.1

|  | Budgeted $ | Actual $ | Changes $ |
|---|---|---|---|
| Payroll costs | 95 200 | 106 350 | (11 150) Unfavourable |
| Payroll hours | 10 942 | 14 770 | ( 3 828) Unfavourable |
| Patient day | 1 517 | 1 890 | ( 373) Unfavourable |

    As the director of nursing of City Hospital you are asked to explain the unfavourable variance of $11 150. You are also required to recommend a course of action for the future. From the above data, it is possible to undertake a thorough variance analysis of volume, efficiency and rate variances.

    It is firstly necessary to calculate the budgeted activity ratio and actual activity ratio, budgeted hourly rate and actual hourly rate, to proceed with the variance analysis.

$$\text{Budgeted activity ratio} = \frac{\text{budgeted hours [payroll hours]}}{\text{budgeted activity [patient days]}}$$

$$= \frac{10\ 942}{1517}$$

$$= 7.2129$$

$$\text{Actual activity ratio} = \frac{\text{actual hours [payroll hours]}}{\text{actual activity [patient days]}}$$

$$= \frac{14\ 770}{1890}$$

$$= 7.8148$$

$$\text{Budgeted hourly ratio} = \frac{\text{budgeted payroll costs}}{\text{budgeted payroll hours}}$$

$$= \frac{\$95\ 200}{10\ 942}$$

$$= \$8.7004$$

$$\text{Actual hourly rate} = \frac{\text{actual payroll costs}}{\text{actual payroll hours}}$$

$$= \frac{\$106\ 350}{14\ 770}$$

$$= \$7.2004$$

The volume variance is calculated as follows:

| | | |
|---|---|---|
| Where earned hours | = | actual activity × budgeted activity ratio (patient days) |
| | = | 1890 days × 7.2129 |
| | = | 13 632.381 hours |
| <u>Volume variance</u> | = | (earned hours - budgeted hours) × budgeted hourly rate |
| | = | (13 632.381 - 10 942) × $8.7004 |
| | = | $23 407.39086 (Unfavourable) |

The efficiency variance is calculated as follows:

| | | |
|---|---|---|
| Efficiency variance | = | (actual hours - earned hours) / budgeted hourly rate |
| | = | (14 770 - 13 632.381) × $8.7004 |
| | = | $9897.740348 (Unfavourable) |

The rate variance will now be calculated as follows:

| | | |
|---|---|---|
| <u>Rate variance</u> | = | (actual rate - budgeted rate) × actual hours |
| | = | ($7.2004 - $8.7004) × 14770 |
| | = | $22 155 (Favourable) |

Thus our analysis has provided the following results:

| | | | |
|---|---|---|---|
| Volume variance | = | $23 407.39086 | (U) |
| Efficiency variance | = | $ 9 897.740348 | (U) |
| Rate variance | = | $22 155 | (F) |
| | | $11 150 | (U)* |

* (Rounding Off)

But what does all this mean?

We see that the total variance is unfavourable as the unfavourable volume and efficiency outweighed the favourable rate variance.

# 4. CONCLUSION

In this chapter several diverse threads pertaining to resource management are investigated. In section one, time management and the various activities undertaken by individuals at various levels of management are discussed. Major obstacles to effective time management are outlined, along with a range of recommended strategies designed to overcome problems.

Section two outlines the importance of human resource management through effective planning, staffing, development of staff, and creation of a harmonious working environment. It indicates that if managers show a genuine interest in and care for their staff, they demonstrate that they value these people and their contributions. This should result in raising levels of morale and motivation, and hence improve performance.

The final section addresses the management of money as a resource. Factors which influence health costs are described, and a range of formulae for determining costs and budget allocations is provided. If the efficient and effective management of these resources is undertaken, a high quality of service provision should result with a concomitant attainment of organisational goals.

# DRYANDRA CASE STUDY

On Wednesday Lesley Linum, Director of Nursing at Dryandra Base Hospital, had interviewed a staff member Barbara Delforce, who had reported on duty in the surgical ward and was sent to her by the nurse manager. The nurse manager told Lesley that Barbara was under the influence as she smelt strongly of alcohol and looked scruffy. Barbara, aged 35, has been a Charge Nurse for the last eight years, all of which have been served at Dryandra Hospital. There had never been any complaints about her work previously although in recent months she has been very prone to absenteeism. Her flatmate had called in on a number of occasions to say she would not be able to attend work. With the shortages of staff experienced over the past 12 months, and especially with the difficulty Dryandra Base Hospital had experienced in attracting and retaining experienced staff, Lesley felt undecided about what would be the best course of action to take regarding Barbara's behaviour.

1. When considering this problem what are the assumptions you may be making in regard to the information available?

2. How could you validate your assumptions?

3. How could you obtain further information regarding this matter?

4. How would you suggest that Lesley handles this problem?

# REFERENCES

Applebaum, S. H. and Rohrs, W. F. (1981), *Time management for health care professionals,* Aspen, Maryland.

Ashkenas, R. N. and Schaffer, R. H. (1982), 'Managers can avoid wasting time', *Harvard Business Review,* 60:99-105.

Bassett, L. C. and Metzger, N. (1986), *Achieving excellence. A prescription for health care managers,* Rockville, Aspen.

Bingham, R. C. (1984), *Economic concepts: a programmed approach,* McGraw-Hill, New York.

Blaney, D. and Hobson, C. (1988), *Cost-effective nursing practice: guidelines for nurse managers,* Lippincott, Philadelphia.

Brief, J. (1979), 'Developing a usable performance appraisal system', *Journal of Nursing Administration,* October, 7-10.

Clark, R. (1988), *Australian human resources management,* Sydney, McGraw-Hill.

Cleverley, W. O. (1986), *Essentials of health care finance,* 2nd edition, Aspen, Maryland.

del Bueno, D. J. (1977), 'Performance evaluation: when all is said and done, more is said than done', *Journal of Nursing Administration,* December, 21-23.

Department of Employment and Industrial Relations, (1982), *A guide on discrimination in employment in Australia,* Canberra, AGPS.

Fries, B. and Cooney, L. (1985), 'Resource utilisation groups: a patient classification system for long-term care', *Medical Care,* 23:2 1985.

Gilchrist, J. M. (1987), 'Unionism and professionalism in nursing', *The Canadian Nurse,* 83:10, November, 31-33.

Harris, M., Santoferraro, C. and Silva, S. (1985), 'A patient classification system in home health care', *Nursing Economics, 3:5, 1985.*

Herzog, T. P. (1985), 'Productivity: fighting the battle of the budget', *Nursing Management,* 16:1.

Hoffman, F. (1988), *Nursing productivity assessment and costing out nursing services,* Lippincott, Philadelphia.

Huang, S. H. and Schoenknecht, H. D. (1984), 'Contracts individualise orientation', *Nursing Management,* 15:9 September, 53-57.

Ignatavicius, D. and Griffith, J. (1982), 'Job analysis: the basis of effective appraisal', *Journal of Nursing Administration,* July/August, 37-41.

Katz, R. (1974), 'Skills of an effective administrator', *Harvard Business Review,* 52, September-October, 90-102.

Lawler, E. E., Porter, L. W. and Tannenbaum, A. (1968), 'Manager's attitudes towards interaction episodes', *Journal of Applied Psychology,* 52:432-439.

Lucas, P. and Austin, B. (1984), 'The nursing officer at work: tried and tested', *Nursing Times,* 80:47-48.

McCarthy, T. E. and Stone, R. J. (1986), *Personnel management in Australia,* John Wiley and Sons, Brisbane.

McConnell, C. R. (1986), *The health supervisor's guide to cost control and productivity improvement,* Rockville, Aspen.

Mahoney, T., Jerdee, T. H. and Carroll, S. J. (1965), 'The job(s) of management', *Industrial Relations,* 4:103.

Mannisto M. (1980), 'An assessment of productivity in health care', *Hospitals,* 54:18.

Margulies, N. and Duval, J. (1984), 'Productivity management: a model for participative management in health care organisations', *Health Care Management Review,* 9:1.

Marks, B. A. and Smith, H. L. (1987), *Essentials of finance in nursing,* Aspen, Maryland.

Megginson, L. C., Mosley, D. C. and Pietri, P. H. (1989), *Management concepts and applications,*

3rd edition, Harper & Row, New York.

Mintzberg, H. (1973), *The nature of managerial work,* Harper & Row, New York.

Morano, V. J. (1984), 'Time management: from victim to victor', *The health care supervisor,* 27:1-2.

Norville, J. L. (1984), 'Improving personal effectiveness through better management of time', *Nursing Homes,* 13:8-12.

Peters, T. J. and Waterman, R. H. Jr., (1983), *In search of excellence,* New York, Harper & Row.

Pincus, J. (1982), 'The shortlist and interview', *Nursing Mirror,* November 17, 39-44.

Rowland, H. S. and Rowland, B. L. (1985), *Nursing administration handbook,* 2nd edition, Rockville, Aspen.

Saul, P. (1987), 'Change: the strategic human resource management challenges', *Human resource management Australia,* 25, 1, 80-89.

Schneider, D. (1979), 'An ambulatory care classification system: design, development and evaluation', *Health Services Research,* 14:1.

Schuler, R. S., Dowling, P. J. and Smart, J. P. (1988), *Personnel/human resource management in Australia,* Sydney, Harper & Row.

Silvers, J. B., Zelman, W. N. and Kahn, C. N. III. (1983), *Health care financial management in the 1980s,* AUPHA Press, Ann Arbor.

Smith, H. L. and Elbert, N. F. (1986), *The health care supervisor's guide to staff development,* Rockville, Aspen.

Sovie, M. D. (1981), 'Fostering professional nursing careers in hospitals: the role of staff development: Part I', *Journal of Nursing Administration,* December, 30-35.

Strasen, L. (1987), *Key business skills for nurse managers,* Lippincott, Philadelphia.

# Outline of evaluation systems for nurse managers

ROBERT MARTIN AND MARJORIE CUTHBERT

After reading this chapter, you should be able to:

**1.** define evaluation;

**2.** provide a global model of nursing service evaluation;

**3.** introduce the basic concepts of evaluation;

**4.** introduce and explain the different approaches in evaluation;

**5.** link evaluation to the practice of nursing unit management.

## 1. WHAT IS EVALUATION?

Evaluation is the systematic intellectual activity of determining the worth of an action or activity in relation to a defined purpose. It arises out of a concern for knowing the merit of organised human actions and activities. Evaluators examine the structure, process and outcome of organisations to find whether their activities achieve an intended purpose.

The broadly understood aim of an organisation is called a mission (Stoner, 1985:118, 129). The structure of an organisation is the design, organisation and utilisation of physical and human resources necessary for mission implementation. The process is the putting into place and carrying out of the activities necessary to achieve mission implementation and accomplishment. The outcomes are the measurable consequences of the organisation's activities when compared to its mission.

## 2. WHY IS EVALUATION USED?

Managers and service providers — health carers in the health care context — ought to be concerned with knowing the merit of their actions if they are concerned with doing good. Merit is judged by examining activities and determining whether they achieve what was intended. Generally, the activities are related back to the organisational mission from which they were derived.

Imbedded in a mission statement are a number of goals and objectives that explicitly define what the mission is and how it is to be achieved (Stoner, 1985: 118, 129). For example, in organised health care the purpose is the maintenance and improvement of wellbeing, or when that is not possible the minimisation of pain, distress and disability. The goals of organised health care imply that activities should be directed at achieving health by 'maintenance', 'improvement' and 'disease minimisation'. These terms basically define relatively exclusive goals that are general statements of intention. Goals form a base for the organisation to plan the activities that will ensure the mission is accomplished. These statements of means are called objectives and define how the goals are to be achieved. Goals are, therefore, statements about what is planned for the health care organisation, and objectives are statements of how those goals are to be achieved. Strategies are the mechanisms for implementing the objectives. The strategies form the basis of the organisation's plan and assist the organisation in adapting to its environment and meeting its mission.

Evaluation provides the means for examining the management and implementation of planned strategies and their consequences in relation to the resources provided. Evaluation establishes whether the mission as defined by goals and objectives has been implemented, and determines if there is a match between what was intended and what actually eventuated. Evaluation also provides a means of checking the validity of the mission in the light of increased knowledge.

# 3. WHY IS EVALUATION IMPORTANT?

It follows that if managers and care-givers are concerned with the merit of their activities, they will want to know their consequences in terms of whether the activities were right or wrong, or good or bad. They will want to correct undesirable and ineffectual activities in the light of increased knowledge to ensure a better fit between the achieved results and what was intended by the mission.

Evaluation in health care determines whether the services provided are appropriately effective and efficient. Effective care may be defined as care which achieves either an improvement in health, maintenance of health status, or the minimisation of pain, distress and disability. Efficient care may be defined as appropriate care that achieves effective care at the least possible cost. Cost in this context relates to all the resources used, human and material, in providing care (Drummond, 1984:10).

If one or other of a health care organisation's services are decreasing a person's or a community's health, or increasing pain, distress and disability, then a match between goals and objectives and services does not exist. If this is the case, there is a reasonable basis for concluding that the organisation's activities are in some way bad or wrong. Evaluation provides a means of identifying inappropriate, inefficient and ineffective care. When evaluators have rigorously examined structure, process and outcome, they are better able to make an informed judgement about the value of the care provided and make recommendations about improvements to future services.

# 4. THE DYNAMICS OF MANAGEMENT EVALUATION

Management dynamics are the forces that result from human thoughts, actions and interactions when enterprise or service is organised. Watson (1986:39) argues that management is 'the pulling together of the various bits and pieces of the organisation and a pulling along of the organisation in some general direction'. Managers are of necessity concerned with the efficiency and effectiveness of their organisation's services. The capacity to control and manipulate resources to a desired end is the hallmark of the managerial process. Evaluation equips the manager with the principles and methods necessary to systematically examine the organisation, activities and outcomes and to compare them with prescribed goals and objectives. If managers cannot provide information about the efficiency and effectiveness of their organisation's service, then they cannot be claimed to be managing. (McFarland et al, 1984; Sullivan and Decker, 1985). In effect, management evaluation is the process of the manager knowing if the service has achieved what it set out to do.

The dynamic elements of this process of management evaluation are:

☐ eliminating or reducing risk of adverse effects related to service organisation and delivery;

☐ minimising cost;

☐ knowing what has been achieved and why;

☐ gaining and providing feedback;

☐ maximising gain and minimising loss;

☐ building on strengths and overcoming weaknesses. In later parts of the chapter, evlauation techniques for each of these elements will be described and explained.

# 5. A GLOBAL MODEL OF EVALUATION PERSPECTIVES

Evaluation arises out of human intelligence. In attempting to discover if defined goals and objectives have been achieved, a number of cognitive processes are focused, either independently or collectively, on the task at hand. These cognitive processes provide perspectives on how evaluation should be performed.

Evaluation can be schematised as a two dimensional matrix divided into four quadrants consisting of rational and intuitive poles on a vertical plane and structural and functional poles on a horizontal plane (see Figure 2.3.1.)

The rational pole is derived from a formalised set of rules that evolved from traditional Western philosophical thought (Gorovitz et al, 1979:3). The rules are public and are formulated to lead to consistent judgement. Rational thinking and *ipso facto* evaluation are concerned with arriving at truth and validity by the consistent ordering of arguments involving analytic or synthetic propositions (Gorovitz et al, 1979:119–134).

FIGURE 2.3.1: Model of cognitive perspectives used for evaluation purposes

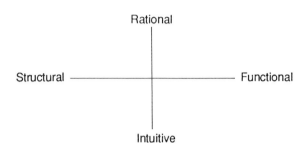

An analytic proposition is one that is true because it is necessarily true. For example, one plus one necessarily equals two. A necessary truth is one that is true because it is defined to be true. Necessary propositions tell us nothing about the state of the world. They only inform us about what has been defined as being from the logical ordering of the argument. A useful explanation is contained in Richard and Commons (1990:140–147).

A synthetic proposition, on the other hand, is one that is true because it is seen, generally over a number of observations, to be true. As such, the truth of a synthetic proposition can be altered by the observation of a negating case. For example, it may have been observed over a long period of time that diet control was a sufficient treatment of maturity-onset diabetes, but if on one occasion, observation showed that diet was not a sufficient treatment, the proposition clearly is no longer universally true. Synthetic truths are derived from the experience of the world and are considered conditional. They are referred to as being objective and are informative about the state of the world. They are, however, dependent upon the continuous testing of their veracity by repeated observations.

Synthetic and analytic propositions are ordered into information-producing sets through rational argument. Such argument can be deductive or inductive.

A deductive argument is made up, in its most basic form, of a necessary and a conditional proposition, and a conclusion (Lessnoff, 1979:13; Chinn and Jacobs, 1983:59–61). The necessary proposition is the major premise of the argument and the conditional proposition is the minor premise. The conclusion is based on a proposition that either conjoins or disjoins the definiens of the necessary proposition to the definiendum of the conditional proposition. A classic example of a deductive argument is:

| All unmarried males are bachelors | (major premise) |
| Joe is an unmarried male | (minor premise) |

| Joe is a bachelor | (conclusion) |

The syllogistic form of the argument is:

| a — b | eg, | a defines b |
| c — a | | c defines a |
| ——— | | ——— |
| c — b | | c defines b |

The conclusion of the argument is deduced from the conjoining of the definiens of proposition one (b: bachelor) to the definiendum of proposition two (c: Joe). Proposition one implies that proposition three is correct, and provided proposition 2 is correct, it is a consistent or valid argument.

Deductive arguments are used extensively in evaluation methodology. Generally when goals are written they are formulated as major premises; that is, they are taken to be necessarily true. If, for example, the goal of a health service is to improve health, it is taken to be unconditionally true that improved health is an intention of a health service. The argument may be more complex than the syllogistic one presented above. It may include the consistent ordering of many objectives and the data collected about them, but the conclusion will always be implied by the ordering of a major premise or premises with a minor premise or premises.

An inductive argument differs in that the major or minor premises are synthetic propositions (Lessnoff, 1979:14; Chinn and Jacobs, 1983:61–63). The argument is entirely conditional and is based on an estimate of the probability of the truth of all its premises. For example:

In airways disease, respirations are decreased by the administration of oxygen.
Joe has airways disease and has increased respirations.

Joe's respirations will be decreased by the administration of oxygen.

Clearly this argument is valid because the conclusion is derived in such a way that the definiens of the major premise is implied by the definiendum of the minor premise. It is not, however, a deductive argument because the major premise is not necessarily true. It is conditional and dependent upon being observed to be true.

Inductive arguments are very common in evaluation methodology. They are used when goals are formulated from conditional statements. For example, take the goal 'tobacco smoking should be reduced to improve community health'. The objectives and the data collected to support the argument may be used to back up the goal of reducing smoking, but its truth is derived from observations that tobacco smoking is bad for community health.

The intuitive end of the vertical pole in Figure 1 is derived from a tradition of human activity that relies upon immediate apperception and emotional reaction as a form of knowing (Christian, 1981:160–161). The most extreme form of studying intuitive knowledge is called phenomenology. This understanding of human knowledge emerges out of a tradition of philosophy that focuses on the subjective as the basis of human existence. The tradition rejects objective science as a means of understanding human experience (Cohen, 1987:31–33). There is no attempt to consistently order premises or to follow the rules of logic in order to arrive at knowing.

In some forms intuition is highly complex because the sensations by which the person is describing and responding form an elaborate schema. The knowledge derived intuitively is taken to be true when it can be demonstrated to be authentic. Authenticity is the hallmark of intuition because it provides knowledge which is in harmony with the state of the world (Warnock, 1979:55–56).

We believe that the test of authentic intuitive truth is the emotional reaction it brings about. If one is disturbed or placed in a state of angst by a phenomenon, then it challenges authenticity. If a human reaction leads to disquiet, correction is necessary to reinstate authenticity. The correction may be entirely practical. For example, the nurse's experience of a patient's expression of pain may be disquieting and result in the administration of analgesia in response to the disquiet and the need to reinstate the nurse's authenticity. The state of knowing is always referred back to the person who is experiencing the phenomenon, in this case, the nurse. Intuition is always a subjective experience which requires the individual who experiences knowledge to search for authenticity and to correct those experiences within oneself which lead to inauthenticity. Caring for others is fundamental to intuitive knowledge because of the relational basis by which human experience emerges. Health care is, therefore, a necessary element of one's search for authenticity.

Another feature of intuitive knowledge is that it is derived subconsciously (Christian, 1981:160). The person who experiences the knowledge may not be able to recall exactly how the knowing was achieved. All that the person may be able to communicate is a solid sense of authentic truth which feels right.

Intuitive knowledge provides a valuable contribution to evaluation. Many novel understandings and solutions to mis-matches between mission and services are brought about because of a subjectively derived insight. Sometimes, these experiences are called 'aha!' or 'light bulb' insights. The understanding of how the knowledge is gained is frequently not immediately known and is referred to as arising subconsciously. An experienced practitioner may frequently suggest that a purpose might be better achieved if a particular activity were introduced, without being able to fully explain why. However, when the activity is tested, the 'aha' knowledge is found in fact to be useful. Much evaluation relies upon the intuitive judgement of carers and the patients they serve.

The structural pole of the horizontal axis in Figure 2.3.1 is determined by an ancient Greek philosophical tradition that can be summarised by the maxim, 'structure governs function'. The maxim has its origins in the physics of Aristotle (Russell,

1980:213–217) where it was thought that the precise description of the building blocks of matter would bring about an understanding of nature, as such universal structural 'forms' were considered to be identifiable and at the basis of all universal activity.

This philosophy has persisted into modern times where it can be identified in the thinking of many physical and social scientists (Burrell and Morgan, 1982:326–364; Watson, 1977:53; Paturi, 1978:13–15). In evaluation theory it takes on the form of an intellectual concentration on how services are designed and resources organised to achieve a desired purpose (Mintzberg, 1983:1–23). If there is mission failure, it is because the 'structure' has in some way been ineffective or inappropriate. For example, early anticigarette programmes were considered to have failed because they could not compete with the prevailing social structure of cheap tobacco, easy availability and prolific advertising. They were made more effective by changing the social structure, by imposing higher excises on tobacco, limiting the amount of cigarette advertisement, and restricting smoking in public transport and workplaces (Bain, 1986; Hill and Gray, 1984).

Structural approaches to evaluation are important because they aid the health manager to examine the way in which physical and human resources are organised and utilised to bring about specific purposes.

The functional pole on the horizontal plane of Figure 2.3.1 arises out of an equally ancient philosophy which has had a scientific re-emergence since the discoveries of Darwin (1964) and Einstein (Calder, 1979). In this case the maxim is 'function determines form' (Burrell and Morgan, 1982:41–117). A functionalist argues that knowledge about the world and its events can best be gained through an understanding of the principles underlying the 'workings' of physical actions, that is, co-operation or conflict as forces for social change. Functionalists assert that function produces the structure of the world. The reason why human beings walk upright on two legs, unlike other animals that walk on all fours, is that human technical function determined that the forelegs had to be free. A more practical example is that the needs of sick patients determine the way in which hospital wards have been designed (Green et al, 1986:4; Glassner and Freedman, 1979:65–74). A functional perspective always focuses primarily on the process of action as being the determinant of events.

In evaluation, the functional perspective is useful because it draws attention to the important place that process plays in the achievement of an organisation's purpose. Functionalist perspectives are criticised because they do not consider the interaction between form and action (Glassner and Freedman, 1979:70–72). The perspectives fail to fully explain the way cause and effect relationships interact with the role that human choice plays in determining the nature of organisations.

## 5.1 EXPLAINING AND EXPANDING THE SIGNIFICANCE OF THE GLOBAL MODEL OF EVALUATION PERSPECTIVES

This model of evaluation is presented to aid in understanding the intellectual activity of judging the merit of human actions. The model does not require a controversial choice, nor does it treat any of the perspectives as being mutually exclusive. Rather, it provides a schema for explaining how different perspectives work when examining the evaluation process. A comprehensive programme of evaluation would, depending on what it aims to achieve, be based on methods and techniques derived from any of the perspectives or their interactions to ensure fair and balanced judgement. This approach to evaluation does not rely on the evidence derived from one perspective. It is pluralist and extracts evidence from as many sources as possible. The evidence, be it objective or subjective, is organised to obtain a clear view of the merit of the service under investigation.

A method used in nursing research called 'multiple triangulation' provides a way of understanding how a number of sources of data provide a means of getting closer to 'truth' (Murphy, 1989). In triangulation, the phenomenon of interest is examined using a number of different methods or techniques which cross-reference objective and subjective measurements with participant observations. When a perspective is gained and corroborated by objective, subjective and participant data sets, then a sound basis for understanding the phenomenon of interest is achieved.

A further clarification is necessary to understand how this model works. In the classic Donabedian (1966, 1968, 1969) model, evaluation is linked to an organisation's mission by the examination of the achievement of goals and objectives for structure, process and outcome. If evaluation only takes account of one element of an organisation, say structure, it is called formative evaluation. As it is only testing the merit of one component of the organisation, it does not explain the full effect and worth of the organisation. Summative evaluation, however, attempts to examine the full scope of the organisation and relate it back to the mission. It is called summative evaluation because it accounts for structure, process and outcome.

The concepts of triangulation, and formative and summative evaluation, are part of a global model of evaluation. The model provides a means for nurse managers to determine the scope and level of evaluation planning that may be necessary to implement an evaluation programme in their unit. This will help provide answers to questions about the worth of the nursing care provided. The manager should be aware of the perspective on which the evaluation is based. Different methods will provide different answers. The more comprehensive and rigorous the methods used, the more likely the answers will reflect the true state of affairs.

# 6. METHODS OF EVALUATING NURSING UNITS

In this section an examination of the areas of nursing practice and management that are amendable to evaluation will be presented. An overview will be given of the systems the nurse manager can utilise to evaluate nursing structures, processes and outcomes in relation to the health service's mission. The overview is not exhaustive but attempts to draw attention to the key features of nursing management.

In this section, evaluation in the nursing context falls into all quadrants of the model presented in this chapter. However, in the authors' Australian experience, the intuitive = structural quadrant has dominated nursing management. It is perhaps over the last 10 years that the influence of the rational-functional quadrant has been observed to be exerting an influence on the role of the nurse manager.

# 7. EVALUATING THE NURSING OF PATIENTS

A key element of nursing a patient is a comprehensively organised clinical information system (Murray and Zentner, 1985:111–153; Long, 1981). In nursing, this system is often made up of a patient history, nursing care plan and nursing progress notes. The basis of evaluation in this information system is the subjective judgement of the practising nurse. As such, it relies heavily on an intuitive perspective, but as a legal document, has to be cross-referenced and corroborated by rational evidence from observation charts, clinical tests, reports and progress note entries by other health professionals. The Australian Council on Healthcare Standards (ACHS) in Standard 3.3, 3.4 (p. 100) requires that a care plan be developed in consultation with the patient and significant others. The plan is to be based on the patient's needs and must include the expected outcomes of nursing care. ACHS also specifies that the plan and other nursing documentation be 'incorporated in the patient's medical record'.

The aim of the nursing clinical information system is to communicate and support nursing decisions through a systematic process of care — called the nursing process. It is logistically derived and is claimed to provide the nurse with a means of systematic care delivery (Kelly, 1981:161). The steps in the process are assessment, diagnosis, planning, implementation and evaluation. The nursing process is a system of formulating care and judging the merit of the nursing care plan and interventions in relation to a defined purpose. The defined purpose is the implementation of quality nursing care which helps to assure that the mission of the health service is achieved. The end stage of the process is evaluation which provides a means of judging the effectiveness and efficiency of operation nursing care (Murray and Zentner, 1985:143; Long, 1981:60–67).

Nursing clinical information systems can be used as a source for formative evaluation but this can be time consuming. A number of criticisms have also been levelled at this process. It requires subjective information from an acutely ill patient (Duberley, 1979:116) or significant others to ensure that the written documentation matches the care given. Further criticisms have been made about the discrepancy between the use of a professionally-oriented model of care and a task-oriented care plan. This discrepancy has resulted in difficulties for the nurse in effective documentation and use of care plans (Costello and Summers, 1985). Another criticism is that the degree of responsibility apportioned to 'novice' nurses in identifying problems in planning and evaluating care may be greater than their level of nursing development permits (Duberley, 1979:117–118).

Care plans are frequently over-generalised. For example the statement 'satisfactory day' as an evaluation provides the oncoming nurse with very limited information about the patient's condition. The language used is vague and no data is provided to back up the statement. Nursing care entries are often not consistent, leading to gaps in information and loss of meaning. Nurses are frequently busy and neglect systematic documentation. When the demands of a patient's immediate condition are great, the imperative to systematically document care can be lost. The documentation process relies on memory and is therefore frequently modified by fatigue and workload pressures.

Care plans are often given a low priority and are written up retrospectively during quieter periods. Their use as a reference for care becomes rudimentary with nursing action being dominated by the institution's routine and doctor's orders, rather than the nurse's rigorous assessment of patient needs. In the authors' experience, quality assurance audits indicate that the assessment of patient needs, and the evaluation of care in relation to the patient's response to nursing interventions, are areas where care plans commonly fail (Cuthbert, 1983:179–180; Martin and Ballard, 1990, unpublished paper).

Another complementary and institutionalised method of evaluating nursing care over short time spans is the handover report. The handover report communicates the successes, failures, problems and difficulties of a previous shift period to an oncoming shift. Although not always a formal system, handover acts as a means of evaluation because outgoing nurses report on what has been achieved and oncoming nurses plan nursing interventions. The handover report can be an invaluable evaluation process because it is based on written and subjective clinical judgement, and involves nurses' observations of patients.

The problems with handover are that the rules used for evaluation are not consistently known or applied. All the factors necessary for sound judgement are, consequently, not given the same weighting by each nurse. Moreover, not everyone at handover report is equally attentive or knowledgeable. It occurs at the end of a shift, involving nurses who are tired and wanting to go home. The evaluation performed, therefore, often does not have clear reference points linked to defined goals. Menon (1990) has raised the issue of the two languages spoken by nurses. Nurses' technical language is brief, abbreviated and requires implicit knowledge by other members of staff. This can be very confusing to new or uninitiated nurses.

A traditional way in which the nurse manager evaluates patient care is by the ward round. The round generally involves a walk round the ward and a brief examination of each patient. It provides the manager with a global view of the patients and their care activities in the ward, and an orientation point for the correction of ineffective and inefficient practice. It is time efficient and aids in the setting of short-term priorities.

The problem with ward rounds is, however, that judgement can become stereotypical, because the final arbiter of the round is the manager. Human judgements, unless challenged for veracity, may become entrenched or inconsistent. Implicit rules about goals and their achievement can also lead to personal preferences being the arbiter of choice. In some cases observations can become selective, leading to ignorance about important issues and over-emphasis of trivial ones.

# 8. EVALUATING NURSES

An essential element of achieving an organisation's mission is the capacity of workers to perform in ways that are advantageous, correct, desirable and legal. It is said that an organisation's greatest resources are its people. However people do err and prejudice their judgements. This may lead to a mismatch between how a worker is performing and what the organisation intended for that person's role. It is therefore necessary for comprehensive evaluation to include appraisal of nurses' work.

The most basic way nursing staff are evaluated is through performance appraisal (Lansbury, 1981; Beck, 1990). This is generally a management-initiated system where the nurse manager examines the competence of nurses. Standards are set by a variety of organisations such as the Nurses' Registration Boards in each state and professional organisations, and specify levels of competence for nurses. Explicit and implicit standards are defined either by expert opinion or by the folkways prevailing within the professional culture. These standards are a guide to the level of performance expected by nurses providing care in health services and should form the basis for performance appraisal (Australian Congress of Mental Health Nurses, 1985; Toth and Ritchey, 1984). However standards are constantly subjected to change as knowledge, skills, abilities and techniques evolve.

Another method is appraisal based on the achievement of the nurse's objectives, and/or the organisation's objectives as identified in the job description, for a stated period of time (Johnson, 1987). Mismatches can occur between the organisation's and the nurse's objectives. When this occurs the appraisal is not necessarily based on the nurse's abilities but on the capacity of the nurse to adapt to the organisation's requirements.

The appraisal is generally performed by the use of a standardised form which allows for judgements to be made on either intuitive or rational indicators, or a mixture of both (Nadzam, 1987; Lawler, 1988). Performance appraisals provide managers with information about an employee's skills, knowledge, behaviour and attitudes. In a more comprehensive assessment, information is also gained about motivation, job enrichment, satisfaction and initiative. The appraisal of commencing and mature employees is seen as complimentary and interactive, providing feedback about performance in relation to the service's purpose and goals. Each type of employee requires an appraisal format geared to their particular level of skill development and needs. Toth and Ritchey (1984) found that 'length of experience was the best predictor of basic knowledge' and there was a significant difference in knowledge between new nurses and more experienced nurses. This finding supports Benner's (1984:38) thesis regarding the five skill-acquisition levels of practising nurses and her observation that 'with expertise and mastery the skill is transformed'.

The problem with performance appraisals is basically that they are formed from subjective judgements which have not been demonstrated to have high rater reliability. All judgements are subject to error. These errors may be systematic where the same error is made on each occasion, and non-systematic where different errors are made on different occasions. Further the rater often is not impartial and therefore is subject to biased judgements which can be based on first or most recent impressions, or the most enduring impression of the employee. A means of overcoming some of the limitations of management-initiated performance appraisal is to have the employee self-evaluate, or to devise a system of peer review. Two other methods are critical incident reviews and management by objectives. Coaching as a method of improving performance has gained prominence since the work of Peters and Austen (1985:324–377) which reviewed organisational cultures achieving excellent results. Coaching, properly used, is non-threatening, encourages co-operative effort and develops the skills and abilities of staff. Another recent development is the linking of new nurses to preceptors who will guide the new nurse until the required standard of competency is achieved (Menon, 1990). Preceptors are experienced nurses who volunteer their services for this role and undertake a course to equip them to carry out the role proficiently. Mentors are executive nurses who recognise the potential of junior nurses and facilitate opportunities for their technical and personal development and career advancement (Puetz, 1983).

The problem with many of these approaches is that they have generally not been scientifically tested for reliability and validity.

# 9. EVALUATING THE FINANCIAL MANAGEMENT OF NURSING

The financial aspects of managing a nursing unit are driven by the basic principles and conventions of accounting and financial management (Rapoport, Robertson and Stuart, 1982). These to some degree limit the achievement of nursing goals by imposing cost controls on the purchase of resources necessary for service provision. The mission of a health service is constrained by the amount of finance the market or the community is willing to invest in health. An imperative for nursing unit management is that cost and budget provisions are monitored and that available resources are distributed in an efficient and equitable manner (Capp, 1988).

Some Australian hospitals have established systems of global accounting or clinical budgeting which give ward managers a much better means of comparing the funds available against what is being expended (Keegan, 1990). Controllable cost reports provide the basis of such accounting. Costs are allocated to cost centres which are split into two kinds, those providing services which produce revenue, and those which are service providers (Donovan and Lewis, 1987). They are an integral component of the information that nurse managers have available to evaluate the effectiveness and benefit of the services in their charge. Some hospitals also cost services by diagnosis-related groups (DRGs) of diseases. This information allows the nurse manager to compare costs with other units treating similar types of patients. DRG costings also enable the nurse manager to examine costs in relation to quality (Cuthbert, 1990).

Other innovations in financial management include time series and variance analysis. Both aim at examining deviance of cost compared to fund supply. Year-to-date statements provide managers with another means of evaluating cost compared to funds supplied. A regular report states the amount of funds expended compared to the budgeted funds for that period. The annual financial statement provides a report on the balance sheet, a profit and loss statement or deficit and surplus statement, and a statement of special purpose fund expenditure. The annual financial report is of limited use to the nurse manager because it only reports on the financial functioning of the organisation and not on individual units. However if the annual report is used in conjunction with global unit reports, it provides an indication of the proportion of funds used by a unit, and it should be read conscientiously so that nursing unit managers are informed of the costs of providing health services.

Many methodologies are available, and are an important resource base for the nurse manager for the evaluation of financial performance. Included are:

☐ financial auditing;

☐ case-mix costing and budgeting;

☐ cost-benefit analysis;

☐ cost-effective analysis;

☐ budget adjustment for inflation, changes in technologies and case-mix;

☐ linking of budgets with patient service data.

However Johnson (1987) emphasises that in US health care organisations, as yet 'concurrence among nurses about the value of costing nursing services does not include agreement about how to cost and price those services'. So far, five methods: 'global, DRG-based, patient-acuity based, procedure based and relative intensity measures (RIMs) are used'.

Financial management falls within the rational-structural quadrant of the model for evaluation and the reader is referred to listed texts for further information. Even though it is important for nursing unit managers to be mindful of costs it is even more important that the relationship of costs to quality is examined.

# **10.** EVALUATING THE QUALITY OF CARE

## 10.1 QUALITY ASSURANCE

One of the most significant advances in health care over the past 10 years has been the advent of quality assurance (WHO, 1989). The concern for assuring quality is directly related to our understanding of the role evaluation plays in service provision and development (Westbrook, 1990). High quality services are the benchmark by which an organisation's mission is realised. If quality cannot be maintained, then the likelihood of mission attainment is reduced. If a nurse manager is to be committed to a health service mission then a detailed knowledge of quality assurance principles and methods is required.

Quality assurance cuts across the structure, process and output of a health care organisation. As it is both structurally and functionally based, and can be realised through both rational and intuitive methods, it is a comprehensive system of evaluation for the nurse manager. Another important feature of quality assurance is that it can be structured as a system of continuous evaluation. In the past, evaluation frequently has been time limited and programme specific, leading to a minimal input in the process by nursing staff.

In quality assurance, unlike pure evaluation, goals and objectives are translated into standards and criteria as a means of evaluating the merit of a service. A standard is a prescribed level of excellence necessary for goal accomplishment. Criteria are the objective elements of the standards by which the merit of the service will be judged. Standards can be defined as necessary truths or as conditional truths. They can be rationally or empirically derived depending on the issue of concern. They can be based on local expectations, or they can be nationally or internationally based. The World Health Organization Working Group on Quality Assurance (1989) states that

four particular components must be addressed in any effort to develop an effective statement of the objectives or content of quality assurance activities:

☐ professional performance (technical quality);

☐ resource use (efficiency);

☐ risk management (the risk of injury or illness associated with the service provided);

☐ patient satisfaction with the services provided.

Generally, in the hospital context, quality assurance measures can be divided into two forms. The first form is performance indicators (Roberts, 1985; Arnold, 1989). These generally are the outcome measures of adverse events — an 'illness or injury associated with the service provided' — occurring in hospitals. They are generally discrete statistics and are reported as incidence rates. The definition of incidence is the new occurrence of an adverse event within a specific time period. The denominator used can either be the number of cases treated or the number of bed days occupied, depending on the type of indicator. Prevalence rates are sometimes used instead of, or in conjunction with, incidence rates when the event may occupy two or more time periods. In such cases it is important, when comparisons are made, that incidence for one time period is not compared with prevalence in another time period. The two sets of rates would give different results with prevalence rates always being higher. Prevalence rates are only useful when it is important to know if a condition is persisting over time. For example, decubiti prevalence rates may be helpful in determining if a particular nursing intervention or medical treatment is working.

The most commonly used performance indicators are:

☐ patient morbidity;

☐ patient mortality;

☐ adverse patient events (ie, falls, medication, administration errors or decubiti);

☐ adverse staff events (ie, needle pricks, stress, or job satisfaction);

☐ staff turnover;

☐ workload (ie, patient acuity or nurse dependency);

☐ infection control (ie, wound acquired infections or hospital acquired infections);

☐ patient complaints;

☐ patient satisfaction.

Performance indicators are useful for determining trends and comparing rates between and within wards against quantifiable standards. They, however, require a rigorous collection system and rely on the care giver to report adverse events to a central agency. They also require that a central agency report trends in an intelligible way to the source of the problem so that corrective processes can be put in place. As such, the report quality can often be low and significant under-reporting can occur.

The second type of quality assurance measures are audits. Audits are a means of measuring standards by asking questions about associated criteria. Two of the best known audits are the Phaneuf audit (Phaneuf, 1976:191–211) and the Rush-Medicus Audit (Jelinek et al 1975). Raters judge structure, process and outcome to assess whether criteria have been met. Audits can be performed retrospectively or concurrently. A retrospective audit is one that is performed 'after the event'. The audit is taken from the medical record and attempts to assess criteria on the basis of historical evidence. Concurrent auditing is performed 'while the event occurs'. The audit can be of the environment, the activities of practitioners, the knowledge of the practitioner, the state of the patient, or the records and clinical measures taken.

Retrospective audits are useful because they enable the identification of standards across a large number of health service units and subsequently allow the setting of reasonable and achievable standards. They are limited because they rely on accurate clinical record keeping. They are expensive as they are time consuming and it is difficult to achieve reliability when untrained raters are used. Another weakness is that the results of the audit are not fed back immediately after the event. This delays negative reinforcement of undesired practices and the positive reinforcement of desired practices.

Concurrent audits have the advantage of communicating results immediately to care givers. They, however, can be adversely affected by the 'Hawthorn effect' (Roethlisberger and Dickson, 1939). This occurs when a subject who is being observed alters behaviour on the basis of what is believed to be expected. Moreover, the auditors may be influenced to change their assessment on the basis of the expectation of an acceptable result by care givers, the 'Rosenthal effect' (Rosenthal, 1966).

Audits are a conventional way of assessing quality, and useful tools if their reliability and validity is established and if both types are counter-balanced so that evidence is corroborated. They can be performed internally within the structure of a health service unit by the nurse manager or a delegated practitioner or they can be performed externally by an expert team. Whatever the chief focus in an organisation, it is important that at regular intervals audits are checked against independent measures to ensure that they are measuring what they are intended to measure: this is called validity. Equally important is the checking of the audit to ensure that it measures the same event consistently between auditors: this is called reliability.

## 10.2 RISK MANAGEMENT

A related development in quality assurance has been risk management. This development emerged out of the highly litigious environment of American health care. Risk management aims to minimise the risk of adverse patient outcomes during a hospital stay (Craddick and Bader, 1983; Pena et al, 1984). It also aims to minimise risks to hospital-employed staff and to visitors. By reducing the possibility of adverse outcomes, it is believed that the cost associated with litigation and workers' compensation claims will be reduced. Risk management is a proactive approach where indicators are used to identify areas of potential litigation and so reduce the danger of adverse occurrences by planning more efficient and effective services. It targets the total health care environment. Quality indicators are used to target unsafe work practices, imperfectly operating equipment, and the organisation of the health service environment to try to ensure safety for all.

## 10.3 TOTAL QUALITY MANAGEMENT

Quality assurance in its most modern form places participatory management as the focus of improving standards. Quality assurance only works when workers have a commitment to improving the quality of their input. This is dependent on an organisational culture that promotes and reinforces leadership through initiative and risk taking. An extension of risk management is the concept of total quality management (TQM) (Sprouster, 1987; Oakland, 1989; Koska, 1990). The essence of TQM is that we all serve one another. We each provide services to our patients, our colleagues and ourselves. We also receive services from others. The provision of a service or a product is a balance between quality and cost. TQM is also based on the concept that continuous improvement is possible.

An essential aspect of the process of TQM is 'variance analysis'. Variance analysis is the evaluation of services against predetermined standards. Services are said to meet customer requirements and to increase satisfaction when there are low system-failure costs. These costs are also known as 'poor quality costs'. When work has to be repeated because it does not meet a standard, costs are increased. Standards are derived by expert opinion and by customer demand. The quantitative comparison of standards against service provides the means for variance analysis. This is a statistical process dependent on reliable data collection. When there is a match between standards and service, quality is high and variance is low. When there is no match between standards and service, quality is low and variance may be either high or low depending on the variability of the services (Figure 2.3.2).

A recent innovation is the concept of quality circles (Adair et al, 1982; Johnson, 1985; Goldberg and Pegels, 1984). They are a means of all workers within a unit meeting regularly to solve a specific problem that has been identified by quality monitoring, or ad hoc problem identification. The aim of the circle is worker participation in problem identification and resolution and the improvement of the efficacy and efficiency of work. The quality circles work well in a system where leadership and initiative are encouraged and reinforced, and where risk taking is promoted. They require workers who have a genuine commitment to improving their work and managers who are prepared to act as 'sponsors' for continuous quality improvement (McLaughlin and Kaluzny, 1990).

A crucial element of quality assurance is that it be generally non-punitive. It aims to achieve the highest possible standard of health care by providing feedback and encouraging practitioners to be actively involved in problem solving. Through the use of quality circles, workers can become actively involved in reaching their own potential as well as positively contributing to their patients' care. Importantly, McLaughlin and Kaluzny (1990) warn that TQM, of which quality circles are a component, represents a 'fundamental paradigm shift' in health care management and this can create conflict in the organisation. These authors present 11 actions for successfully managing the

FIGURE 2.3.2:   The relationship between variance and satisfaction with services

|  | | Service satisfaction | |
|---|---|---|---|
|  | | High | Low |
| Variance | High | False quality | False disquality |
|  | Low | True high quality | True low quality |

implementation of TQM and theirarticle is suggested reading for all interested in this issue.

# 11. PROGRAMME EVALUATION

Until now we have examined the nature and purpose of evaluation and looked at the ways nursing unit managers can evaluate a nursing unit. A more formal type of evaluation that has not yet been explored in this chapter is programme evaluation. When planners decide that a particular health service programme is to be implemented, it is generally based on some form of needs identification, service requirement deficiency or vested interests. Needs are generally identified from the opinions and scientific investigations of experts in the field. For example, it may be the opinion of surgical experts that a cardiac surgery programme is needed because of the high incidence of angina within a community. Service requirement deficiency is generally based on a demand for a service, which can come from scientific opinions of experts or from the community groups who lobby for the service because it appears to have a high value for that community. This demand may be seen to be rational or irrational depending on the perspectives of those concerned, for example, demand for neonatal ICU beds as opposed to concern for the conditions which result in neonates requiring ICUs.

Groups with vested interests work through the media, formal and informal networks, and liaisons with political parties to have their valued programme implemented. Whatever the case, planners and funding agencies are keenly interested in knowing whether the planned programme will be effective, beneficial and efficient. Therefore, part of the planning process includes a systematic assessment of a programme's worth.

This form of evaluation is referred to as one-shot evaluation. Before funding can be provided for a new programme, it is necessary to assess its merit (Craig, 1978). The steps in programme evaluation are the same as those with any other form of evaluation. A mission is identified, goals and objectives are stated and refined, and resources are allocated. The programme is implemented and its merit is judged through the examination of structure, process and outcome to determine if there is a match between what is achieved and what it was intended to achieve.

# 12. THE LINK BETWEEN EVALUATION AND NURSING UNIT MANAGEMENT

Nurses function in a health care culture that is changing at a rate faster than it ever has in the recorded history of humanity. The explosion in knowledge that has occurred in the biological and social sciences has made health care services more efficacious and complex. The opportunities for improvements in health in western industrialised societies have never been greater. Many diseases that once were life threatening are now relatively easy to cure or control.

Public health measures have done much to bring about this dramatic improvement. The context in which the nurse mainly works, the hospital, has also benefited from advances in health care science and technology. Modern surgical and medical techniques have reduced the invasiveness of many treatments. Patient stays in hospitals have been dramatically reduced so that illness treatment only minimally disrupts a patient's personal and social functioning.

However, while the vast majority of individuals experience improved health, a number of disease states and risk groups continue to present a challenge for health service provision. These disease states are coronary heart disease; lung, bowel and sexual organ cancer; arteriosclerosis; cerebral vascular accidents; trauma; diabetes; hypertension; mental illness and arthritis. The risk groups are individuals with underdeveloped or impaired psychomotor abilities; cigarette smokers; alcohol abusers; youthful motor vehicle users; obese people; consumers of high fat diets; and the frail aged. Many of the factors associated with these disease states and risk groups are amenable to preventive and public health strategies. Unfortunately many are also associated with an ageing population and continue to have a high prevalence in modern societies. Public Health is discussed in more depth in chapter 2.4.

Nursing as a professional health care discipline has a responsibility to respond to the changing nature of community health needs. It also has a duty to develop the personal potential of members within the profession. These responsibilities are best achieved by meeting social and personal health care needs in a dynamic, fully functioning and caring organisation. To achieve this with a high level of competence and proficiency, the profession must be involved in the planning and evaluation process that is part of managing health care organisations.

It has often been claimed that knowledge is power. Intuitively, this proposition has great appeal. If we examine those professional disciplines that command the greatest influence in our society then it can be reasonably deduced that power does truly come from knowledge and its application. However, scientific knowledge about the need for nursing care, the way in which nursing care is delivered and the effect of nursing care is limited. Nurses have always been practical people responding to patient needs through the commands of doctors, administrators and the dictates of routine. Limited scientific investigation and a practical orientation have restricted the power and influence of nurses in the health care system (Turner, 1985; McCoppin, 1989).

The inception of the nursing process was an attempt to elaborate on nursing practice by implanting a logistic framework. Studies into the efficacy of the process are, however, limited and it is still difficult to determine whether nursing care has any impact on improving the health of society. Nurses have not been required traditionally to demonstrate the efficacy of their work. It has been taken as given that nursing is in some way beneficial. Commonsense dictates that nursing care is a necessary and important component of health and illness care. In fact patients only stay in hospitals when nursing care is indicated. If nursing is to be recognised as a highly qualified profession, then systematic research and evaluation are required into what nurses do that makes a difference to health care outcomes.

If nursing is a response to the much larger human need, to be cared about and to be provided for when not capable of providing for oneself, then its value may be intrinsic. This, however, is a 'motherhood' notion of nursing. Humans grow, function, recover from illness, and respond to disability, distress and death when a caring other is present to plan and implement care. Nursing is part of a continuum of human benevolence that commences with the mothering of infants and ceases with the acceptance of death. Nursing, therefore, emerges out of the need for human societies to organise care for those who are not able to meet their own needs.

One of the features of modern technological societies is that cultural demands have fragmented the role agrarian family support played in the fulfilment of the need for care.

Consequently the demand for nurses and their care has exponentially grown. The nursing organisation has not, however, been considered an independent discipline. It has largely been under the direction of the medical profession, which has been the basic source for the contract between the patient and the health system. Given this professional dominance, nursing has been viewed as having no specific scientific focus of its own. The responsibilities for the great discoveries in health have been left to the doctors. Not surprisingly the medical profession has prospered and grown as a result. It has not, however, entirely been without costs and losses. Nursing has tended to lose its control over its own density. The access to the spirit of enquiry and discovery has been reduced by a profession whose only requirement was to follow orders.

A feature of the management of the health care system in the past has been its highly regimented approach to organising nurses. Nursing administrators and educators rigorously trained young impressionable women to follow orders regardless of personal thought and values. 'Mine is not to question why, mine is but to do or die' epitomised the call of nurses. As subservient female inferiors, no trust could be accorded to these young women. The regimentation of hospitals through medical command and managerial edict has, in the past, limited a nurse's capacity to actively participate in the planning of health services.

Improvements in the liberties of women and changes in nurses' educational status have meant that health service organisations are examining means of increasing nurses' input into the planning process. A chance now exists for nurses in leadership positions to become involved in assessing and evaluating the service they co-ordinate. This opportunity will only be realised, however, if nursing unit managers become committed to systematic evaluation.

Questions of the efficacy, effectiveness, cost, benefit and appropriateness of nursing care cannot be ignored. We cannot simply rely on a traditional role in health care without demonstrating that what nurses do is of a special nature and high merit. These questions require diligent consideration and a commitment to a rigorous process of inquiry to ensure truthful and valid answers. Nurses have always demonstrated a capacity to create novel solutions to difficult problems. The responses of many patients are testimonies to the intrinsic values of nursing. However, ask nurses to explain what it is that they do that helps a patient and you will receive varied answers, many of which are opinions not verified by evidence from systematic inquiry.

This difficulty in examining the merit of nursing has been explained away by allusions to the contextual and intuitive nature of nursing. However, it is believed that nursing increases comfort and promotes healing. There is no reason to believe that, if this is the case, nursing cannot and should not subject itself to systematic enquiry based on the principals and methods of evaluation. Health care by its very nature is multi-disciplinary, and consequently, it is difficult to extract the nursing care process and examine it in isolation from the work of other health professions. Nonetheless, until nursing is extracted and examined in isolation, the relative weight of its contribution to health care will not be known. Therefore enquiry that focuses on the value of nursing care is a professional responsibility. If the value of nursing can be demonstrated, it will provide nurses with the confidence required to attain resources and shape the type of health care that will be provided in the future (Tierney et al, 1990). Increased automony and professional recognition are potential gains for nurses. More importantly, patients stand to gain from improved nursing care resulting from discarding poor practice and improving sub-standard practice.

Evaluation principals and methods provide the nurse manager with a means of examining and understanding the care that is being provided. If applied systematically and rigorously, they will help in determining the merit of nursing's contribution to health. Evaluation should not, however, be implemented as a means of point scoring or doctor bashing. Nursing occupies a symbiotic relationship with the patients, doctors and other carers in the health system. The mission of a health service organisation can only be completely fulfilled if the relationship is allowed to mature and fully function.

The nurse manager has the potential to play an integral role in the attainment of effective patient outcomes. As the co-ordinator and potential evaluator of patient care services, the nurse manager integrates the services of the nurse, the doctor, other health professionals and the health care organisation so that optimal care is achieved. This is a very powerful position that is easily abused when decisions are based on unfounded opinions.

The models and methods of evaluation presented in this chapter equip the nurse manager with the tools to be an informed planner and decision maker. Therefore evaluation is a means of ensuring that the management of health care systems at the unit level remains a nursing initiative.

# SUMMARY

Evaluation using the Donabedian model of structure, process and outcome is described in this chapter. An explanation of what evaluation is, why it is used and its importance to nursing care is included. The evaluation process equips the manager with information on the efficiency and effectiveness of the patient care services provided. It is suggested that there are four evaluation perspectives, the structural, the functional, the rational and the intuitive and their effect on the construction of knowledge and the evaluation process is examined. The methods of 'multiple triangulation', formative and summative evaluation and their contribution to global evaluation is discussed. The issue of performance appraisal and its advantages and disadvantages in staff assessment is raised. Within the hospital the two prevalent forms of quality assurance, performance indicators and quality audits, are discussed in depth as is the relationship of risk management to the quality assurance process. Risk management is seen as a proactive approach which is part of a total quality management programme which when properly implemented reduces the possibility of accidents and adverse outcomes to patients, staff and hospital visitors. The importance of all nurses being actively involved in evaluating the service they provide is emphasised throughout the chapter.

# MALLEE CASE STUDY

You are the Director of Nursing of a major teaching hospital and have been asked to evaluate the nursing division of Mallee District Hospital, a 250 bed hospital in a large country town. Mallee Hospital has 120 general medical/surgical beds, an accident and emergency unit, a paediatric ward, intensive care unit, adolescent, maternity and rehabilitation units and a day only ward. The hospital is situated in a growth area because of the recent opening of a carpet factory which plans to use the coarse wools grown in the surrounding countryside. The factory has attracted many of the smaller farmers and farm-workers who have moved into town to join their workforce. The increase in population has also led to the expansion of the shopping centre and the provision of new amenities such as an indoor bowling and recreation centre. It has also created a demand for increased health care services and has resulted in the addition of 50 beds and the building of a Community Health Centre adjacent to the hospital. As a result of the additions to the hospital a paediatrician, a second obstetrician and a geriatrician, all of whom have only recently gained their specialist qualifications, have been attracted to the town.

The Director of Nursing of Mallee Hospital, Miss P. Pritchard, was appointed 19 years ago. You have met her several times at seminars and at the Annual General Meetings of the Institute of Nursing Service Administrators. She has always seemed to you to be very dogmatic, as evidenced by the eager way in which she voices her opinions at these meetings, even though much of what she has to say is not backed up by supportive evidence. You have heard rumours recently that there has been open conflict between the new CEO and the Director of Nursing.

The CEO is a much younger man who replaced the retiring administrator, Mr Bill Boulder, 10 months ago. The CEO, Mr Lo Pang, graduated with you 12 months before with a Master of Health Administration degree. This is his second appointment as a CEO. The first appointment was to Crowea, a 60 bed hospital in a small country town of the same name which is noted for its fine Poll Hereford cattle. Despite strong initial resistance from the townspeople to his appointment, they were sorry to see him go as they were grateful for the improvements, such as the rehabilitation department, day centre and nursing home, that he had been instrumental in getting for Crowea Hospital. Lo Pang had also served diligently on the parents and citizens, church, Apex and Rotary committees and his efforts for the organisations would be sorely missed. Since coming to Mallee he had been encouraged to join similar organisations and only last month was elected president of the Mallee High School parents and citizens association.

You have heard from the Regional Nursing Officer, who agreed to Lo Pang's request for a consultant to undertake an evaluation, that Lo Pang has been dissatisfied with Miss Pritchard's performance as a director because of her inability to present any data from which the executive of the hospital can obtain information to make decisions. The CEO is also having similar difficulties with the Administrator of Medical Services, Dr Davids, who is close to retirement. There is no Quality Assurance or Peer Review Programme at the hospital and when Lo Pang asked to view the policies and procedures manuals at a recent executive meeting he found that these were disorganised and outdated. Dr Davids and Miss Pritchard have been close friends for many years and consider they have been running their divisions as well as could be expected with limited funds. Recently they have received a number of complaints from the newly appointed specialists and their registrars regarding

outmoded and poorly maintained equipment. The CEO has also complained about the size of the ambulance bill for transport of patients to the city, 104 kilometres away, for CT scans, haemo-dialysis and the like. The Department of Health has also recently notified all CEOs that DRGs are to be introduced by July 1993 as a management tool and as a first step costing centres must be established for each department.

The Regional Nursing Officer had also received a complaint from the CEO that there appeared to be few, if any, nursing care plans or nursing histories written, the nursing budget was overspent by $800 000 and the length of stay in the intensive care ward had increased by 2.4 days. The doctors and patients were also complaining about the delays in the outpatients department and in the admission of patients to the wards. The doctors were blaming the nurses whom they said were poorly organised and appeared to have little knowledge of recent innovations in either medicine or nursing. The nursing staff at Mallee comprised one third RNs and two thirds ENAs and the greater proportion of them had served the hospital for many years, many of them having trained at Mallee when it was a registered nurse training school.

---

1. Describe in no more than 4000 words how you would carry out the evaluation of the nursing services over a three day period. Include the time frame you would allow for each stage of the project, the people you would talk to, the records you would investigate, where you would carry out your investigations and what recommendations you would make to the CEO and the Board of Mallee Hospital.

# REFERENCES AND FURTHER READING

Adair, M., Fitzgerald, M., Nygard, K. and Shaffer, F. (1982), *Quality circles in nursing,* National League for Nursing, New York.

Arnold, C. (1989), 'Performance indicators — can you afford not to have them? Royal Children's Hospital a structured approach', *Australian Health Review,* 219–231.

Australian Congress of Mental Health Nurses (1985), *Standards of mental health nursing practice,* ACMHN, Greenacres, SA.

Bain, C. (1986), 'Cardiovascular disease: a preventable epidemic', *Community Health Studies,* 10:310–403.

Beck, S. (1990), 'Developing a primary nursing performance appraisal tool', *Nursing Management,* 21 (1):36–42.

Benner, P. (1984), *From novice to expert: excellence and power in clinical nursing practice,* Addison-Wesley, California.

Burrell, G. and Morgan, G. (1982), *Sociological paradigms and organisational analysis: elements of the sociology of corporate life,* Gower, Aldershot, England.

Calder, N. (1979), *Einstein's universe: the layman's guide,* Penguin, Harmondsworth, England.

Capp, S. (1988), 'Economics, dollar and nursing practice', *Australian Health Review,* 11, 186–196.

Chinn, P. L. and Jacobs, M. K., (1983), *Theory and nursing: a systematic approach,* C. V. Mosby, St Louis.

Christian, J. L. (1981), *Philosophy: an introduction to the art of wondering,* 3rd edition, Holt, Rinehart & Winston, New York.

Cohen, M. Z. (1987), 'A historical overview of the phenomenological movement', *Image,* 19:31–34.

Costello, S. and Summers, B. Y. (1985), 'Documenting patient care: getting it all together', *Nursing Management,* 16 (6):31–34.

Craddick, J. W. and Bader, B. S. (1983), *Medical management analysis: a systematic approach to quality assurance and risk management volume 1: an introduction,* Joyce W. Craddick, California.

Craig, D. P. (1978), *Hip pocket guide to planning and evaluation,* Learning Concepts, San Diego.

Cuthbert, M. (1983), 'Patient classification for nurse staffing', No. 52 in *Australian Studies in Health Service Administration,* School of Health Administration, University of NSW, Kensington.

Cuthbert, M. (1990), 'Utilisation of clinical costing, *Proceedings of effective health care management conference,* 8 November, Sydney.

Darwin, C. (1964), *On the origin of the species by means of natural selection,* Harvard University Press, Cambridge, Mass.

Dewar, D. L. (1980), *The quality circle guide to participant management,* Prentice-Hall, Englewood Cliffs, NJ.

Donabedian, A. (1966), 'Evaluating the quality of medical care', *Millbank Memorial Fund Quarterly,* 44:166–206.

Donabedian, A. (1968), 'Promoting quality through evaluating the process of patient care', *Medical Care,* VI, 2:181–202.

Donabedian, A. (1969), 'Part II — some issues in evaluating the quality of nursing care', *American Journal of Public Health,* 59, 10:1833–1836.

Donovan, M. I. and Lewis, G. (1987), 'Costs of nursing services. Are the assumptions valid? *Nursing Administration Quarterly,* 12 (1):1–12.

Drummond, M. F. (1984), *Principles of economic appraisal in health care,* Oxford University Press, Oxford.

Duberley, J. (1979), 'Giving nursing care', in Kratz, C. R. (Ed), *The nursing process,* Baillière Tindall, London.

Glassner, B. and Freedman, J. (1979), *Clinical sociology,* Longman, New York.

Goldberg, A. M. and Pegels, C. C. (1984), *Quality circles in health care facilities,* Rockville, Aspen.

Gorovitz, S., Hintikka, M., Provence, D. and Williams, R. (1979), *Philosophical analysis: an introduction to its language and techniques,* Random House, New York.

Green, J., Adams, A., Nelson, S. and Aisbett, K. (1986), 'Evaluating hospital ward designs in use: report of a comparative study of the effects of hospital ward design on nursing staff performance and user satisfaction', No. 58 in *Australian Studies in Health Service Administration,* School of Health Administration, University of NSW, Kensington.

Hill, D. and Gray, N. (1984), 'Australian patterns of tobacco smoking and related health beliefs', *Community Health Studies,* 8:307–316.

Jelinek, R. C., Haussmann, R. K. D., Hegyvary, S. T. and Newsman, J. F. (1975), *A methodology for monitoring quality of nursing care,* U.S. Department of Health, Education, and Welfare, Maryland.

Johnson, L. (1987), 'Performance appraisal', Forceps, Snippets & ACORN News, June, 21–26.

Johnson, S. (1985), 'Quality control circles: negotiating an efficient work environment', Nursing Management, July, 16 (7):34A–34G.

Keegan, C. J. (1990), 'Implementation of clinical budgeting in a public teaching hospital — first steps', *Australian Health Review,* 13 (1): 45–51.

Kelly, L. Y. (1981), *Dimensions of professional nursing,* 4th edition, Macmillan, New York.

Koska, M. T. (1990), 'Quality watch — adopting Deming's quality improvement ideas: a case study', *Hospitals,* July 5: 58–64.

Lansbury, R. D. (1981), *Performance appraisal,* Macmillan, Melbourne.

Lawler, T. G. (1988), 'The objectives of performance appraisal — or "where can we go from here?"', *Nursing Management,* 19 (3):82–88.

Lessnoff, M. (1979), *The structure of social science: a philosophical introduction,* (Studies in Sociology: 7), Allen & Unwin, London.

Long, R. (1981), *Systematic nursing care,* Faber & Faber, London.

Marker, C. G. S. (1988), 'Practical tools for quality assurance. Criteria development sheet and data retrieval form', *Journal of Nursing Quality Assurance,* 2 (2): 43–54.

McCoppin, B. (1989), 'The use and abuse of industrial power — the profession's dilemma', in Gray, G. & Pratt, R. (Eds), *Issues in Australian nursing 2,* Churchill Livingstone, Melbourne.

McFarland, G. K., Leonard, H. S. and Morris, M. M. (1984), *Nursing leadership and management: contemporary strategies,* John Wiley & Sons, New York.

McLaughlin, C. P. and Kaluzny, A. D. (1990), 'Total quality management in health: making it work', *Health Care Management Review,* 15, 3, 7–14.

Menon, M. (1990), 'Migrant nurses: cross cultural understanding or misunderstanding', Paper delivered at the Nursing Research Conference, Adelaide.

Mintzberg, H. (1983), *Structures in fives: designing effective organisations,* Prentice-Hall, New Jersey.

Murray, R. B. and Zentner, J. P. (1985), *Nursing concepts for health promotion,* 3rd edition, Prentice-Hall, New Jersey.

Murphy, S. A. (1989), 'Multiple triangulation: applications in a program of nursing research', *Nursing Research,* 38: 294–297.

Nadzam, D. M. (1987), 'Documentation evaluation system: streamlining quality of care and personnel evaluations', *Nursing Management,* 18 (11): 38–42.

Oakland, J. S. (1989), *Total quality management,* Heinemann, Oxford.

Paturi, F. R. (1978), *Nature, mother of invention: the engineering of plant life,* Harmondsworth, England, Pelican Books.

Pelletier, L. R. and Poster, E. C. (1988), 'Part 1: an overview of evaluation methodology for nursing quality assurance programs', *Journal of Nursing Quality Assurance,* 2 (4), 55–62.

Pena, J. J., Hoffner, A. N., Rosen, B. and Light, D. W. (1984), *Hospital quality assurance: risk management and program evaluation,* Rockville, Aspen.

Peters, T. and Austin, N. (1985), *A passion for excellence: the leadership difference,* Fontana/Collins, Glasgow.

Phaneuf, M. C. (1976), *The nursing audit: self-regulation in nursing practice,* 2nd edition, Appleton-Century-Crofts, New York.

Puetz, B. E. (1983), *Networking for nurses,* Rockville, Aspen.

Rapoport, J., Robertson, R. L. and Stuart, B. (1982), 'Economic evaluation of health programs', in *Understanding health economics,* Rockville, Aspen.

Renwick, M. and Harvey, R. (1989) 'Quality assurance in hospitals: report of a survey, Canberra', Australian Government Publishing Service.

Renwick, M. and Harvey, R. (1989), 'The organisation of quality assurance in Australian hospitals', *Australian Health Review,* 12 (3), 16–27.

Richards, F. A. and Commons, M. L. (1990), 'Post formal cognitive-developmental theory and research: a review of its current status', in Alexander, C. N. and Langer, E. J. (Eds), *Higher stages of human development,* Oxford University Press, New York.

Roberts, R. (1985), 'Hospital performance indicators: development of an index of hospital performance using negative outcomes', thesis submitted for the Degree of Master of Public Health, University of Sydney.

Roethlisberger, F. J. and Dickson, W. J. (1939), *Management and the worker,* Harvard University Press, Cambridge, Mass.

Rosenthal, R. (1966), *Experimenter effects in behavioural research,* Appleton-Century-Crofts, New York.

Russell, B. (1980), *History of western philosophy: and its connection with political and social circumstances from the earliest times to the present day,* Unwin paperbacks, London.

Sprouster, J. (1987), *TQC-Total Quality Control: the Australian experience,* Second Revised edition, Horwitz Grahame, Cammeray.

Stoner, J. A. F., Collins, R. R. and Yetton, P. (1985), *Management in Australia,* 2nd edition, Prentice-Hall, New Jersey.

Sullivan, E. J. and Decker, P. J. (1985), *Effective management in nursing,* Addison-Wesley, California.

Tierney, M. J., Grant, L. M. and Mazique, S. I. (1990), 'Cost accountability and clinical nurse specialist evaluation', *Nursing Management,* 21 (5):26–31.

Turner, B. S. (1985), 'Knowledge, skill and occupational strategy: the professionalisation of paramedical groups', *Community Health Studies, IX, (1):38–47.*

Toth, J. C. and Ritchey, K. A. (1984), 'New from nursing research: the Basic Knowledge Assessment Tool (BKAT) for critical care nursing', *Heart and Lung,* 13, 272–279.

Warnock, M. (1979), *Existentialism,* Oxford University Press, Oxford.

Watson, J. D. (1977), *Molecular biology of the gene,* 3rd edition, W. A. Benjamin, California.

Watson, T. J. (1986), *Management, organisation and employment strategy: new directions in theory and practice,* Rutledge & Keegan Paul, London.

Westbrook, J. (1990), 'Quality assurance in Australia and NSW in 1990: we have come a long way', *AQA Newsletter,* 1, 6–8.

WHO Working Group. (1989), 'The principles of quality assurance', *Quality Assurance in Health Care,* 1, 79–95.

# Care in the community

SHIRLEY SCHULZ

In this chapter it is intended to discuss:

1. the major challenges inherent in caring for people in the community;

2. ways in which nurses (managers and practitioners) might encourage self care and autonomy;

3. the significance of age and culture in providing care in the community;

4. the importance of establishing professional/community networks;

5. relationships between carers and recipients of care;

6. analysis of how community resources might be established and/or utilised by health care workers.

> There are three kinds of people;
> Those who make things happen;
> Those who watch things happen;
> Those who wonder what happened.
>
> Anonymous/F.V.R.

This chapter has three major aims: (1) to outline issues of concern to community nurses who seek to provide a quality service to those individuals, families and communities with whom they work; (2) to discuss the implications for nurses of primary health care, and (3) to suggest ways in which nurse managers (that is, leaders) can provide an environment that supports nurses in their attempt to promote health in keeping with the principles of 'health for all by the year 2000'. For general ease of expression the term 'nurse' will be used throughout. The issues, save those directed specifically at community nursing contexts, are relevant to all nurses.

# 1. EXPANSION OF COMMUNITY CARE

In Australia, community nursing has focused on the needs of the aged, the very young and women of child-bearing age, providing personal or clinical services for the aged, screening for school children and babies, and health education for mothers. With the trend to deinstitutionalisation and emphasis on care in the community, the services expanded in the 1960s to include people with developmental disabilities or chronic mental illness, and their families. Emphasis was given to the needs of chronically ill and disabled persons. Services for the different client groups were administered separately (and often paternalistically) until the 1970s when a national community health programe was introduced, emphasising service integration, the development of multi-disciplinary teams and a change in orientation towards community participation, self care and prevention.

As governments and health services respond to demands for community based care and attempt to limit costs, there will be an increasing number of people being maintained at home or discharged from hospital, yet requiring nursing care. The needs of this new clientele for complex nursing care, often technical and possibly long term, will need to be addressed. The question facing nurse managers, regardless of where or with which population they work, will be how best to use the human and financial resources available to them to improve the health of populations. Central to this question is the need to address the current confusion and divergence of thought regarding the dimensions of community nursing practice. This issue is especially important as the need for community nurses will increase (Mahler, 1981) and more nurses lacking experience or knowledge of community nursing will be required to practise in this area. In the future, nurse managers will bear responsibility for managing resources and providing staff with the leadership and professional support required to practise effectively as community nurses within an environment of limited financial resources and increasing requests for nursing care. Nurse managers thus have a responsibility for managing a service to meet the needs of two communities: the community in which they are based, and their staff.

For many nurse managers, the concern will be whether to continue to provide personal clinical services or whether to focus on health promotion and disease prevention, seeing the question as requiring a decision in favour of one approach or the other. Others, coming to the decision that both clinical services and health promotion are essential, will find that another issue arises: which activity is to be given priority? Clinical services, aimed at individuals and families, or health promotion which focuses on the whole community? These questions simplistically reflect the confusion and divergence of thought that exists regarding the scope of community nursing. Such questions are therefore significant and need to be addressed by individual teams, as the answers influence the practice-orientation of nurses employed in a particular service. Assistance in exploring these questions can be gained from the World Health Organisation's (WHO) 'health for all' (HFA) policy which both poses a challenge and points to a way out of the confusion for nurses and nurse managers.

# 2. HEALTH FOR ALL: A FRAMEWORK FOR COMMUNITY NURSING

In 1986 the World Health Organisation, in recognition of the increasing disparity in health status between and within nations, declared that the main goal for all governments would be 'health for all by the year 2000'. Primary health care, outlined in the Declaration of Alma Ata in 1978, was identified as the key to achieving this goal. This concept is based on seven principles:

☐ the right and duty of individuals and communities to become self-reliant and participate in matters concerning their health;

☐ that health programmes reflect and evolve from the unique social, economic and political situation of each country;

☐ that health programmes address the main health problems and integrate preventive, curative and rehabilitative services;

☐ that health workers work as a team to respond to the expressed health needs of populations;

☐ that programmes are based on relevant research findings;

☐ that governments and health professionals have a responsibility to provide information about health to the public; and

☐ that primary health care relates to other sectors of national and community development (WHO/UNICEF cited by International Council of Nursing 1986:4).

According to Mahler (1981:7–8), the three prerequisites for primary health care are 'a multi-sectoral approach, community involvement and appropriate technology. A multi-sectoral approach recognises that health issues are embedded in questions of social conditions. For instance, people's health is endangered by such conditions as 'unemployment (and underemployment), poverty, a low level of education, poor housing, malnutrition and lack of will and initiative to make changes for the better'. Health requires removal of such restraints. In identifying the principles of primary health care, the Alma Ata declaration re-affirmed health as a fundamental human right and a desirable social goal. The WHO defined health as 'a state of complete physical, mental and social well-being, and not merely the absence of disease or infirmity'. Far from implying that all persons will be well, this definition recognises the social nature of health, acknowledging that achievement of health requires action on the part of all sectors of society; social, economic, environmental and health.

The thrust of primary health care is that health services need to emphasise health rather than illness. Given the curative, illness orientation of health services in Australia, implementation requires a reorientation of our thinking, from the present disease (medical) focus to one which recognises that environment, individual behaviour and socio-economic conditions are major determinants of health. This broader view is reflected in the emphasis primary health care places on health promotion and disease prevention, the adoption of appropriate technology, the integration of all aspects of care, and co-operation between professionals and communities. Using such a model, individuals, families and communities form the basis of the health system and primary care workers become the central health workers (Mahler 1981:7). As a signatory to the Alma Ata Declaration, Australia has a commitment to achieve health for all and to advocate health, equity and intersectoral co-operation.

The International Council of Nursing, supportive of the principles of primary health care, has affirmed the commitment of nurses to effect changes in 'nursing education, practice and management' necessary for implementation. This implicitly broadens nurses' responsibilities to include involvement in health planning and decision making (ICN/WHO 1979 cited in ICN 1986). Opportunities therefore exist to redefine the role of nurses and increase their scope of practice. As Styles argued at the International Congress of Nursing's 17th Quadrennial Congress in 1981, primary health care is relevant to nurses, being

> a universal concept with infinite adaptability to any region, any culture, any stage of development. It appeals to us because it speaks a common language, it represents values long held by nurses, and it is immensely practical ... Primary health care begins with the admission that the prevalent pattern which emphasises sophisticated and costly tertiary institutions and highly specialised professionals does not work. This dissatisfaction must be coupled with a national will to bring about change. Primary health care proceeds by involving all sectors of the community, those dealing with health, the environment, social welfare, labour, transportation, agriculture and the media to create a partnership among the family, health professions, and government agencies. Together, these sectors focus upon major health problems and the appropriate technology and personnel for their solution in each setting (Styles, cited by ICN, 1986:3).

## 2.1 NURSING AND THE ACHIEVEMENT OF HEALTH FOR ALL

The importance of nurses to the acceptance and implementation of primary health care becomes obvious when one examines the structure, organisation and staffing of health services. Representing roughly half of health personnel resources (Palmer and Short, 1989), nurses are considered by Mahler (1985) and Seivwright (1988) to be key personnel in implementing changes essential to the acceptance and expansion of primary health care. Similarly Maglacas (1988) considers nurses to be the occupational group best placed to realise the social goal of health for all. Before this can occur, however, the confusion of divergent approaches currently plaguing the profession must be solved. Despite endorsement and support from various international and national nursing organisations including the International Council of Nursing, Australian Nursing Federation and the Australian Council of Community Nurses, support for primary health care from nurses in general has, according to Maglacas (1988), been ad hoc. This lack of cohesive support should not be surprising. As the International Council of Nursing points out, the education and professional experience of nurses directs them towards involvement in, and therefore understanding and support of, the existing curative, technical, medically-orientated health system. While this may change in the future, nursing's past and the placement of educational programmes in service settings, has had a profound and sustained effect on nursing practice.

The function of hospitals, be it caring for acutely ill persons or those requiring long-term custodial care, has determined the education and training received by nurses (ICN 1986:5). Other influential factors are the status, prestige and thus the funds accorded primary health care services. Highly specialised, technical areas are accorded higher status, considered more useful to a society's health, and seen as providing a more desirable career option. This is so even though it is now acknowledged that emphasis on curative services does little to promote the health of the population as a whole. If nurses are concerned with promoting health it is time to question the part they play in maintaining the current illness orientation of health services, and the cost of this orientation, both social and fiscal, to society. (For more information, consult criticisms of health care services by Navarro, Milio and the WHO; various reports from the Commonwealth and State governments are also useful references.)

Maglacas (1988) has argued that nursing requires 'leaders who can motivate and mobilise others, and who can help orient health care systems towards health promotion and sickness prevention, while at the same time achieving a balance between institution and community, treatment and prevention, management and cure'. A similar point is made by Donoghue (1978). What is being suggested is a change in values and ethos, a return to a view of health which recognises that the conditions in which people live affect their health. As Tansey and Lentz (1988) point out, the focus of nursing practice is helping people cope with physiological, psychological and social stress and upheaval by providing a supportive environment and helping people's innate abilities to repair and heal themselves. Similarly, Nightingale emphasised assessment and the promotion of health status, assets and potential of people regardless of age, nationality, race or circumstances (Watson 1979). Nursing, it can be argued, has in some ways lost its direction: concerned with professionalism, it has emulated medical practice and in the process become preoccupied with illness and disease. The concepts of health for all and primary health care provide a path for returning to the basis of nursing, caring and enabling. Before examining how primary health care principles can be integrated into community nursing practice it is necessary to identify differences and commonalities between hospital and community nursing practice.

## 2.2 COMMUNITY NURSING

Simplistically, community nursing blends nursing practice and public health practice. An added dimension is that people are considered in terms of the larger family and community rather than in isolation. It is this emphasis on aggregates as well as individuals that theoretically differentiates community nursing from other spheres of nursing. Therefore, while the skills gained working in a hospital are essential, they are not sufficient for community practice. The difference in clientele and the degree of autonomy and accountability mean that some nurses may find that the attitudes and expectations effective in a hospital environmental hinder their ability to work as a community nurse.

In a hospital, nurses care for persons confined by four walls — some bedridden, many acutely ill, and others requiring long-term institutionalised care. Care focuses on their immediate needs, determined by their current medical condition. Although some psychiatric hospitals, residential care facilities and nursing homes conduct programmes that focus on development or maintenance of skills, the immediate needs remain the prime concern. While holistic care is advocated, and attempts are made to provide it, the function and organisation of hospitals limits the possibility of achievement. Emphasis on the disease or disorder, and task allocation and roster changes limit the degree to which nurses are able to get to know and understand the people they care for (Menzies, 1970; Masson, 1988). Caring for the whole person, as Masson points out, is difficult when one has little knowledge of who the person is, where she/he comes from or where she/he will return upon discharge. The consequence of focusing on the disease or disorder underlying each episode of illness according to Sax (1989:105) is that it leads to neglect of the multiplicity of causative factors as well as fundamental problems. Consideration of psychosocial, environmental and/or socio-economic factors relevant to health are therefore overlooked.

Such environments do not encourage nurses to consider why the person became ill, how they might promote health or prevent a recurrence of illness for a person during a period of hospitalisation, or how that person's illness might affect their family or community.

Hospitals are highly structured, hierarchical, predictable and increasingly specialised environments within which professionals' roles and responsibilities are limited as well as being clearly defined (Menzies, 1970; Mechanic, 1978). Like other professionals, nurses are cast as, and assume the position of, experts who provide care to persons who are passive recipients rather than active participants in their own care (Waring and McLennan, 1979). Overtime, contact with persons who are passive and ill leads to the development of a distorted perception of the causes, incidence and prevalence of illness as well as of people's ability to be self-reliant and make decisions regarding their own health.

As well as limiting patients' participation in their own care, the organisation of hospitals also limits the autonomy of nurses, who are given responsibility but at the same time denied control over their practice. According to Menzies (1970) and Mechanic (1978), success and promotion depend on individuals' ability to curb their initiative and conform to existing practices, including deferring to medical staff. While nurses are responsible for carrying out medical instructions and implementing care, they are not ultimately responsible for decision-making regarding patient care. While the degree of contact nurses have with patients would in many situations make them the most appropriate care co-ordinators or case managers, this role officially is assigned to medical officers, who have limited and intermittent patient contact and often informally delegate the role to nurses. Nurses have then responsibility but no power (Mechanic, 1978:361). The hierarchical structure of hospitals and their emphasis on disease or disorder limits nurses' practice and their ability to be active advocates for patients. It makes them responsible for implementing medical instructions while at the same time denying them authority and limiting their autonomy and accountability (Masson, 1988; Menzies, 1970; Mechanic, 1978). This situation has contributed to poor co-ordination of patient care and poor care as well as to nurses leaving nursing, learning to survive by curbing their initiative and playing the necessary game, or (as a way of gaining greater professional autonomy) entering specialty areas including community health nursing (Menzies, 1970; Mechanic, 1978; Schulz, 1992). The move to specialisation may thus be seen as a way of gaining professional autonomy rather than a statement of commitment to a particular area of practice (Schulz, 1992).

In contrast, community nurses care for persons with self-limiting conditions, chronic illnesses or disabilities in a less structured, more isolated and less predictable environment (Mechanic, 1978:480). Professional boundaries are blurred so that in rural or disadvantaged areas nurses often take the place of medical practitioners (Cramer, 1987). As Mechanic points out, in addition to the lack of structure, roles are less defined, while goals are often unclear, multiple and at times conflicting. The majority of clients have chronic conditions of a physical, psychiatric or social nature. Cure is unlikely, and progress is often slow or limited. Working with such clients is often difficult and requires skills different from those required to work with persons with acute illnesses. Yet the education system fails to prepare nurses for such work (Australian Health Ministers Advisory Council, 1988; Health Commission of NSW, 1977; Seivwright, 1988; WHO, 1988). Professional education and experience focuses on acute illness, often in one area such as general, psychiatric or developmental disability. Little experience is gained in community settings.

Hospital training and experience does, as Waring and McLennan (1979:16–17) point out, provide nurses with some important qualities; a view of themselves as a helping person, a valuing of high quality care, a systematic approach to problem solving and knowledge. Yet as Menzies (1970) argues, nurses also learn to avoid making decisions by delegating upwards; are discouraged from forming therapeutic relationships; and are considered interchangeable as individual skills are not recognised. Moreover they learn to work within the framework of existing practices (Mechanic, 1978). Educationally the skills, knowledge and attitudes required to work within a primary health care framework are absent from nursing programmes. Some colleges and university based diploma and degree programmes prepare graduates for community practice, while for others the only change is a change of venue, not course content or orientation. (Seivwright, 1988:101). Seivwright argues that skills in comprehension and analysis, and questioning and development of attitudes and values, are ignored while development of cognitive skills, such as rote learning, enabling recognition and recall of unsynthesised information and the psycho-motor skills required to carry out procedures, are emphasised. Compare this situation to that in Britain and the USA, where courses are available and in some instances necessary for employment in community nursing. In Korea and Indonesia, community experience is part of the basic course and in-service programmes are run by the Health Department for employees.

The consequences of this lack of preparation, compounded by limited access to courses and qualifications in community nursing and nurses learning 'on the job', are clear. Most community nursing services have become an extension of the personal care services offered in hospitals, in a more accessible and acceptable structure (Donoghue, 1978; Schulz, 1992). Obviously lacking, as Donoghue (1978) argues, is a community focus. What is maintained in an outreach mode is the individual curative focus of the traditional health services. What is not obvious is the effect of this lack of preparation on community nurses, their clients and communities.

Nursing services have emphasised provision of follow-up care to people after discharge. With the exception of baby health and school medical services, which focus on screeing in an attempt to identify existing problems early, nursing services have emphasised provision of care to already ill people to prevent their admission or readmission to hospital. Thus rather than focusing on prevention, habilitation, rehabilitation, and increasing each individual's, family's or community's abilities, resources and autonomy, the illness focus of the hospital system has remained. Achievement of the goal of health for all requires nurses to reach beyond their view of themselves as providers of individually oriented clinical services. Clinical services are essential but inadequate if placed in a narrowly curative context.

The introduction of the National Community Health Programme in the 1970s was an attempt to reorient health services, and emphasise prevention. On humanistic, social and economic grounds the change was needed. Many health problems can be prevented, and it is reasonable to expect professionals to use their knowledge and skills to ensure that this occurs. Because the combined expertise of various disciplines is required to comprehend complex health issues, multi-disciplinary centres were established to provide general primary care services, reduce fragmentation, increase access, promote self-reliance and improve continuity of care (Health Commission of NSW, 1977; National Hospitals and Health Services Commission, 1973). It was expected that nurses would establish and provide appropriate clinical services and work with local communities to promote health. The programme failed to focus on health promotion and illness prevention as a review of the community health programme demonstrated (Australian Community Health Association, 1991). Like other health professionals, nurses continued to provide personal care services to individuals but did not work in interdisciplinary mode. According to Gibson (1984), lack of leadership, implementation strategies and education for community practice, as well as previous professional socialisation, all played a significant part. Rotem (1984), Wellard (1990) and Schulz (1990) point out that the lack of goals, along with lack of experience of working in a team, also led to development of intra- and inter-disciplinary rivalries and friction over professional boundaries. These problems Rotem considers symptomatic of the lack of guidelines concerning roles, goals and procedures (1984:14). By maintaining a curative focus, community nurses have maintained an approach which fails to address the health needs of communities because it emphasises one component of nursing (clinical practice) at the expense of public health practice.

The focus of nursing needs to change from concern with how to service increasing numbers of clients to one which seeks to identify ways in which nurses can work with other health professionals and community groups to promote health. A preoccupation with illness and treatment merely perpetuates what Donoghue (1978) describes as 'downstream practice'. That is, practice which emphasises 'episodic crisis orientated care' and thus perpetuates client demand. Nurses need, so Donoghue argues, to participate in 'up-stream practice' by making time to identify determinants of ill health and adopting appropriate counter measures to promote health and prevent illness. Personal care services to the already ill need to continue; but rather than being episodic, they need to focus on continuity of care, prevention and health promotion, and on encouraging people to improve and take increasing control of their health. Special attention should be paid to the needs of people with limited access to resources.

## 2.3 SKILLS REQUIRED FOR COMMUNITY NURSING

According to the International Council of Nurses, generalist rather than specialist skills are required to practise within a primary health care framework. These include a good understanding of common health problems and therapies, human behaviour and new technology, as well as skills in encouraging and promoting self-help and community self-reliance, problem solving, research, communication, management and leadership (International Council of Nurses, 1986:5). In addition to having clinical skills, nurses in primary health care practice must be able to act as teacher, supervisor, team worker, epidemiologist, investigator and collaborator. Preparation for using a primary health care framework in community settings requires curricula which emphasise development in students of a 'team spirit, a spirit of inquiry and assertiveness and perhaps most important of all an ability to solve unforeseen problems and be responsible for their own life-long learning' (International Council of Nurses, 1986:5). As already mentioned, the education received by most community nurses sought to prepare them for practice in hospitals (be they general, psychiatric or developmental disability), so changes in practice are required. This implies rethinking and questioning accepted values, beliefs and attitudes about health, nursing, people and the health system, since these all influence practice as well as learning, thinking and motivation (WHO, 1983-B).

Moving from hospital to community nursing thus requires a change in orientation, focus and practice: from illness to health, from individual to family and community, from reactive to proactive. New skills, knowledge and attitudes need to be developed to enable the nurse to work confidently in a new environment. In the past as Schulz (1990) points out, community nurses have been left to their own devices, receiving neither orientation nor guidance. Consequently old assumptions and practices are often retained for reasons of security rather than because they are appropriate to the new situation. Faced with new problems in a less structured, less predictable environment, feelings of powerlessness and self-doubt sometimes develop (Schulz 1990). All community nurses interviewed by the author spoke of the difficulties they experienced in working out what they were expected to do and how to manage clients. Nurses new to community health practice require access to the support, guidance and skills of more experienced nurses while they learn to participate effectively as team members. This requires clinical skills to be integrated with the new skills needed for public health practice. These are not separate domains but should rather be viewed as a continuum, each reinforcing the other, as nurses focus on the health needs of people and on the environments in which they live, play and work. In this context, individual health issues need to be considered in relation to their effect on, or consequences for, families and communities and vice versa. New skills and perspectives are best developed in an environment that encourages critical debate, provides support and clearly works towards achievement of team goals.

Some community services are administered in such a way that nurses are allocated a list of clients with a list of tasks and required to complete those tasks within a set time. Little account is taken of increased dependency or an episodic personal crisis occurring for the patient which requires more of the nurse's time. However, in general, community nurses work autonomously; individual nurses decide who fit the organisation's criteria and so receive services, as well as the nature of those services. This involves deciding which response is appropriate: referral, a weekly or monthly visit, health education, community action or no action. By virtue of their isolation, community nurses have greater control over the nature, orientation and quality of their practice and thus the service they provide. Judgemental assumptions are possible if community nurses lack insight into the multiple factors that contribute to ill-health and thus take a stance that individuals are responsible for their own health problems. This raises issues both of teamwork and of accountability. Awareness of other services, other carers and a willingness to refer or co-operate is essential. Accountability issues emerge because services provided in homes are not open to the scrutiny of others and thus the quality and appropriateness of care is hidden. As in any service, evaluation and quality assurance programmes are essential components of any community nursing service. (This is discussed further in Chapter 2.3.) The Community Health Accreditation and Standards Program (CHASP), developed specifically for community health services, provides a method of maintaining standards and evaluating services.

Managers need to consider how they might work to achieve the goals of health for all and establish a commitment to the principles of primary health care in their area. Concentrating on the groups mentioned below is focal to this task, for all have been identified as requiring action to improve their health. Of concern for these groups are issues of equity and access to resources, and a focus on health rather than illness. As the health issues for all are complex, achievement requires action in many sectors (health, employment, housing and environment) and by various health professionals. The task of hospital managers is to ensure optimal care of acutely ill people within hospitals, and to work with community services to ensure that appropriate after-care is available. For managers of community services, the task is somewhat different. They must ensure that appropriate services are available to meet the needs of their community, and also work to establish a supportive environment and develop policies which promote health and increase the availability of healthy options and environments which are physically, emotionally and socially supportive of health.

# **3.** GROUPS WITHIN THE COMMUNITY

To promote health, nurses require knowledge and awareness of factors which contribute to, or are detrimental to, the health of individuals. Also required is an understanding of the needs of specific groups or population aggregates. It has been emphasised that community nurses work with individuals and communities and need to be aware that what affects individuals affects families and communities and vice versa. A primary health care framework requires nurses to be knowledgeable about indicators of health; to be able to identify and reduce inequality; to act to reduce (where possible) existing and potential risks to health; and to respond to changing health needs. It is not possible to discuss all of the health problems or all the groups which one will encounter working as a community nurse. It is possible, however, to identify specific population aggregates or groups for whom health services are currently less than adequate and who would benefit from an emphasis on health promotion and disease prevention. These include women and children; persons with chronic or long term health problems and/or disabilities; and those with acute illnesses who participate in early discharge programmes. Because of its increasing significance, the use of technology in community nursing will also be discussed briefly.

## 3.1 WOMEN AND CHILDREN

Women and children have traditionally been the concern of community nurses. Baby health clinics, school medical services, family planning, midwifery, aged care, mental health and services for the developmentally disadvantaged have been, and continue to be, provided by nurses. These domains of practice are either combined in the role of generalist community nurse or maintained as specialist services. Regardless of how services are arranged, community nurses work with women as clients, relations of clients and peers. An understanding and awareness of women's health issues is required because doing something for women means doing something for children and families (Kickbush, 1989).

Recent concepts of health emphasise its positive nature. For instance Watson (1979:219) suggests that a healthy person has 'a high-quality, balanced life, a sense of happiness, and the ability to adapt to change'. Mahler (1981:6) refers to 'a sense of personal wellbeing ... that enables a person to live a socially and economically productive life'. Such criteria are to a degree subjective and therefore difficult to measure. For this reason, indicators of health such as morbidity and mortality rates, expected life span at birth, neonatal death rates, level of education, quality of housing, employment opportunities, income and access to health care are used to ascertain health status and health potential of individuals, families and communities.

As a group, women fare poorly on many of these scales. They are more likely to have low levels of education, poor housing, low wages, receive poorer quality health care and be more dependent than are men. It should therefore not be surprising that rising morbidity rates and access to opportunities and services are of concern. Studies of modern societies indicate that while men die earlier, women have higher morbidity rates (Broom, 1989:122). Even allowing for increased consultation during their reproductive years, women consult more frequently and take medication more frequently than do men. Contributing to this situation is the fact that, unlike men, women are likely to suffer from chronic diseases and conditions related to child bearing and child rearing rather than the major killer diseases (Broom, 1989:123–125). Common health problems include genito-urinary conditions, breast and cervical cancer, use of alcohol, cigarettes and prescribed drugs, and chronic disorders (Davis and George, 1988:296–7). Because they experience different patterns of illness, men and women consult, use and experience the health system differently (Broom, 1989:125).

It is, however, well documented that although women consult more frequently, they are more likely to receive inferior treatment and be incorrectly diagnosed (Wyndam, 1982; Furler, 1985; Broom, 1989). This has negative effects, since the health of women also affects the health of families and communities. Women are carers for children and the dependent elderly and act as educators and cultural transmitters of knowledge, attitudes and values about health (Davis and George, 1988:298). As Kickbush (1989:5) argues, 'women are the primary health promoters the world over and most of this work is performed without pay or for a minimum wage'. If they receive poor health care, have limited knowledge and are unable to improve their own health, there is little chance of them improving the health of their families.

In Australia, 60-70 per cent of adults living below the poverty line are women. Families headed by women (single mothers) are most likely to live in poverty. The opportunities accorded women therefore limit the opportunities and health of their children. Health is affected by life chances as well as individual behaviour and this is reflected in different morbidity and mortality rates. For instance, the health of Aboriginal women is still poor. They suffer higher than average death rates from pneumonia and other infectious diseases, alcohol related problems, mental stress arising from poverty and domestic violence (Davis and George, 1988:298). Similarly migrant women's access to services and employment is limited by language and cultural barriers. Interpreters have in some areas made access easier, but many health problems of these women are related to their employment in low-paying repetitive jobs where their risk of injury is compounded by language difficulties (Davis and George, 1988:298).

The Australian government has developed a women's health policy, the fundamental objective of which is to increase equity and the health of families and Australians in general. The most immediate concerns for women's health, according to Newby (1989:94) are reproduction, mental health, nutrition and eating disorders, as well as preventive health strategies such as breast and cervical screening. In the last decade, as a consequence of campaigns by various consumer and women's groups as well as research, various services have been established: women's health clinics, screening programmes, sexual assault centres, educational programmes aimed at reducing the abuse of alcohol and prescribed drugs, and programmes to increase community awareness of crimes such as domestic violence and sexual abuse. Services have also been established to cater specifically for the needs of migrant and Aboriginal women. However all these services have developed in an ad hoc fashion, funded and administered by various levels of government and different government departments. As a consequence, accessibility and service co-ordination often rely on the interest, co-operation and goodwill of individual workers. Lack of knowledge on the part of health and welfare workers of available services limits the access of clients, depriving them of options.

Fragmentation of services not only limits access, it also means that women with several problems need to consult different services in different locations at different times. This presents problems for all women, but has greater difficulties for those who are isolated, poor or otherwise disadvantaged by their particular circumstances (for example, carers for young children or the elderly).

Even when nurses do not see themselves as 'women's health nurses' they have a contribution to make to the health of the women with whom they work. In a community, nursing opportunities arise to gain an understanding of the health problems faced by women in specific communities. Issues can be raised and acted on by teams in whatever manner is considered appropriate from a health promotion perspective. Services need to be evaluated in relation to their appropriateness, relevance and accessibility to all women. While it is not clear to what degree women's health problems are related to their role as carers, it is agreed that some relationship exists. Health services alone therefore will neither prevent nor significantly reduce morbidity or mortality rates, which are related to the social and political situation of women. However access for women to information, health education and opportunities to participate in increasing their own and their families' health, as well as access to services which focus on their needs, can have positive effects.

Women's health needs change throughout their lives. Often issues pertaining to their reproductive capacity or their role as carers bring women into contact with nurses even when they are not ill. Advice is sought on contraception, sexuality, pregnancy, menopause, child rearing, childhood illnesses or crises relating to children, partners and elderly relatives. As Stott (1983) points out, all one-to-one situations regardless of their purpose provide opportunities for promotive and preventive activities such as providing information, health education, identification of vulnerable (or at risk) persons, screening, identification of problems requiring referral or counselling, as well as for maintaining continuity of care when appropriate. These contacts enable identification of constraints and barriers to health, and thus lead to recognition of potential community development activities aimed at increasing the health of a group of persons. Educational and social interventions, as well as clinical responses, are thus available (cf Jackson et al, 1989; Stott, 1983:59).

Several periods lend themselves readily to opportunistic care, both in prevention and in health promotion; these are childhood, adolescence, pregnancy and middle years (menopause). Access to schools and work environments present opportunities for nurses to interact with healthy people at periods in the person's life when they might benefit from health education and health promotion programmes, screening and clinical services.

Pregnant women have universal educational, physical and emotional needs. The first pregnancy is for most women and their partners a time of excitement and concern. Improved care during pregnancy, birth and the postnatal period has reduced mortality rates for women and also mortality and morbidity rates of infants. (Another significant factor is access to contraception, thus limiting the number of pregnancies.) Prenatal care has been demonstrated to decrease neonatal morbidity and mortality especially for those considered to be at risk for reasons of age, previous history, low income or ethnic background, yet not all women avail themselves of prenatal and postnatal care (Davis and George 1988:80; Holtzman, 1979). Prenatal classes convey information on pregnancy, nutrition, contraception and child development, as well as allowing discussion of the effects on the mother of caring for a new baby. As the success of programmes depends on relevance and participation, classes need to cater for different groups of women, for instance those with partners, single women, and ethnic minorities (using an interpreter when necessary). The participants should also be involved in programme development. Ideally, services for women and children including prenatal care and education, child health clinics, school screening, women's health, home nursing and mental health services, are provided locally by staff in one centre. As well as increasing accessibility and continuity of care, such an arrangement provides opportunities for nurses to work with other disciplines and the local community in order to learn more about the needs and concerns of local women and their families. Nurses providing clinical services should be aware of other agencies and self-help groups providing services to women, and develop links with them. When providing information, practical assistance and support to women, such services are an essential resource; they include child care associations, stillbirth and miscarriage support group (SAMS), sudden infant death support group (SIDS), groups concerned with childbirth education, single parents, family support, women's refuges, nursing mothers and mothers of handicapped children, sexual assault centres, mothers of twins' clubs. Other health professionals such as counsellors, clinical nurse specialists and consultants in maternity and paediatric units, general practitioners, drug and alcohol services, paediatricians, obstetricians, social workers, are also to be considered, as are government departments such as Family and Community Services, Housing and Social Security.

During childhood the foundations for good health are laid. To develop normally, children require good nutrition and nurturing, as well as access to reasonable housing, education and health services. Neonatal mortality rates are an important indicator of community health. Australia, while having a higher rate than the Scandinavian countries, compares well with Britain and the USA with 7.6 deaths per thousand (Davis and George, 1988:78). However, the rate for Aboriginal children of 19.1 per thousand demonstrates the poor health of these infants and their mothers. It is in child health that the disparities in health status and the need for preventive activities on the part of health, welfare and social services are most obvious and most easily addressed. Health education, immunisation and school screening have been shown to be beneficial, as have increasing access to health services and providing income and social support for disadvantaged women and their families (Townsend and Davidson, 1986; Milio, 1975, 1981).

The major causes of morbidity and mortality in children under 14 years include perinatal conditions, mainly congenital abnormalities, accidents and cancer (Davis and George, 1988:78). Accidents, a major cause of mortality and morbidity in children, are mainly preventable and related to environmental risks. While poisonings and drownings account for many accidents, motor vehicle accidents in which the child is a pedestrian account for the greatest number (Davies and George, 1988:78).

Adolescents in general have limited contact with health services and unless they have an acute or chronic illness in early childhood, most are healthy. The major causes of morbidity and mortality for this group include accidents, suicide and cancer (Davis and George, 1988:78). Emotional turmoil seems to be considered normal, as does a preoccupation with sexuality, relationships and asserting one's independence from parents. This latter creates difficulties for both children and parents. The provision of nursing services in high schools might be beneficial, making information on health issues, including mental health and sexuality, more readily accessible. Nurses could act as resource persons to teachers and students, both formally and informally.

One concern is the almost unchanging rate of unplanned pregnancy in teenagers. While a higher incidence of teenage mothers is to be found in working class and poorer communities, this does not reflect differences in sexual activity but differences in access to contraception, abortion and life options (Clark, 1984). Women can now choose to continue a pregnancy or have a termination, but either decision is difficult. Continuation of a pregnancy is more likely where young women have few goals and consider motherhood as a career option. Although the availability of government benefits makes it somewhat easier for young mothers, an interrupted education while having a child to care for when employment opportunities and child care facilities are limited means that most live in poor circumstances. As well, they are more likely to deliver low birthweight infants, experience complications and suffer greater social and emotional isolation than other mothers (Clark, 1984). Where mothers are poorly educated and dependent on welfare, both they and their children are more likely to experience poor health. This has implications both for individual families and for communities where a high proportion of women and their families are dependent on welfare.

In the workforce women, like men, experience various occupation related injuries. However, despite the dual role (worker and carer), it is suggested that work is beneficial for a woman's health. Studies have demonstrated that working women consider themselves to be healthier than women who remain at home, who indeed have higher morbidity rates (Broom, 1989). Women who remain at home often lack support and experience geographic and social isolation, limiting their ability to cope with the needs of their children. Mental health, as the high incidence of depression and use of tranquillisers indicates, is a significant issue for women. Although changes are occurring, women still bear major responsibility for children and the care of infirm or elderly relatives. For some, this leads to stress, anxiety and poor health.

For the working woman there are several concerns, such as access to affordable child care and reasonable working conditions. Where child care is unavailable, children may be left in the care of siblings or neighbours or in other less than adequate situations before and after school. This poses problems for their health or safety and points to a need for services such as pre- and after-school care. As well, the working conditions of women, especially migrant women, are often poor with low pay, poor conditions and unhealthy environments. Such conditions contribute to deterioration in women's health and have immediate consequences for the health of families as well as longer term significance for the woman's ability to be healthy and self-sufficient in her old age.

In later adulthood, the responsibility of caring for elderly or ill relatives or spouses again falls to women. Where constant attention is required, social contact for carers may be limited. As in the early years of parenting, dependence of relatives and demands of physically caring for another may lead to physical and emotional exhaustion, thus decreasing the ability of the carer to cope with demands placed on her. When changes in the woman's life such as menopause, retirement (of self or partner), or changes in the life of her children coincide with increasing demands for care from relatives, adjustment may be even more difficult. Unfortunately the rising demand for services means that assistance may not be easily obtained from the public sector. Moreover, a lack of understanding means that requests for assistance related to women's biological and caring roles are often trivialised or dismissed by health workers and support and practical assistance withheld.

To work effectively with women and their families, to promote health and prevent illness, an understanding of the constraints and demands placed on them in contemporary Australian society is required. Ways need to be identified whereby nurses, as health workers, might make services more relevant, accessible and appropriate to women, thus reducing current inequities. This requires nurses to come to terms with their own experiences and to become aware of the social and political factors contributing to the poor health of many women. As the high level of morbidity appears to be related to the relatively powerless and dependent position of women, health promotion requires nurses to encourage development of independence and self-reliance. As a group, women are poorly served by the health services, and nurses as the largest body of health professionals need to give consideration to how this might be changed.

## 3.2 CHRONIC ILLNESS

While health services and professional education programmes concern themselves with acute illness, chronic conditions (often preventable) are increasing (Stott, 1983; Strauss and Corbin, 1988). One concern is the incidence and prevalence of chronic or long-term illness and disability, and the question of whether prevention is possible. Another concern is identifying ways of assisting individuals and their families to achieve or continue satisfactory lives. Yet another is the availability of community resources. People of all ages experience chronic illness, mental and physical, and have varying degrees of disability; a significant number of these problems are the result of work-related injuries including back injuries, repetitive strain injury, asbestosis, carcinoma, and stress or other mental health problems (Davis and George, 1988:89).

> 'Chronic illness' refers to any impairment interfering with an individual's ability to function fully in the environment ... (and is) generally characterised by relatively stable periods, often interrupted by acute periods requiring medical attention or hospitalisation. Prognosis varies from normal life to unpredictable early death. Chronic conditions are rarely cured, but are managed through individual or family efforts (Thomas cited by Hanson, 1987:12)

Chronic illness and disability often go hand in hand although they are not synonymous. 'Disability' refers to 'any restriction or lack of ability to perform an activity in a manner considered normal for a human being' (WHO cited by Palmer and Short, 1989:245). For some people and their families disability, be it deafness, blindness or intellectual, psychiatric or multiple, may mean economic, physical, psychological and social dependency.

In 1977-78, 6.5 million people, 45 per cent of the population, suffered from a chronic illness, with nearly half of them having more than one chronic condition. Although often associated with the elderly, chronic illness actually occurs most in young adults in the 24-44 year age group (Grant and Lapsley cited by Davies and George, 1988:88) thus affecting adults who are likely to be responsible for families during their working years. According to the Australian Bureau of Statistics, the number of persons with a disability was 1 942 200 in 1984. While the majority had physical disorders, a substantial proportion were persons with mental disorders and children with developmental or physical disabilities. Approximately 300 000 members of the population, including some 25 485 handicapped children, were dependent on some form of pension (Davis and George, 1988:88).

What concerns people with disabilities is the 'disability, distress or dependency' that arises as a consequence of their condition (Health Commission of NSW, 1977:7). Another concern is the attitude of other people towards them. During the International Year of Disabled Persons (IYDP) in 1981, people with disabilities sought to make the community aware of their needs. The central issue was that people's abilities rather than their disabilities should be recognised and accepted. Access to education, employment, and health and welfare services to enable independent living were the other major issues (Palmer and Short, 1989:245).

Although the number of people with chronic illness and/or disability is increasing, the present health system is poorly equipped to assist with either their condition or their concerns. Arising from multiple physiological and, at times, psychological changes, chronic illnesses are partially incapacitating and rarely curable. On the other hand, many disabled persons are not ill. Unfortunately the current health system prefers and operates most effectively with curable conditions, and fails to attend in any meaningful way to the social and emotional problems experienced either by individuals with chronic disorders or disabilities, or by their families. The same orientation possibly also contributes to the poor care received by women. Unless they work specifically in child health, community nurses work mainly with people who have a chronic illness. Given however the prevalence of occupationally related conditions and disabilities, all nurses at some time will have contact with those affected by chronic illness or disability. Like other health professionals, nurses are poorly equipped educationally to work with this population in ways that encourage and promote independence, and they lack access to appropriate support and resources (HC NSW, Book 1, 1977:7). This can lead to loss of interest and reduced commitment to the job.

Differences exist according to the manner in which chronic illness manifests itself. Different individuals respond differently, with factors such as race and ethnicity affecting occurrence and response to chronic illness. Families have to cope with crisis prevention, management, control of symptoms, disruption to their life style, and sometimes social isolation, during the course of the illness (Hanson, 1987). For the person or family affected by a chronic illness there is the risk that disability and dependency may follow. Community services therefore are required which are easily accessible and promote independent self-care. Further, a continuum of services is required. Failure to provide services is costly both for governments, in funding accommodation, and for the women and children who cope with inadequate support services while caring for relatives (Palmer and Short, 1989:251). Carers receive little respite, yet seek to maintain a normal existence. The degree to which this is achieved depends on how symptoms are controlled and on how well the individual or family can establish or maintain social contact and support.

Health professionals' preoccupations tend to focus on 'the condition' while the concerns of persons and families are with the risk of disability. Fear of dependence, pain, separation from family, changes in social role and loss of one's identity are common and realistic. Chronic illness for some means experiencing social stigma, social isolation, family disruption, marital discord and alteration of domestic role (Strauss and Corbin, 1988:5). While the degree of impairment varies over time as well as with the nature of the illness and the degree of disability, individuals and their families may find themselves fluctuating between a state of crisis and non-crisis. If the course of illness is gradual the family may have time to adjust to any decline in ability, whereas with conditions arising from acute illness or accident the crisis is immediate. Families faced with chronic illness or disability need flexibility to respond to the changes occuring over time. Different strengths, attitudes and changes are required at different times (Rolland, 1987:37–39). In many instances pain is a feature of chronic conditions. If this is poorly controlled (by either behavioural methods or medication) this can lead to depression, difficulty in coping, drug and alcohol abuse, sexual problems, and alterations in communication patterns.

Persons with a chronic condition have long-term although sometimes intermittent contact with health workers and community services. In hospitals, nurses care for people during periods of exacerbation of their illness; in contrast community nurses see them at home and may have extended contact over weeks, months or years. This has both benefits and pitfalls. On the positive side it provides opportunities for continuity of care. Client and nurse have time to develop a therapeutic relationship, with the client taking increasing control of their own care. It is also possible that the person becomes dependent, giving up their right to make decisions while relying on the nurse. Constant contact and familarity may mean the nurse becomes complacent, resulting in inadequate observation. This is most likely where a person's condition remains stable over time and changes are subtle, the person is passively dependent, and other clients have more acute and immediate needs. To prevent this occurring, it is essential that each contact be used to assess progress, and that each client and family is encouraged to participate in decision making about the care required and the effectiveness of care received. Education about the illness, promotion of independence and encouragement of appropriate use of resources such as counselling or self-help groups by clients is essential. Where other organisations are involved in providing care, communication must be established and maintained to ensure that goals of care are understood by all.

It is particularly important when unqualified persons are involved in providing personal care that the concept of developing and maintaining independence is understood.

Like most people with a chronic illness or disability, the majority of aged people (90 per cent) live at home; only a small number live in hospitals, nursing homes and homes for the aged (Palmer and Short, 1989:249). Most people, especially men, living at home receive assistance from their families, especially from wives and daughters (Kinnear and Graycar cited by Palmer and Short, 1989:249). Women, outliving their husbands, tend to live alone. This accounts for the higher proportion of women requiring institutional care or assistance from health and welfare services (Davis and George, 1988:269). Almost 70 per cent of elderly persons living alone are women (Maglacas, 1989), many of them living in poverty. People who remain at home could benefit from nursing or other services, as ageing and degenerative conditions often mean immobility and many aged people as a consequence experience incontinence and poor hygiene (Palmer and Short, 1989:250). Those who require hospitalisation do so because of factors such as inadequate housing, low income, physical disability, transport difficulties and lack of social support. While a small percentage of aged people require hospitalisation, the majority live, or could live, at home with support — yet the major proportion of aged care funding (80 per cent) goes to nursing homes which cater for the minority (4 per cent) of the relevant population. This contrasts with low funding for community based services.

However, some gains have been made. The Home and Community Care Programme (HACC) for instance, was established in 1985 by the Federal Government to assist the frail aged and people with disabilities to live independently (Palmer and Short, 1989:251). The services provided include home nursing, meals-on-wheels, paramedical services, home care, assessment services, day care, sitting services, respite care and transport. This programme goes some way towards providing a comprehensive integrated service.

Long-term hospitalisation was considered appropriate and desirable for persons with psychiatric illnesses until the 1960s. People with a mental health problem experience similar difficulties to any other person with a chronic illness or disability, but the social stigma is greater, and because they are sometimes less able to participate effectively in their own care or maintain a social network, they are vulnerable to exploitation. The trend to de-institutionalisation of previously hospitalised persons concerns many people working with this group of clients. It is particularly important that living conditions and access to services are maintained, since it may be quite difficult to ensure continuity of care and prevent deterioration in these clients, many of whom are dependent and lacking in living skills.

Most people with chronic illnesses and disabilities live with, or maintain social contact with, their families. Where people with a mental illness have experienced repeated lengthy periods of hospitalisation, family relationships often break down. If illness develops during teenage or young adult years, developing and maintaining close relationships is difficult. Parents anxious to protect their children are often over-protective, limiting their ability to establish independence. Living away from home, obtaining and maintaining suitable accommodation poses problems for people with disabilities of any sort. It is more difficult for those with mental illness. Governments provide only limited accommodation, and many live in private accommodation, hostels, half-way houses, and boarding houses of varying standards (Moore et al, 1982; Bailey and Brodaty, 1982).

The amount of support and assistance received by individuals depends on the availability of services, the relationships between various agencies, and the knowledge of health and welfare professionals. As with all chronic conditions, medical treatment is of limited value, and yet the most common treatment is still medication. Difficulties often arise when lack of understanding or unpleasant side-effects mean that compliance with treatment (especially medication) is poor, leading to the exacerbation of symptoms and further reducing social contact. The importance of maintaining and regaining social contact and social skills cannot be over-emphasised. It was for this reason that self-help groups and living skills centres were established, aimed at assisting individuals to understand their illness or disability and to learn or relearn the social and practical skills essential for independent living (Baily and Brodaty, 1982; Moore et al, 1982). A risk exists for them, as for other persons with chronic illnesses, that all responses or symptoms are attributed to their illness rather than being a valid response to their current circumstances, or to a particular experience or sickness. It is therefore essential that the person rather than the condition be the focus of interaction and planning care. This is often difficult, for as Mechanic (1978:480) points out, working with chronically mentally ill persons is not easy. People regress rather than progress and experience frequent crises. This takes its toll. Staff become tired, or smug, and lose their sensitivity and commitment to their work.

A particular feature of chronic illness is the disruption experienced as a result of hospital admissions. A cycle of re-admission and then discharge may become the norm, leading to what is termed 'the revolving door syndrome'. This may occur when a person is unable to cope with daily events outside the protected environment of the hospital. Minor problems may be sufficient to precipitate a crisis requiring hospitalisation. While hospitals need to provide support for people who are hospitalised, it is not their place to provide a support system for those who are isolated. The need is rather for communities to develop alternative support systems.

It is essential for a person's wellbeing that a complete assessment is carried out during hospitalisation, and that discharge planning occurs, to prevent a pattern of re-admission and discharge developing. Where nurses are involved with these people, each contact needs to be considered within the context of planned care rather than becoming episodic 'interventions'. Continuity of care is often difficult but is nevertheless desirable in the case of persons with chronic illnesses. With discharge planning, a well documented history and a plan of care, continuity of care is more likely to be achieved, since this planning provides an opportunity for problems to be anticipated and prevented. The aim of working with any person with a chronic illness is to prevent deterioration and increase the person's independence, thereby reducing the likelihood of re-admission to hospital. It is not that hospitalisation is to be avoided when essential, but rather that action needs to be taken to reduce it occurring needlessly. To assist in the transition from hospital to community, it is essential that communication links with hospital staff are established and maintained.

Practitioners concerned with mental health disagree about the increased emphasis on community-based care. Some argue, correctly, that the negative aspects of hospitalisation, de-personalisation, isolation, separation from family and regimentation still occur: only the setting has changed. Concern also exists over the lack of community support and understanding of mental illness (Palmer and Short, 1989:241). While these concerns are valid, the answer lies not in increasing periods of hospitalisation but in developing accessible community services whereby assessment, early intervention and family support can be provided and the general public educated about the needs of people with mental health problems (cf Moore et al, 1982). Greater awareness, while not ensuring better understanding, goes some way towards improving community attitudes to these issues.

Coping with a chronic illness ordinarily requires knowledge of the process and prognosis of the condition. Inability to cope and the subsequent development of a non-adaptive behaviour is likely to lead to a further deterioration in health, commencing generally in the early crisis period. Early interventions providing access to information about the illness, self-help groups and counselling enable individuals and their families to cope better with what has happened and to prepare themselves for the likely future. It is essential that health workers consider the psychological and social needs of individuals and their families.

Community nurses work with individuals and families providing direct care, co-ordinating services or acting as a resource person, as well as providing ongoing support for families following the hospitalisation or death of a client. Family support must be organised, especially when care has been extended over a long time or been very demanding. Carers may lose contact with families and friends and require support to rebuild or re-establish their lives.

The major role of the nurse working with chronically ill people is to assist them to develop the skills to care for themselves (with appropriate assistance from family, friends and self-help groups), and to act as advocate to increase their access to services. At all times the emphasis is on assisting people to develop skills which will enable them to take responsibility for themselves, and to utilise when required the assistance of health professionals.

Although community-based services have sought to cater for persons with a chronic illness, in many areas they are insufficient and inadequate, focusing on immediate needs rather than on restoring and promoting health and co-ordinating long-term care. Moreover, factors contributing to the development of chronic illness and disabilities are ignored by providers of health services and others. Increasing demands for care for those with more acute problems may give rise to competition for resources, resulting in care of persons with chronic illness taking second place, so that the demands on care-givers are increased. As the needs of acutely ill people are more in keeping with nurses' professional experience and education, there is a risk that staff will choose to work with the population with whom they feel most comfortable. This could lead to a redistribution of services away from care for the chronically ill, or a handing over of care to less qualified persons. Where pressure is applied to services because of increasing needs of the acutely ill, extra staff should be provided rather than handing over the care of chronically ill persons to less qualified people or otherwise neglecting their needs.

## 3.3 ACUTE CARE, EARLY DISCHARGE

The trend towards early discharge, that is, returning people to their homes and families as soon as possible following hospitalisation, is a recent development which will increase for reasons of client preference, appropriateness and cost. This development raises several issues including increased demands for service, the safe management of technology in the home, and establishing mechanisms to ensure that nurses, clients and carers can manage therapies (Barkauskas, 1990).

Like those with chronic illnesses, the needs of acutely ill persons change over time. Care needs upon discharge may be minimal, increase over time, be intensive throughout the period of contact, or vary between self-sufficiency and intermittent periods requiring intense assistance. Needs are determined by the pattern of illness and stability of the condition, and the abilities of that individual and family to cope with the situation and take reponsibility for care. For some, daily or twice-daily visits may be required, for others monthly visits may be adequate. Some may be able to take responsibility for almost all care, administering medication, changing dressings, using aids, therapies and hygiene, while others require assistance with the simplest care. When assistance is requested it is necessary to assess what is required, for approximately how long, and what the person and family can reasonably attend to themselves. Feelings of incompetence, anxiety, dependence and fear may limit what can be done. Initially dependence may be necessary until confidence is gained regarding the care required. In all instances, assessment has to include the ability of those concerned to cope with their situation, the degree of social support, the actual physical environment, and resources accessible to them. They should be educated about their condition, prognosis, complications and significant changes before discharge. This information can then be reinforced following discharge and if necessary modified as required to suit the environment. Encouraging participation helps ensure compliance and the development of safe practices. As Waring and McLennan (1979) indicate, the role of expert is not appropriate when encouraging people to participate in their own care and ultimately to take responsibility and control, while still seeking assistance as required. Rather, the nurse needs to assist with care so as to become a resource person rather than the ongoing provider of care.

The concerns of nurses and the people with whom they work may differ, especially in relation to the acceptability of specific regimes. Working with people requires compromises on the part of both parties and thus care needs to be negotiated. An attempt has to be made to understand the client's point of view, whether in relation to personal care or specific community issues. As the community nurse carries a client load and acts as case manager, precise documentation is needed. It is especially important that the circumstances and reasons contributing to decisions are clearly documented. Records would include, for instance, the person's current condition, care provided and reasons why aspects of care were refused or altered. This information is essential both to ensure continuity of care and to fulfil legal requirements.

## 3.4 TECHNOLOGY IN THE COMMUNITY

The use of technology is increasing in all areas of nursing. Community nursing is no exception. Increases in early discharge programmes and home maintenance of acutely ill persons has meant complex medical equipment, various therapeutic techniques, paging systems, data collection and data storage systems being used outside hospitals. Technology is used to provide treatment, diagnose problems, maintain contact between centre, staff and clients, provide access to services, monitor client progress and store and analyse data.

Whether these developments are seen as a challenge (adding a new dimension) or a problem depends on the resources available, whether nurses have prior experience with the technology they are required to use, and their particular view of what constitutes community nursing. An important aspect of nurses using technology in the community is their willingness and ability to teach people how to use, monitor and manage the technology they need. The other issue is the degree to which individuals and their families can take responsibility for managing their own care and using specific therapeutic systems. Regardless of the purpose or complexity of the technology being used, knowledge, understanding and confidence are required. Nurses are not constantly in attendance, nor can they be, so both users and the nurse need to feel confident about each other's abilities. This is especially the case when technology is used intermittently as symptoms dictate. In all instances where technology is used, people need knowledge of the effects of non-use, misuse or over-use, as well as of the maintenance required. Over time the best judge of what is required is often the client, but assistance, support and encouragement are initially required to ensure that confidence develops and appropriate decisions about usage are made.

As in hospitals, there is a risk that equipment may be used incorrectly or inappropriately. If nurses are to encourage people to take responsibility for their own care, they must have confidence in their ability to do so. Anxiety on the part of the nurse can limit or delay the person's ability to develop skills and confidence. As the use of incorrect methods may give rise to complications, nurses need to be vigilant in ensuring that equipment is not used inappropriately or incorrectly, or therapies incorrectly administered. The solution is to ensure that the individual and family concerned receive adequate education. Time therefore needs to be taken before and after discharge to identify any existing anxieties, concerns, misinformation or false perceptions of either the person's illness or the purpose and effect of whatever technology is being used. This applies whether one is concerned with administration of medication, use of ventilators, oxygen therapy, specific behaviour techniques or specific observations. Where people are educated and encouraged to participate in understanding and planning their care, they are more likely to comply with the suggested regimes. Issues such as unpleasant side-effects, interference with lifestyle, misunderstandings and financial cost all contribute to people's refusal to carry out treatments. While this may be interpreted by nurses as lack of interest in their own health, for some people the benefits of treatment are outweighed by the disadvantages experienced. For instance the effects of psychotropic and cardiac drugs on some people may be such that they refuse to take them. Nurses therefore need a thorough understanding of the side-effects and complications to ensure that these issues are explored initially on discharge. To be of assistance, and to participate in health promotion, nurses need to be aware of how people feel about their illness and the care prescribed.

Discussions with clients and their families enable nurses to gain some understanding of their concerns and needs. Where differences of opinion arise between nurse and client regarding the most appropriate means of care, nurses have an obligation to ensure that clients are aware of the possible consequences of their decisions. Professional judgement is needed, but nurses also have to be aware of their own attitudes and values and how these might influence their decisions. If recommendations and advice are rejected, this should be respected if the decision was made with a full awareness of the likely outcomes. Refusal of treatment may have major or limited outcomes, leading for instance to unpleasant and foreseeable consequences such as death or an increase in hallucinations. If individuals and families are able to make decisions they have the right to do so. Only when their decision would cause harm to another, or if their condition or circumstances render them incapable of making valid decisions, should a nurse act on clients' behalf. Nurses have a responsibility to act as advocates for those they work with regardless of whether they agree with their decisions or not. Where decisions conflict with the nurse's own beliefs and values, discussion with a colleague may help. If such a situation is unresolvable, one should refer. The nurse should be aware of legal consequences of action taken, or not taken.

Client records and information about a community require the use of technology. Records form the basis on which individuals are assessed, care planned and interventions recorded and evaluated. Computers may be used to analyse information to enable a broader understanding of a community's health and a centre's activities. Information should include who is referred, by whom, for what purpose, where clients live, which areas receive or do not receive services, which age groups are served, which age or other groups of people are not being contacted, the incidence and prevalence of specific illness, which staff provide which services, and what problems are referred to other agencies. Comparisons could then be made of the activities of various centres, and existing services compared with needs using morbidity and mortality statistics and indicators of health as a guide. Such analysis would demonstrate which health problems were being addressed, and which needed attention. Data collected by health services could be used in conjunction with identified community concerns for the purpose of evaluation and identification of team goals as well as in discussions with various groups, preparation of reports, submissions for resources and planning how a service might be extended or altered. With adequate data, community nursing services would be able to begin identifying existing and anticipated community needs, plan projects to increase health and decrease illness, and anticipate increased (or decreased) needs for staff, as well as areas for ongoing staff education.

# 4. MAINTAINING A COMMUNITY PERSPECTIVE

A tension often exists in community health between the immediate needs of individuals and the long-term needs of population groups. This tension needs to be addressed at a management rather than individual worker level. Where it is not, the needs of those with existing health problems are likely to take precedence over health promotion and prevention activities. This is not to suggest that the choice is one of either-or, but rather that concerns about an individual's health should be intertwined with concerns about the population's health. As Fowler argues, prevention and cure are not alternatives but complementary activities. This unity is demonstrated in the concept of 'anticipatory care' which combines 'health promotion and maintenance, disease prevention, treatment and continuing care' (Fowler, 1986 in Fry and Hasler, 1986:69). The education of health professionals, however, prepares them to care for the immediate short-term needs of people who are ill or in crisis. The immediate needs may be physical, psychological or social depending on the discipline of the health professional concerned. Thus psychiatric nurses, psychiatrists, psychologists and social workers working in mental health, like their counterparts in the general system also focus on individuals (and families) and their immediate problems. This is a role which provides immediate personal rewards, and is comfortable since suffering is reduced, the person gets well and a sense of accomplishment is experienced. In contrast, working with persons with chronic illnesses exacerbated or caused by their lifestyle (including occupation and living conditions as well as their behaviour) or promoting the health of populations provides few and infrequent rewards.

Change or improvement in the health status of populations as a result of health promotion may take years or fail to occur at all. The attempt to establish or demonstrate a need for a new service is also a long-term project. When clinically-oriented nurses receive multiple requests for assistance from people who are acutely, chronically or terminally ill, together with requests for health education at schools and reports on area needs and service gaps, conflicts arise. While recognising that all activities are important, clinical demands more often than not are the ones responded to. There is often a failure to recognise that other services, including volunteers and home care aids, may be able to provide care safely, with the support and guidance of a registered nurse. Yet only people knowing the resources and health problems of an area can carry out the other health promotion and illness prevention activities.

Where demand rather than policy determines the allocation of resources, demands are perpetuated, and there is no examination of how best to utilise the available skills and resources for the purpose of improving the health of the community. Individual services, whether offered in clinics or in homes, are essential and appropriate. Equally important is identification and documentation of the health problems of the area, identifying groups who might require assistance or who are likely to develop an illness sometime in the future unless some intervention occurs. Where services respond to requests without ascertaining the overall needs of a community, or fail to advertise services for fear of being overwhelmed, access to services is limited and the needs of some people are neither identified nor addressed. Currently it is fashionable to espouse a commitment to primary health care. What is more important is establishing primary health care principles as a foundation for practice within an organisational framework.

It is not possible to improve the health of populations and support health promotion and illness prevention while providing a curative service, in which community nurses are judged by the number of people to whom they provide services. Pressure to carry a heavy case load limits flexibility and time available to individual clients, as well as professional autonomy, thus replicating conditions existing within hospital services for both nurses and their clients. Such pressures on time lead to provision of individualistic care which focuses on clients' 'conditions' rather than identifying their potential or anticipated needs. Care thus becomes task oriented and routine. The structure of services with emphasis on the number of home visits limits the ability of nurses to act as co-ordinators of care, or to undertake their preventive and supportive care activities. As Stott (1983:13) argues, each one-to-one contact can be used as an opportunity for health promotion. He suggested a framework of four interrelated areas on which to focus to enable this process to occur:

1.  management of presenting problem;

2.  modification of health seeking behaviour;

3.  management of continuing problems; and

4.  opportunistic health promotion.

This framework encourages looking at the presenting problem as well as other actual or potential problems. It also addresses the prevention of problems which the nurse can anticipate on the basis of clinical knowledge, current research and knowledge of the individual and family involved.

How health promotion and prevention activities are undertaken will depend on the perspective of those persons working in a particular service; that is, the understanding by the health professionals involved of what is meant by health, the causes of ill-health, and who is considered responsible for individual health. It has been suggested that in adopting a PHC perspective community nursing services need to adopt a social view of health and in doing so look beyond the needs of individual clients with existing health problems. Certainly, as Fowler (1986:157) suggests, we invest too little attention in preventive measures to pretend that we are working towards becoming a 'healthy nation'.

Barriers to the implementation of primary health care with its emphasis on health promotion and prevention are significant. They include the curative orientation inculcated by the health care system, which is supported by the current style of community nursing. A belief, widely held by health professionals and communities, is that sophisticated health services are synonymous with the attainment of health. Interrelated with this is the belief that people are passive recipients who are unable to take responsibility for themselves or participate actively in maintaining their own health, so that health professionals should make decisions for people about what they need. Another barrier is the emphasis on specialist services rather than generalist ones based on interdisciplinary teamwork. Some nurses see primary health care as a threat to professional workers' knowledge and skills (Van den Bergh-Braam, 1988:134), not only because it emphasises participation of communities but because roles for different groups of health professionals are blurred. Thus the concept of primary health care with its aim of decentralising care to benefit the public cuts across established professional interests (Van den Bergh-Braam, 1988:135).

The major goal of community nursing is to improve the health of the community served: it can only be achieved by identifying those factors that contribute to health and illness within a given community. This includes identifying major health problems and at-risk groups, and providing clinical services for people with specific health care needs. It also involves working to remove or reduce stresses that adversely affect the health of a population as well as developing individual and community strengths to resist the impacts of stresses (Waring and McLennan, 1979:130). Mahler (1981:9) argues that health and social awareness go hand in hand and that those who understand that poor health is not inevitable and that political, economic, social and environmental factors contribute to health, should make others aware of that fact. Similarly Kickbush (1989) points out that public health is about 'social justice, social change and social reform'. This approach, Kickbush believes, has been replaced by 'behavioural blaming' (1989:3). Many health problems arise in response to social, economic or environmental circumstances. The solutions require nurses to become involved in developing health policy, decision-making and writing reports and submissions to bring to the attention of health boards, local and state governments the effects of specific environmental or social issues affecting the health of populations with whom they work. At a local level, this means assisting people to establish self help or lobby groups, or food co-ops, as well as developing more accessible and appropriate services.

## 4.1 ORGANISATION OF SERVICES

The orientation of health care is more important than how much is spent or whether nurses are organised to care for specific groups. Is it narrowly focused on individual curative issues? Are the social, economic and environmental factors that contribute to health, or its absence, taken into account and acted on? Is the service accessible geographically, financially and culturally? Does it work with other organisations to promote health in communities for which the nurse has a responsibility? Does the nurse actively seek out people who may be at risk or require assistance? Does the service involve recipients of care, and the general community, in discussions about health issues that concern them? Or does the health centre merely provide a service to those people who request care for specific medical conditions? This is the difference between primary health care and conventional nursing services.

A primary health care model, unlike the passive curative model, is proactive rather than reactive, and includes case finding, ambulatory care, delegation and shared commitment. It makes care accessible, has a long term focus, encourages self reliance, fosters non-dependent relationships, initiates education projects, integrates health, and questions and influences the health system and national health policy. Health professionals are not educated in a manner that equips them for such practice (Stott, 1983). However, while education is an important influence, the orientation of the organisation in which staff work is equally important (Milio, 1981). It is essential that managers ensure that the organisation philosophically and structurally supports these activities. While education is needed for post-graduate students, if organisational structure fails to support a preventive, promotive orientation such values are unlikely to underpin the practice of nurses.

Nurse managers in community services are faced with problems similar to those of their colleagues in other areas of the health service, including 1) ensuring the provision of quality care to clients, and 2) providing an environment that ensures that health professionals are both accountable and capable of providing the service required. Allocating specific geographic areas to individual nurses may take little account of the characteristics of the population, the nature of people who require or are likely to require services (for example, aged, chronically ill), the availability of other services, socio-economic status, dominant occupations, the number of young families or new housing developments in a given area, or population density. Similarly, focusing on the number of home visits ignores the complexity of care, differences in resources, need for co-ordination, referral and the sheer unpredictability of home care (Barkauskas, 1990:400). Working away from a main headquarters means nurses have infrequent contact with colleagues, and thus have greater control over the nature and quality of the services provided (Waring and McLennan, 1979; Barkauskas, 1990). While the goals of nurse managers in all settings are similar, the organisational structure, day to day routine, fixed resources and diverse clientele means that significant differences exist between hospital and community nursing. In a hospital, extra staff can be requested as patient numbers or needs increase. This is generally not possible in a government operated nursing service. The unpredictable nature of community nursing may mean deciding who manages without assistance on a particular day or within a particular week. It may mean working extra time, with or without pay, in order to see a family with a difficulty tangential to their initial problem. Data collection and systems have to be established which enable recording of extra activities. It means working at night to have contact with community groups. Working effectively therefore means having the autonomy to make decisions about one's practice and time allocation. One also needs time to reflect on what one is doing and to respond. For example, if services are unavailable, denied or inaccessible for whatever reason to various persons, one needs to document this and set out the consequences of the situation. One needs time to work with people to promote health, and this may mean saying 'no' to demands which deflect one from this purpose.

It has already been emphasised that managers need to be able to articulate the relevance of primary health care to team members. For only when the principles are clearly understood can they be integrated into a team's philosophy, forming the basis on which team goals, strategies and services can be developed and evaluated. The role of management is to achieve the organisation's goals. It is important that management practices reflect and support the principles and values articulated. Thus participatory leadership and decision making are required. Given the community emphasis, it is important that knowledge and experience is shared with the public. Public support is necessary. Kleczkowski et al argue that primary health care 'begins with community and individual priorities and local environmental situations. It is not a blueprint or plan to be applied in a standardised way, but a dynamic and flexible approach to be adapted to each set of local needs and circumstances' (1984:15). A flexible management approach requires decentralisation of planning, decision-making and financial responsibility. Managers become responsible for choices and the allocation of resources in a region (Kleczkowski, 1984:15). The difficulty experienced by nurse managers is that while popular support exists for their services, allocation of resources, human and financial, favours acute care services rather than comprehensive services for chronically ill or disabled persons. As well, support for health promotion and illness prevention is limited. As Fabb (1986:157) argues, since many of Australia's health problems relate to lifestyle, more rather than less time needs to be spent on prevention if a healthier nation is desired, and primary health care workers such as nurses are in a position to carry out this work.

# 5. NETWORKING TO BUILD COMMUNITY RESOURCES

In keeping with a health rather than illness orientation is a management strategy that includes working with communities, other professionals, government and voluntary agencies to promote community participation in planning, implementing and evaluating health services, thereby increasing the community's ability to care for itself. It has been suggested that to improve health, nations require national goals. However, as different regions have different resources and serve different communities with different health needs, regional goals are also required. While national goals have been established by the Better Health Commission, there is no integrated policy as to how these goals might be achieved (Fabb, 1986:166). Services are therefore fragmented and unco-ordinated. Different regions need to establish goals relevant to their communities. The introduction of Area Health Boards and regional projects provides an opportunity for a regional perspective to be developed. Area health services, unlike hospital boards, have a responsibility to improve the health of regions rather than providing services to those who present for care. Thus the health problems of regions should be examined and service development should reflect the health needs of the community rather than individual professionals' interests. Taking a social view of health means recognising that it is affected by industry, transport, housing, welfare and social services as well as health services. These are factors which interrelate, and are more easily dealt with at a regional level. Networks need to be established to assist health services achieve their goal of improving the health of the population. Collaboration between various sectors may lead to a more effective co-ordination of services and referral structures and act also as a catalyst for co-operative ventures between members of different groups or organisations. Where various sectors emphasise the needs of communities rather than the interests of specific services and professions, benefits accrue to people living in that area. As co-operation between various sectors of the health services increases, there are further benefits in improved access to services and more appropriate referral procedures. Involvement of community members can assist in the evaluation of services and increase health professionals' understanding and awareness of the concerns of local people. When community members are invited to participate, care needs to be taken to ensure that they are involved in such a way that they are able to contribute. Health or its absence arises as a response to a complex array of interactions. The existence and upgrading of health services is important. However, many issues need to be resolved at a political level as they are beyond the scope of individual nurses and nursing services. Concerns about specific issues need to be raised in the appropriate manner and forum, with the appropriate people or organisations.

# 6. CONCLUSION

Over the past decade, the health care system has changed to emphasise cost containment, community care for the elderly and those with a chronic or terminal illness, early discharge programmes for mothers and babies and persons following surgery, and deinstitutionalisation for persons with a chronic mental illness or developmental disability. This has placed increasing stress on community nursing services. These services do not appear to be expanding at the same rate as the demands placed upon them. Managers of community nursing services are therefore faced with the onerous task of working to improve the health of the whole community within an environment of limited growth. An individual constraint is that health professionals lack an education that prepares them for community practice, so that nurse managers have responsibility for managing a service in such a way that it meets the needs of two populations: their staff, and the community in which they are based.

Strategies directed at promoting health for a community need to come to terms with health problems faced by all sections of a community as well as health policy and environmental issues. Nurses seeking to improve the health of individuals and families need to examine ways of providing care that where necessary promote continuity of care and deal with episodes of illness as they occur. As well, community nursing services require a structure that views clinical, promotive and preventive activities as a continuum, supporting all rather than considering them to be mutually exclusive domains. Such a view requires a rethinking of nursing practice; a change in emphasis from treatment of illness to health promotion focused on people's strengths rather than weaknesses, on what is possible rather than what is. To focus on either treatment or promotion and prevention limits the opportunities available to community nurses to contribute to improving people's health in keeping with the policy of health for all by the year 2000.

The WHO has indicated that prevention of illness and promotion of health are major components of health care. Additionally Mahler (1981) has emphasised the actual and potential contribution of nurses in these spheres. In Mahler's view, nurses can lead the way to the development of health services that best meet the health needs of communities. As the largest group of health professionals, nurses are in a position to influence and change the health care system for the better. Those working outside hospitals gain the most opportunities in this regard. Community nurses are aware of how their clients live, play and work, and this enables them to thoroughly assess their environment. However, for community nurses to work in such a way as to optimise the opportunities afforded them, they require an organisational structure that explicitly supports the philosophy and goals of health for all and primary health care and encourages adherence to, and achievement of, those stated goals.

# COMMUNITY HEALTH CASE STUDY

You are the newly appointed Team Leader for a multi-disciplinary Community Health Centre at Bogen Dale. Building of the centre has just been completed. Until now the staff in this area were considered to be a sub-team of Clackton, 50 kilometres away, and were responsible to the team leader there. It was decided to establish a separate team as the population at Bogen Dale has increased and is projected to double over the next 10 years.

Currently the 60 000 population is diverse. There is a large established elderly population. The major area of population growth is young families, that is young married couples with young children. In addition there is also a small population of young adults who moved here prior to the recent housing development because it was relatively easy to find cheap accommodation. Most of the working population in the area work in suburbs and the city some distance from Bogen Dale. In many instances the travelling time is between one and one-and-a-half hours in each direction. The staff at the new centre consists of one social worker, three community health nurses, a part-time speech pathologist and a receptionist. You have been told that you might draw on regional specialists, based at Clackton, for support.

As the new team leader you have been asked to carry out an analysis of the needs of the area and the priorities for service development. Your brief included the need to include development of clinical services as well as health promotion. At present the staff working in the area are providing clinical services to aged and mentally ill persons, baby health centre service, child and family counselling, and school medical. Some community development projects have also been undertaken and for instance, play groups have been established. The area manager believes in managers being proactive rather than reactive.

1. What would be your plan of action?

2. How would you begin to address the health needs of the area?

3. In what way would you involve the team in this undertaking?

4.  How would you manage already existing clinical services while addressing the needs of the area?

5.  How would you evaluate existing community development projects?

6.  What strategies would you use to ensure that team members provide the clinical services identified as needed and participate in community development and health promotion?

7.  What difficulties would you anticipate encountering in establishing this team?

# REFERENCES

Australian Community Health Association, (1991), *Manual of standards for community health: community health accreditation and standards program,* 2nd edition, Australian Community Health Association, Bondi Junction.

Australian Health Ministers Advisory Council (1988), *Continuing education for primary health care in Australia: Report and recommendations.*

Australian Nursing Federation, (1990), *Primary health care in Australia, strategies for nursing action,* ANF, Melbourne.

Bailey, M. and Brodaty, H. (1982), 'At the periphery. Life after hospital: trials of a boarding house "mother"', *Australian and New Zealand Journal of Psychiatry,* 16, 289–292.

Barkauskas, V. (1990), 'Home health care: responding to need, growth, and cost containment', in Chaska N. L. (Ed), *The nursing profession: turning points,* 394–405, C.V. Mosby, St Louis.

Broom, D. (1989), 'Masculine medicine, feminine illness: gender and health', in Lupton, G. M. and Najman J. M., (Eds), *Sociology of health and illness. Australian readings,* 121–134, Macmillan, Australia.

Clark, M. (1984), *Facts, myths and stigma: a report on teenage pregnancy and parenting,* Health Promotion Resource Centre, Parramatta.

Cramer, J. (1987), 'Commentary: A blind eye: community health services in remote areas of Australia', *Community Health Studies,* Vol. 2.2. 135–138.

Davis, A. and George, J. (1988), *States of health: health and illness in Australia,* Harper & Row, Sydney.

Donoghue, P. (1978) 'A Sense of Community; the Pivot of Community Nursing', Paper presented at the National Congress of the Council of Community Health Nursing, Sydney.

Fabb, W. E. (1986), 'Australia', in Fry, J. and Hasler, J. C. (eds), *Primary health care 2000,* 151–169. Churchill Livingstone, Edinburgh.

Fowler, G. (1986), 'Prevention', in Fry, J. and Hasler J. C. (eds), *Primary health care 2000,* 65–83. Churchill Livingstone, Edinburgh.

Furler, E. (1985), 'Women and health: radical prevention', *New Doctor,* 37, September, 1985, 5–8.

Gibson, D. M. (1984), 'Rosy goals reactive practice: interpreting programme failure', in *Australian and New Zealand Journal of Sociology,* Vol. 20.2. July. 218–232.

Hanson, S. M. H. (1987), 'Family nursing and chronic illness', In Wright, L. M. and Leahey, M. (Eds), *Families and chronic illness.* 2–32. Springhouse, Pennsylvania.

Health Commission of NSW (1977), *Community health: book 1–6,* Health Commission of NSW, Sydney.

Holtzman, N. (1979), 'Prevention: rhetoric or reality', *International Journal of Health Services.* Vol.9.1. 25–39.

International Council of Nurses, (1986), *Mobilising nursing leadership for primary health care,* ICN, Geneva.

Jackson, T., Mitchell, S. and Wright, M. (1989), 'The community development continuum', in Miller, M. and Walker, R. (eds), *Health promotion: the community health approach,* Australian Community Health Association, Sydney.

Kickbush, I. (1989), 'Health in Public Policy', in Miller, M. and Walker, R. (eds), *Health promotion: the community health approach,* 1–10, Australian Community Health Association, Sydney.

Kleczkowski, B. M., Elling, R. H. and Smith, D. L. (1984), *Health system support for primary health care: a study based on the technical discussions held during the thirty-fourth World Health Assembly, 1981,* World Health Organisation, Geneva.

Maglacas, A. M. (1988), 'Health for all: nursing's role', *Nursing Outlook,* Vol. 36.2. 66–71.

Mahler, H. (1981), 'The meaning of "health for all by the year 2000"', *World health forum,* 2 (1), 5–22.

Mahler, H. (1985), *Nurses lead the way,* World Health Organisation News Release, June, 1985, Geneva.

Masson, V. (1988), 'If new graduates went to the community first', *Nursing Outlook,* Vol. 36.4. 172–173.

Mechanic, D. (1978), *Medical sociology,* The Free Press, New York.

Menzies, E. P. (1970), *The functioning of social systems as a defence against anxiety,* The Tavistock Institute of Human Relations, London.

Milio, N. (1975), *The care of health in communities. Access for outcasts,* Macmillan, New York.

Milio, N. (1981), *Promoting health through public policy,* F. A. Davis, Philadelphia.

Moore, et al. (1982), 'Insane accommodation: accommodation needs for the emotionally and psychiatrically disabled', *New Doctor,* No. 27, 18–21.

National Hospitals and Health Services Commission (1973), *Interim report a community health program for Australia,* Australian Government Publishing Service, Canberra.

Navarra, V. (1976), *Medicine under capitalism,* Prodist, New York.

Navarro, V. (1986), *Crisis, health and medicine,* Tavistock, New York.

Newby, L. (1989), 'Equity for women in health. Developing national policy for women', in *Health promotion. The community health approach,* 93–97, Australian Community Health Association, Sydney.

Palmer, G. R. and Short, S. D. (1989), *Health care and public policy: an Australian analysis,* Macmillan, Australia.

Rolland, J. S. (1987), 'Chronic illness and the family: an overview', in Wright, L. and Leahey, M. *Families and chronic illness,* 33–54, Springhouse, Pennsylvania.

Rotem, A. (1984), 'Development of effective health teams', *New Doctor,* 34, 1984, 12–14.

Sax, S, 'The politics of health in Australia', (1989), in Lupton, G. M. and Najman, J. M. (eds), *Sociology of health and illness: Australian readings,* 101–117, Macmillan, Australia.

Schulz, S. A, 'Working Happily in Community Health', *Australian Community Health Association. Third National Conference Proceedings,* for publication ACHA 1992.

Seivwright, M. J. (1988), 'How to develop tomorrow's nursing leaders', *International nursing review,* 35.4, 99–106.

Short, S. and Sharman, E. (1989), 'Dissecting the current nursing struggle in Australia', in Lupton, G. M. and Najman, J. M. (eds), *Sociology of health and illness: Australian readings,* 225–235, Macmillan, Australia.

Stott, H. H. (1983), *Primary health care: bridging the gap between theory and practice,* Springer-Verlag, Berlin.

Strauss, A. and Corbin, J. M. (1988), *Shaping a new health care system: the explosion of chronic illness as a catalyst for change,* Jossey-Bass, San Francisco.

Tansey, E. M. and Lentz, J. R. (1988), 'Generalists in a specialised profession', *Nursing Outlook,* Vol.

36.4, 174–178.

Townsend, P. and Davidson, N. (1986), *Inequalities in health in the Black report,* Penguin, Middlesex.

Van den Bergh-Braam, A. (1988), 'Dispelling nurses' fears about primary health care', *International Nursing Review,* 35.5, 133–136.

Waring, J. E. and McLennan, J. P. (1979), *Community health nursing: helping with health,* McGraw-Hill, Sydney.

Watson, J. (1979), *Nursing: the philosophy and science of caring,* Little Brown, Boston.

Wellard, R. (1990), 'Decision making and teamwork. Issues in community health centres', in *Health promotion. The community health approach,* 229–232, Australian Community Health Association, Sydney.

World Health Organisation, (1985), *A guide to curriculum review for basic nursing education: orientation to primary health care and community health,* WHO, Geneva.

World Health Organisation, (1988), *Learning together to work together,* Technical Series Report 769, WHO, Geneva.

World Health Organisation, (1983-B), 'Report: expert committee on manpower requirements on the achievement of health for all by the year 2000', WHO, Geneva.

Wyndham, D. (1982), '"My doctor gives me pills to put him out of my misery": women and psychotorpic drugs', *New Doctor,* 23, March, 1982, 21–25.

# CHAPTER 2.5

# Links between nursing research and nursing management

ROBERT MARTIN AND MARJORIE CUTHBERT

After reading this chapter, you should be able:

1.  to identify the links between nursing research and nursing management;

2.  to identify the role of research in improving nursing practice, nursing education, nursing management and patient care;

3.  to define the role of the nurse manager in initiating research, in monitoring the research process and in implementing research findings to improve patient care, ward management and staff development;

4.  to define the differences between research and other methods of problem investigation;

5.  to demonstrate techniques for critiquing research;

6.  to enable the nurse manager to understand and identify the resource implications of research projects carried out in the ward or unit;

7.  to describe the different types of research and their application to care provided by nurses;

8.  to identify the links between research and standards.

This chapter is not a chapter about how to do nursing research. There are a number of excellent books available to the nurse manager on this topic including Polgar and Thomas (1991), Wilson (1989), Sarter (1988), Polit and Hungler (1991), LoBiondo-Wood and Haber (1986) and Holm and Llewellyn (1986). This chapter is designed to assist the nurse manager to recognise the important part that research plays not only in patient care but in the way in which nurses deliver and reflect on the care they provide.

Nursing managers are responsible for the operational management of a health service unit. They provide organisational support for the day-to-day operation of nursing activities and the interactions with other health care professionals. The first-line nurse manager is responsible for seeing that the nurses provided to the unit are used in the most effective and efficient way. Knowledge is needed about the patient population, casemix, dependency and resource requirements. Other responsibilities include using the skills of individual nurses appropriately to ensure the highest standard of care possible, and arranging rosters so that workloads are fairly distributed and meet patient needs. The needs for motivation and reward among staff must be met in a compassionate and caring fashion. Caring for the sick is often stressful and unrewarding and the nurse manager needs to be aware of distress in staff and implement appropriate strategies to relieve work induced strain.

Communication skills are essential for the nurse manager (Porritt, 1990). Listening to patients, nursing staff, doctors and other health professionals to ensure requests for care are clearly known is the most rudimentary of skills required. Setting up structures, whereby effective communication occurs at all levels of staffing, from the most junior to the most senior, is a key responsibility. Meetings, handovers and case reviews are organised to ensure that the right information reaches the right individuals at the right time. In effect the key features of the nurse manager's role are organisation, motivation, and communication. The basis, however, for all management action is technique knowledge.

The question that requires an answer then, is how are aspiring nurse managers to equip themselves with the necessary knowledge required to perform their duties. Knowledge can be gained in a number of ways. It can be acquired by trial and error through experience. However, continual exposure to patterns of unchanging behaviour may lead to entrenched and erroneous assumptions about future behaviours. If such assumptions are not tested by information derived publically and systematically then one is prone to continue to labour under false assumptions which leads to ineffective learning.

Science, on the other hand, provides a forum for the testing of assumptions. Over three centuries the research process known as the scientific method has developed. This method is a planned systematic method of investigating a question or assumption in order to draw a rational conclusion based on the evidence obtained from the data collected. The scientific method and its conventions (the accepted set of practices followed by researchers using this method) have developed from a set of cognitive values and normative assumptions shared by adherents to that perspective. Scientific disciplines have been built up on an accumulation of knowledge collected using this method. This method tests the assumptions of the researcher through the formulation of hypotheses or propositions which are either supported or not supported by the evidence collected in the research study. The nurse manager as a leader and as a professional sets an example by adopting a scientific approach to knowledge development.

As nursing has developed professionally it has acquired its own body of knowledge regarding its organisation, education and practice. Broadly speaking this body of knowledge has been acquired through the traditions of practice and the science of the western world. As it became evident that medicine did not have many of the answers about the organisation and well-being of nurses, the profession turned to the social sciences for guidance (Young-Kelly, 1985:285). In the USA during the 1950s most of the research into nursing was about nurses and performed by social scientists. As educational achievements improved and more nurses acquired the education required to do their own nursing research, the scope of nursing science increased to include nursing practice.

Currently nurses are engaged in a range of research activities surrounding the essential nursing role. Research may be performed in a collaborative context with the more established medical, biological and social science disciplines addressing an issue which is mutually interesting, or it may be performed independently by a nurse or a group of nurses addressing an issue only of particular relevance to nursing.

The fact that nurses are investigating themselves and their practice, sharing in medical research and interested in social scientific investigation has led to a proliferation of information about nurses and nursing, and the role of nursing in the organisation and delivery of health care. This body of knowledge contributes to the historical and public development of nursing as a professional discipline.

The nature of a professional discipline can be schematised by Figure 2.5.1.

**FIGURE 2.5.1:**   Nature of a professional discipline

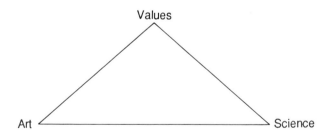

In the left corner is the practice or the doing side of nursing called 'art'. This is performed by any nurse be they practitioner, educator, manager or researcher. It is the sum total of innate capacity, education, practical experience and initiative; the skills by which a nurse performs nursing. The upper corner 'values' defines the agreed moral code to which nursing subscribes. 'Values' covers the questions of what 'ought a nurse do' in myriad contexts in which they practise. Values are often very personal, linked to culture and are metaphysically based. For example, the caring demeanour adopted by a 'good' nurse is based on the altruistic value and a belief that no matter what the human condition, care is warranted and should be delivered in a kindly and respectful manner.

In the right corner is 'science' which is the description and explanation of the what, how and why of nursing. It is a set of methods fundamentally based on the concept of falsifiability; if a proposition is true then it will only hold to be true if it cannot be demonstrated to be false. Conversely, if a proposition is not true then it can be demonstrated to be false. Science provides nursing with the structure and methods necessary for answering questions and testing the truth of assumptions. As assumptions underlie both the values and art of nursing, science therefore takes a prominent role in the shaping of progress in the profession.

Science is characterised by three essential features: first it is an investigative process, second it is systematic and third it is open to public scrutiny. This provides it with immense power for if it reveals truth and provides understanding, it enables the development of values and art that are guided by knowledge. It enables the assumptions on which art and values are based to be tested and either falsified or verified.

A nurse manager therefore, to be truly a leader and co-ordinator of nursing, must lead from a position of science. If the best possible care is to be provided to patients then the nurse manager is responsible for knowing what the best care is, why it must be provided, how to organise it and how to ensure that it is delivered and evaluated by members of the nursing team.

# 1. THE STRUCTURE OF THE SCIENTIFIC METHOD

In the western world what is known as the 'scientific method' has come to be respected as the most powerful means of problem solving available. While it is not expected by the health care organisation that a nurse manager be an expert and active scientist, it is reasonable to expect that a nurse manager would be capable of critiquing research publications on nursing and related health service issues and of evaluating requests to perform research into or about nursing or other care provided in their particular area.

Research has an important role in the general management of the ward or unit and in the education of nurses. For the nurse manager who has had no previous exposure to research and research methods the literature can be confusing. Research has been classified in a number of ways such as basic and applied research; qualitative and quantitative research; and according to the discipline of the researcher, that is, epidemiological research, historical research, psychological research, sociological research or nursing research to name a few. There have even been arguments as to whether in these areas the terms research in psychology, research in sociology or research in nursing may be more appropriate in certain circumstances.

As knowledge in an area of research increases, models are developed and tested to determine whether they are worthwhile in practice. When a model is shown to apply to a number of different groups of people or subjects the model is said to have good 'generalisability'. If the models are supported by replication or repetition of the research in other settings and with other subjects then a theory is developed and the theory shapes practice.

Advances in research using the scientific method have been made when there has been disagreement between scientists. These disagreements have arisen because of differing cognitive values, different methodological approaches and standards being used, and the inability to completely prove or refute a theory with any certainty (Laudan, 1984; 13–22, 54–57, 136–137).

The structure and form of the scientific method are quite precise and can easily be schematised:

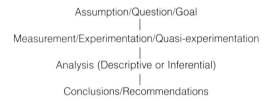

The starting point of any research is either an assumption which requires testing to determine its truth, a question which requires observation to determine an answer, or a goal that has been defined as worthy of achievement which requires measurement and analysis to determine its outcome. In this context research is thought to be objective because measurement, experimentation and quasi-experimentation are performed on events or objects which are taken to be independent of the observer. The implementation of a research design and the analysis of its results can be simple or highly elaborate.

When research is driven by a simple question, for example about the prevalence of limb contractures in immobilised patients, simple frequency counts and percentage distributions may only need presenting to indicate the extent of the problem. Converting numbers of contractures occurring to a percentage of all immobilised patients treated in the period of time during which the frequency count was taken is a process of standardisation. It allows different periods of time to be compared even though there may have been more or less immobilised patients in each period investigated.

In the case of more complex assumptions about cause and effect relationships, for example the prevention of limb contractures by provision of exercise for profoundly immobilised patients, the experimental method may need a control group of similar patients who do not receive exercise to allow for comparisons between the groups to occur. The comparisons would be carried out by a formal test of statistical inference to determine whether there are any significant differences between the two groups after the treatment has been given. If there is a significant difference and an improvement is shown in the experimental group (the group receiving the treatment) then the association between the treatment and the assumed outcome allows conclusions to be drawn and recommendations to be made which will influence future care of similar patients.

A simple caution must be issued to the reader regarding the nature of scientific knowledge. It is often argued by hard nosed positivists that the only true form of science is that based on experiment. This is a hotly contested viewpoint and not the only one that is held. Science to that end can be broadly divided into two schools. The first, and perhaps the oldest, school is called 'emic' science (Research Unit in Health and Behavioural Change, University of Edinburgh, 1989:30–31). This form of science relies on the powers of observers to describe their experience which for the purpose of the investigation is within a circumscribed time period. The method seeks through descriptive language to increase knowledge of the context in which human and interaction occurs. This method is often referred to as 'qualitative' research.

The second school is called 'etic' science and is generally that performed by most modern western scientists. In this form the investigator seeks to find explanations for casual relations or to discover interventions which will alter an undesirable effect. The most rigorous approach to science in this form is the controlled experimental trial. This method uses a 'quantitative' approach. However, it is strongly argued that, depending on what the investigator is concerned to discover, both approaches are legitimate for investigating issues in nursing.

No matter what the approach, the scientific method aims to be precise and factual. Because scientists are attempting to demonstrate new knowledge, the reporting of research is highly schematised and an awareness of the required format is essential. When published a report is generally structured in the following way.

## 2.1 THE TITLE

A research report title conveys to the reader the problem of interest specifying the variables being investigated and the relationship requiring testing. As the title is the first part of the report to which the reader refers, and often the only part to appear in a search of the literature on the topic, it must convey sufficient meaning for readers to know if the report is of interest.

## 2.2 ABSTRACT

The abstract is a succinct summary of the body of the report and is generally between 100–250 words long. Its purpose is to convey in very general terms the problem being investigated, the assumptions made by the investigators, the data collection and analytic methods used, the findings, conclusions drawn and implications of the study. The abstract provides a very good overview of the report and may be the only part read by a generally interested reader who is skimming a range of related articles, particularly if the report is in a foreign language.

## 2.3 INTRODUCTION

This is the first substantive part of the research report. The introduction provides the reader with a detailed description of the background to the problem being investigated by either describing its salient features or by enunciating the component variables and any implied relationships. It should give the reader a very good understanding of the concerns of the investigators. When the investigators are performing research where an hypothesis is being tested, the hypothesis is explicitly stated. If a question is being asked or if goals are to be achieved, they are also explicitly stated so that important terms are defined and explained.

## 2.4 LITERATURE REVIEW

The literature review provides supportive evidence for the problem under investigation. It is not intended to be a general review of the subject to which the problem is attached. Rather it provides the reader with an explanation of how the problem has been investigated in the past, the strengths and limitations of previous research efforts, the substantive findings of previous research and questions left unanswered. In this way it sets the stage for the research problem and justifies the importance of the research being reported.

## 2.5 METHODS

Along with the results section, the methods section is probably the most important section of a research report but the least read and the most misunderstood. Particular attention should be paid to this section of a research report because it states how the investigator went about addressing the research problem. It should first define the target population if the research is studying a group of people, or define the case study or the sample to be used. The rationale for the selection and the technique used is clearly defined. In experimental studies, subject assignment to treatment or control groups is explained fully as is the technique that is being applied – allocation according to a set of random numbers or matched pairing, for example. The method of measurement is explained and the reliability and validity of the instrument clearly detailed. Reliability refers to the ability of the researcher or researchers to use the survey tool or the instrument in the same way on repeated occasions of use. In order to do this the instrument used must be clearly worded and unambiguous and the researchers and subjects should not be affected by weather, moods, fatigue or other factors. Similarly subjects involved in the research will respond in the same way if tested at different times and in different settings. If an instrument is valid it is actually measuring what it is designed to measure. It is possible for an instrument to be valid when used in one setting but not in another and without reliability there is no validity.

In experimental studies the research design is set out so that the reader knows exactly what treatments are being applied and how error and bias are being controlled. Both error and bias affect the degree of reliability and validity achieved. Analytic methods that have been applied to provide descriptions or to draw inferences are also clearly explained so that somebody who wanted to replicate the research could do so.

## 2.6 RESULTS

In this section the findings of the investigation are recorded in sufficient detail to provide the reader with enough evidence to corroborate conclusions. Generally this section describes what was found by the researchers. If the research is contextual then a verbal description is provided. If the study is numerically descriptive then tables and graphs along with statistical and verbal descriptions may be provided. If the study has used statistical tests to draw inferences, their results may be presented in numerical, graphic and verbal forms.

## 2.7 CONCLUSION

This section is where the investigators present what they believe are the major findings of the research project. This section should link the introduction, research problem, methods and results together, in general terms, so that the reader can judge the validity and accuracy of the inferences drawn.

## 2.8 DISCUSSION

This section follows on from the conclusions and puts the research into context by stating how it is linked to the literature cited previously. Major advances, strengths, limitations and weaknesses of the current investigation are stated to aid the reader in judging the value of the research. Any problems or unanswered questions are raised and recommendations for future research suggested.

## 2.9 REFERENCES

All literature cited in the report is listed so that the reader can refer to it if there is the need or the wish to check the context of the references.

The major characteristic of scientific investigation is the desire to know and to understand what is true. This is highlighted by the rigour of the method be it etic or emic and the requirement of a high level of precision in publishing results. Nurse managers have an integral role to play in being aware of major developments in science and the profession of nursing and in promoting this awareness to their staff so they can judge the strengths of various published reports.

# 2. MANAGING SCIENTIFIC INVESTIGATION AT THE UNIT LEVEL

Increasingly nurses are being exposed to health services research in action. Doctors, biological and social scientists, allied health professionals and nurses are interested in increasing their knowledge about health, sickness and how to care for those in need. Knowledge about health, illness and its treatment and health service delivery is not complete, requiring updating and challenging so that it grows and produces better results. Science in this context is dynamic and like any other human process requires management to maintain quality and efficiency. In this information era the nurse manager will be required to deal with requests from nursing colleagues and from other health professions.

It is recommended that in all but the most trivial requests some formal mechanism for judging the merit of the research proposal be in place. In larger hospitals, generally all requests are required to be vetted by a research and ethics committee. In smaller hospitals the responsible committee may be the patient care committee. Most institutions have a formal written policy about how proposals should be judged and approved, and how research is to be conducted. It is a nursing unit manager's responsibility to be aware of and follow such a policy. Moreover, on many occasions, requests will be made for the unit to be involved in some form of research; if that research is to be planned and implemented in a sound manner, precise management will be required. Any budgetary implications for conducting the research require careful consideration and negotiation with the principal researchers.

The research proposal serves as the basic medium for stating the plan of research. If research is being planned on the ward or if requests are being made to perform research, the nurse manager will require knowledge about research proposals if their merit is to be assessed.

The following presents an outline of what should be contained in a well-thought-out proposal. The structure is similar to a research report in the sense that it will have an introduction, a statement of the problem, literature review, methods section and a section on how the researcher plans to analyse the data collected. Preferably a copy of any instruments to be used should be included so that the nurse manager and staff can assess the likely affects on patients and workloads. In addition the nurse manager should ensure that the following information is included.

1. Included in the introduction should be a definition for any technical or idiosyncratic terms used. If relationships are being measured or tested then both the independent variable and the dependent variable should be operationally defined. The independent variable is the variable which is manipulated by the investigator while the dependent variable is the variable which is being measured. In a study carried out by Hodge et al (1990) to investigate the effect on nursing practice of the introduction of the Norton Scale as an early warning system for prevention of decubitis ulcers, the Norton Scale used in care planning is the independent variable. Skin assessment linked to types and times of nursing interventions are the dependent variables. The researchers specified the days and times on which the patients' Norton scores and skin assessments were to be carried out and the level of experience required of the nurses undertaking the assessments.

2. The validity and reliability of any measurements being used should be clearly stated. This is important because the investigators must be able to demonstrate that what they want to measure is what they actually are measuring. They must also be able to demonstrate that the measure can be used consistently by different observers and that it can measure the same observation in the same way over time. The measure used should also be able to obtain similar results as another instrument designed to measure the same variable. A four year study by Prescott et

al (1991) describes the complexities involved in assessing validity of nursing intensity systems. The researchers used a variety of statistical tests, staff estimates and observational studies to assess the validity of the instrument used to measure the levels of nursing intensity required for patient care. Both LoBiondo-Wood and Haber (1986) and Holm and Llewellyn (1986:126, 129) provide checklists which the nurse manager can use to help assess the worth of research proposals. The latter authors also provide guidelines for the level of involvement in research of nurses with different educational levels (Holm and Llewellyn, 1986:220).

3. The research design must also be valid for the type of problem that is being addressed. An internally valid research design is one that endeavours to hold constant as many extraneous factors as possible and thus prevent the likelihood of an alternative explanation for results obtained. These extraneous variables, also known as confounding or intervening variables, are factors which the researcher may not have considered and could affect the relationship between the independent and dependent variables. Such factors as time of day, lighting, heating, background noise, degree of privacy etc may produce false positive or false negative results. Extraneous variables which cannot be controlled should be spread randomly across the study in order to eliminate any biases present. Cook and Campbell (1979) identified a number of extraneous variables which may affect nursing research. The most likely to occur are:

☐ **selection:** subjects ought to be selected in an impartial and fair way. The researcher has to be cautious not to select subjects that will bias the outcome towards the desired result. This can sometimes be a problem if volunteers are used;

☐ **history:** variables change as time progresses. Subjects are affected by their experience over time: if the study is longitudinal, that is, tests are repeated over a period of time, then subjects may be affected by events to which they are exposed between tests;

☐ **maturation:** just as time has an influence so does ageing, so subjects need to be grouped according to their different ages and/or experience. Rivalry, boredom, fatigue, are other factors which also occur with maturation;

☐ **instrumentation:** wear and tear affect material objects so instruments need to be calibrated before each use. Individual differences in response times and idiosyncratic methods of use can also affect measurements obtained so it is important to check both inter-rater and intra-rater reliability levels;

☐ **statistical regression:** in nature there is a tendency for high and low measures to move towards the average score, especially if subjects are being measured on more than one occasion;

☐ **loss of subjects:** in complicated and time consuming studies, subjects may drop out, changing the characteristics of the sample and biasing the results.

Equally important is external validity which is exclusively concerned with generalisability of results. The results of a study ought to be applicable to other settings (known as 'ecological validity') or to other people ('population validity') than those from which the problem arose (Huck, Cormier and Bounds, 1974). Many of the problems associated with external validity are due to poor study design. They are fully described by Holm and Llewellyn (1986:264) and are related to the ability of other researchers to repeat the study from the description of the variables and their measurement supplied by the author of the study. Other problems relate to the way in which the personality, bearing, cultural background or authority of the researcher can affect the subjects' responses (the 'Rosenthal' effect) or simply through subjects' responses being influenced because they are participating in a study. This is known as the 'Hawthorne' effect and has led to control subjects in drug trials being given a placebo to counter the effect of taking part in a study. A study design which is limited by the subjects selected, the instruments used and the methods applied will lead to results which cannot be validly applied beyond the context of the investigation. It is a shame when researchers or nursing staff invest large amounts of time and resources only to find that their results are limited because of poor design. Empirical research requires rigorous planning and preparation to ensure external validity.

4.  A statement of the resources required to perform the investigation. Research takes time and human effort. New and novel treatments are often expensive. A good research proposal details the time and resource cost, providing wherever possible a dollar value. If co-operation and help is required from staff, it is best stated as this then permits the nurse manager to make a much better assessment of staff involvement required and its implications for staffing. Sources of funding are listed and if subjects or staff are to be paid, the amount is detailed. When studies are performed on recovering patients their rest time is intruded upon and their recovery may be affected in ways not intended. McCarthy, Ouimet and Daun (1991) when reviewing the literature on noise stress found that it had the potential 'to alter the course of wound healing'. If recovery is delayed this adds to the costs of overall treatment of patients with financial implications for hospital, patient and patients' families.

5.  A time plan indicating how long the study is likely to take is provided. This includes the expected commencement and completion times.

6.  Ethical considerations are clearly detailed. The method of obtaining consent from subjects should indicate voluntary agreements. A statement of how any dangers involved in treatment or measurements applied are to be communicated to subjects in plain language prior to the investigation's commencement are to be clearly detailed. Measures taken to protect the interest and safety of staff, visitors and patients not involved in the research, along with that of the subject, are identified in the proposal. No matter how well the research is planned on paper, when it is implemented it will intrude into the usual activities of the unit. Special consideration

will be required for the investigators and every effort made to ensure that the study conditions remain the same and that the results obtained are not accidentally damaged, falsified or biased. An important function for the nurse manager is communicating with staff and all the people involved so that every caution is applied.

# 3. SIMILARITIES BETWEEN QUALITATIVE AND QUANTITATIVE RESEARCH

Many hospitals and health services are not used to receiving qualitative research proposals. However similarities will be present in proposal applications. Qualitative proposals will still have a purpose and a set of objectives and these should be stated in simple, clear language. If the nurse manager does not understand any terms used then the researcher can be asked to explain them so they can be communicated to staff. The research method, the time frame and the resource implications can all be provided. Morse (1989:249–250) suggests that the most appropriate form of consent for an ongoing qualitative study is a 'process consent' which 'offers the opportunity to actualise a negotiated view and to change arrangements if necessary'. Nursing staff do need to be aware that at times interviews may result in emotional responses from the person involved and they may have to support both the patient and the researcher if this occurs. The nurse manager also needs to consider whether there are beneficial effects to be derived from the research to justify the involvement of patients and staff.

# 4. PROMOTION AND ENCOURAGEMENT WITHIN THE WARD OR UNIT

In the previous study mentioned by Hodge et al (1990) the researchers found that in general nurses were 'reactive rather than proactive to pressure area care' and 'demonstrated little understanding of the theoretical principles involved' in the prevention and treatment of decubitus ulcers. Holm and Llewellyn (1986:216–219) consider there are a number of difficulties nurse managers face in implementing research in their wards or units. Listed among these are 'failure of researchers to communicate findings', lack of researcher role models, the problem of research which is not linked to nursing theory, lack of replication of studies to validate clinical research, and the bureaucratic difficulties associated with the implementation of findings into clinical practice.

Some of the strategies that other nurse managers have found useful are to encourage staff to join the research special interest groups. Staff can also be encouraged to enrol in courses providing education in research methods. Nurses undertaking degrees can be provided with the time and the support required to undertake the research required as part of their course work. Inservice sessions can be held weekly at appointed times when staff together assess patient care problems occurring on the ward and decide who will be responsible for undertaking the research required for this problem. Nurses can be encouraged to join multi-disciplinary research teams or collaborative research teams with staff from universities (MacKay et al, 1991; Pittman et al, 1991). Provision and distribution of relevant articles can also be arranged. Researchers who have carried out research in the ward or unit can be invited back both during the research and on completion to give a report, answer questions and promote discussion.

Nurse managers are in a powerful position to change nursing practice and research is a powerful tool for change.

# SUMMARY

This chapter introduces the nurse manager to nursing research and its importance to the improvement of nursing care. It identifies the links that exist between nursing research and the management of patient care. A model is provided which describes the art, science and values of nursing and its relationship to nursing research is discussed. The structure of the scientific method is described. The different forms of nursing research are discussed and techniques suggested for critiquing proposals submitted to the nurse manager. Included is a discussion of the many factors affecting reliability of instruments or survey tools and the validity of the research. The role of the nurse manager in facilitating, reviewing and monitoring research and in implementation of results is identified. Finally strategies are suggested for promoting and encouraging research in the nursing unit.

## DRYANDRA CASE STUDY 3

On Tuesday, at the Nursing Executive Meeting, Lesley Linum, Director of Nursing of the Dryandra Base Hospital, had noted that the report from the Assistant Director of Nursing on the Quality Assurance Programme had identified an alarming increase in the number of medication errors and patient accidents. The ADN had also reported concern at the numbers of drugs being prescribed for some of the elderly cardiac patients. One patient was reported to be on more than 30 different drugs a day.

1.   As the nurse unit manager, how would you deal with the problems identified by the ADN Quality Assurance?

# REFERENCES

Cook, T. D. and Campbell, D. T. (1979), *Quasi-experimentation: design and analysis issues for field settings,* Rand McNally, Chicago.

Hodge, J., Mounter, J., Gardner, G., and Rowley, G. (1990), 'Clinical trial of the Norton Scale in acute care settings', *Australian Journal of Advanced Nursing,* 8, 1, 39–46.

Holm, K., and Llewellyn, J. G. (1986), *Nursing research for nursing practice,* W. B. Saunders Company, Philadelphia.

Huck, S. W., Cormier, W. H. and Bounds, W. G., Jr. (1974), *Reading statistics and research,* Harper and Row, New York.

Laudan, L. (1984), *Science and values: the aims of science and their role in scientific debate,* University of California Press, Berkeley.

LoBiondo-Wood, G. and Haber, J. (1986), *Nursing research: critical appraisal and utilisation,* C.V. Mosby and Co., St Louis.

McCarthy, D. O., Ouimet, M. E., Daun, J. M. (1991), 'Shades of Florence Nightingale: potential impact of noise stress on wound healing', *Holistic Nursing Practice,* 5, 4, 39–48.

MacKay, R., Cruickshank, J. and Matsuno, K. (1991), 'Developing a hospital nursing research program', *Australian Journal of Advanced Nursing,* 8, 2, 10-14.

Morse, J. M. (1989), *Qualitative nursing research: a contemporary dialogue,* Aspen, Rockville.

Pittman, L., Warmuth, C., Gardner, G. et al, (1991), 'Developing a model for collaborative research', *Australian Journal of Advanced Nursing,* 8, 2, 34–40.

Polgar, S. and Thomas, S. A. (1991), *Introduction to research in the health sciences,* 2nd ed, Churchill Livingstone, Melbourne.

Polit, D.O'H., and Hungler, B. P. (1991), *Nursing research principles and methods, 4th edition,* Lippincott, Philadelphia.

Porritt, L. (1990), *Interaction strategies: an introduction for health professionals, 2nd edition,* Churchill Livingstone, Melbourne.

Prescott, P. A., Ryan, J. W., Soeken, K. L. et al (1991), 'The patient intensity for nursing index: a validity assessment', *Research in Nursing and Health,* 14, 213–221.

Research Unit in Health and Behavioural Change, University of Edinburgh (1989), *Changing the public health,* John Wiley and Sons, Chichester.

Sarter, B. (1988), *Paths to knowledge: innovative research methods for nursing,* National League for Nursing, New York.

Wilson, H. S. (1989), *Research in nursing, 2nd edition,* Addison-Wesley, California.

Young-Kelly, L. (1985), *Dimensions of professional nursing, 5th edition,* Macmillan, New York.

# Outcomes: their measurement and management

MARJORIE CUTHBERT

This chapter aims to:

1. provide an understanding of casemix and its use as a payment system;

2. describe the benefits of casemix for management of quality patient care;

3. identify the links between care planning, documentation of care and the outcomes of care.

On 28–29 August, 1984 the Commonwealth Department of Health held the first conference on casemix and diagnosis related groups of diseases (DRGs) at the Park Royal Hotel in Canberra. Initially only about 16 invited persons were expected to attend. The interest was so great however that around a hundred researchers, academics, information system managers, and health care personnel were present. Now, seven years later, the Australian Casemix Development Programme is in its third year and major changes have been made to the management of information in many hospitals throughout the country.

The casemix development programme is a five year Commonwealth-funded programme of research to examine options for allocation of funds to health care services. Expenditure on health care services has grown over the past 20 years, mainly due to the increases in biotechnology, nuclear medicine, radiology, pharmaceuticals, and staffing costs. The health services workforce increased 7 per cent overall per 10 000 population between 1976 and 1986 but the government has managed to contain the growth at around 7.5 per cent to 8 per cent of the gross domestic product (Grant and Lapsley, 1991:152, 103). Much of the containment has been possible because of the shifting of a portion of the costs to the consumer and to the insurers.

Health care organisations are big business and are usually one of the largest employers in a town. Like any big business, health care requires careful management and a good information system can assist greatly in that process.

Although the Commonwealth provides the bulk of the funds for health care in Australia, with supplementary funds provided by direct state grants, the funding arrangements to health care organisations differ from state to state. Broadhead (1991) describes the three commonly used approaches which are 'historical funding, population-based allocation and output-based payment'. When funding is based on past requirements over a period of time the funding provided often shows little relationship to the needs of the area served. Vocal lobby groups, political expediency and geographic location can affect the funds provided and consequently inefficient methods of care delivery are often perpetuated. NSW, Tasmania and Queensland currently use population-based funding and while this is certainly an improvement on historical funding it does not guarantee equity of access to health services because within the regions, or areas, the mix of services provided may still be historically based rather than needs based (Broadhead, 1991).

A variety of output-based or fee-for-service payment systems are in use. Hospitals in NSW were formerly funded on the number of patient days in a given period. This method does not account for the intensity or complexity of care provided and does little to promote efficiency.

# 1. DIAGNOSIS-RELATED GROUPS (DRGs) AND CASEMIX

Although there are a number of different casemix systems, the one which has received the bulk of research funding in Australia is DRGs and its variants. This system was developed at Yale University by Robert Fetter and associates in the 1950s. Originally it was planned as a quality assurance system but has also proved useful as a casemix management system especially for health maintenance organisations and as a prospective payment system for Medicare and Medicaid patients in the United States of America.

In a DRG casemix based system, patients are categorised into 477 groups according to a set of medical criteria which includes their principal diagnosis, whether they have had a surgical procedure, presence or absence of other conditions or complications, in some instances age and/or sex, and whether the patient survived. Patients' records on discharge are first coded in the medical record department using the ICD-9-CM system and the cases are then grouped into DRGs using special computer software of which there are a number of different versions. The new market place terminology describes this process as defining a hospital's products, and like the products we see on the supermarket shelves each product has a different production cost.

Two different methods of allocating costs are presently on trial in Australia: 'clinical costing' where costs incurred by each inpatient are recorded, and the 'Yale cost model' developed by the Health Systems Management Group at Yale University (Palmer et al 1991). The Yale cost model requires the allocation of direct, indirect and fixed costs to patient care cost centres. The estimated proportional amount of resources used is allocated to each DRG from each of the patient care cost centres so that an average cost per DRG per day and per episode of care is obtained. At the present time research is endeavouring to discover the best way of assessing the resources used by psychiatric (Meehan, 1991) and paediatric patients and newborn infants (Phelan et al, 1990). Work is also progressing on the grouping of day-only patients and outpatients (Jackson, 1990).

In recent years research at the Centre for Hospital Management and Information Systems Research at the University of New South Wales has led to the development of an Australian version of the software used to group patients into DRGs and to the refinement of the DRG categories to account for case complexity or disease severity and resource use within each DRG. However, refining the DRGs and grouping them into more homogenous classes according to severity usually results in a smaller number of cases in each RDRG (Refined Diganosis-Related Group). Consequently a much larger volume of data is needed to draw useful conclusions for utilisation review and quality assurance purposes (Reid et al, 1991). Administration costs are also increased with the greater complexity making it difficult to justify the refinements.

Once patients are grouped into similar categories the DRG data can be used to provide useful information for a variety of professionals. If the information is to be used for funding purposes or for comparison of costs within or between hospitals, then a standardised system of allocating costs to cost centres according to patient resource use is required (Palmer et al, 1991). The method usually used for distributing nursing costs is according to nursing dependency or nursing intensity (the terms are used synonymously). In the studies conducted in Australia, Palmer et al (1991), when looking at seven teaching hospitals in NSW, used the nursing weights developed in the US by Fetter et al (1987), while in a Victorian study Abernethy, Magnus and Stoelwinder (1990) used data collected using three different dependency systems to cost nursing services.

A number of researchers have emphasised the need to develop a set of local weights for nursing services (Cuthbert, 1990; Fletcher, 1990; Abernethy, Magnus and Stoelwinder, 1990). These researchers also recommended that the reliability and validity of both the nursing dependency systems and the DRG model be improved.

## 2. VALIDITY OF THE PAIS MODEL

The PAIS nursing dependency system is now used in over a hundred hospitals throughout Australia. It was developed by Hovenga (1985) in community hospitals in Victoria for the Health Department Victoria. It is widely accepted by nurses in this country because of its simplicity, ease of use and because it appears to discriminate between groups of patients on the basis of their nursing requirements.

Because this system is so widely used a study of the validity of the PAIS system for a major teaching hospital was funded by the Faculty of Professional Studies at the University of New South Wales, the National Health and Medical Research Council and the NSW Department of Health (Cuthbert et al, 1989). This study followed one conducted at three different types of hospitals comparing five different nursing dependency studies. Results of the comparative study indicated that there were a number of problems with the dependency systems in use, that nurses were writing similar types of statements for each patient rather than individualising care, and what was written was often not translated into action. Not all care plans were retained as a permanent part of the patient record, making it difficult to undertake clinical nursing research. The researchers concluded that the care plan should become a permanent record. There are legal implications as a result and the nurse is more accountable for care planning and delivery. This led to the move to link care to standards.

Results from the validity study showed that lower dependency patients were receiving less time than was allocated for their care while higher dependency patients were receiving more. This indicates how nurses set priorities for care and it does not necessarily mean that a lower standard of care is given. A further finding was that the PAIS model's assumption that patients over the age of 60 required more care was not supported. This result corroborated those of Cuthbert (1983) who also found in a study of patients' dependency that stratification according to age 60 was not warranted.

A further issue raised in this study which is of relevance to the nurse manager is the time used for handover. All staff members attended handover which could last up to 55 minutes with an average of 13 minutes. It is up to the nurse manager to ensure that this time is used productively. It can be a learning time or boring, wasted time. It is a time when staff members, if all are present and if encouraged to do so, can offer constructive criticism of patient care. It is a time when successful interventions can be identified and later tested through research. It is a time when problems can be identified which would be suitable for quality improvement projects.

## 2.1 DEVELOPMENT OF THE NURSING DATA BASE AND ACTION PLAN

In order to maintain the reliability and validity of the PAIS system on an ongoing basis, the author who at that time occupied a joint appointment as a senior lecturer at the University of New South Wales and as ADN Quality Assurance, and the Nurse Educator Ann Murphy jointly developed a care plan based on the PAIS indicators.

The new name of nursing data base and action plan was chosen for the care plan as it was thought to more closely identify its purpose. The purpose of the care plan was to streamline nursing documentation, ensure that patient events such as radiology, diagnostic tests or IV line changes could be notified in advance so that they would not be inadvertently omitted, and facilitate evaluation and nursing research as the care plan was to become a permanent part of the patient record. The Nursing Quality Assurance Committee of St Vincent's Hospital Sydney formed working parties to develop a set of standards for each of the indicators (see Appendix to this chapter). It is possible for the standards to be printed in pocket book size as a handy reference for the beginning nurse. The nursing data base and action plan was trialled for one month in three different types of wards in three different sections of the hospital. Orientation meetings were held with nursing staff at the commencement of the project and regular meetings were held with the nursing staff to obtain their valued comments. A number of changes were made as a result of this input before the final version was accepted by the Nursing Quality Assurance Committee (see Figures 2.6.1 and 2.6.2).

The standards have now been modified to form the basis of an evaluation tool which is available on application to the hospital. An example of the tool is shown in Figure 2.6.3.

The Nursing Information System also includes statistical data bases for the clinical indicators mentioned Chapter 2.5.

The original Nursing Data Base and Action plan as shown in Figures 2.6.1 and 2.6.2 has the pages printed back to back on A3 paper and when folded it is A4 size and fits into the nursing care folder. The front page contains the demographic data, the patient history and an overview of the basic nursing care required so that the nurse can see immediately the patient's requirements. Discharge planning, separation of the patient, instructions for completing the data base and the approved PAIS technical activities are included on the back page. When opened out the middle page shows the initial plan of care and a column for daily evaluation and revision of the care plan. Scheduled appointments can be written in for the appropriate day of the week as can IV line changes. A major advantage is that the nurse and other health care professionals can easily monitor the patient's progress and thus ensure that the desired outcome is achieved.

The care plan has recently been modified for the Wodonga District Hospital in Victoria. It is possible to incorporate minor changes without affecting the format and its purpose.

# 3. LINKS TO CLINICAL COSTING AND DRGS

When costing nursing services it is important to remember that there is only the amount of funding allocated to patient care available — no more and no less. This can only buy a certain number of nursing hours. The other variable which affects costing is the grade of nurse employed. The nurse manager determines the skills required and hopefully is able to employ nurses at that level. A balance of highly skilled and expensive nurses to less experienced and less expensive nurses is required. As demonstrated in the validity study (Cuthbert, Hawkins and Goodwin, 1989) nurses' priorities determine how much care patients receive.

A casemix clinical costing system can provide a variety of useful information for the nurse manager. DRG average lengths of stay are now available for most states and nurse managers can compare DRG information for their unit with the state averages. Costs can be obtained for ward inpatient care, for theatre and for pharmaceuticals for each DRG for each unit, allowing comparisons between units and an assessment of which patients require the most nursing resources and which the least. These can be monitored over time. If the averages change due to say the presence of an increasing number of complications such as pulmonary embolus or deep venous thrombosis then the nursing data base can be a valuable research tool. DRGs permit performance indicators such as these to be monitored on a regular basis and in one teaching hospital has led to greater use of calf compressors and rapid recognition of at risk patients (Figure 2.6.4).

Pharmacy costs can also be monitored in relation to certain illnesses and determined as a proportion of other costs. DRGs and clinical costing enable the nurse manager to examine why certain patients require more resources and provide a ready explanation for cost fluctuations. The extent of the information which can be extracted to explain patient outcomes is only limited by the questions asked by the clinicians and the nurse manager. Explanation of previous patient outcomes assists in identifying actions to be taken to ensure the best possible patient care in the future.

**DISCHARGE PLAN**

Proposed date of discharge ............ Actual date of discharge ............

Comment

| | Yes | N/A | Comment |
|---|---|---|---|
| Social Worker arranged | ☐ | ☐ | |
| Occupational Therapist arranged | ☐ | ☐ | |
| Community care organised | ☐ | ☐ | |
| Patient teaching commenced | ☐ | ☐ | |
| Physiotherapist arranged | ☐ | ☐ | |

**SEPARATION OF PATIENT**

Destination on discharge ............

Escort required ☐ Not required ☐ Arranged ☐ Name of escort person ............

Means of transport - Private car ☐ Taxi ☐ Ambulance ☐ Hospital Transport ☐ Other ☐

Comment

| | Yes | N/A |
|---|---|---|
| Referral letter | ☐ | ☐ |
| Medical certificate | ☐ | ☐ |
| Discharge medications - ordered | ☐ | ☐ |
| - obtained | ☐ | ☐ |
| - explained | ☐ | ☐ |
| Valuables returned to patient | ☐ | ☐ |
| Clothing returned to patient | ☐ | ☐ |
| Private X-Rays returned to patient | ☐ | ☐ |
| Follow-up appointments made | ☐ | ☐ |
| Location for appointments explained | ☐ | ☐ |

Continuing problems on discharge ............

Discharge nurse ............ Name, Signature, Designation ............ Date ............

**INSTRUCTIONS FOR USE OF THIS FORM**

This form is commenced on admission and used for seven days. It is a permanent legal record of nursing care.

On Admission - complete the -
· top section of the front page
· PAIS indicator assessment column, p.2
· 'Day 1' column on front page
· 'Initial plan of care', p.2
· Every box must be filled in
· Every entry must be dated and signed

Day 2-7 (every day)
· Complete every box of appropriate columns on pages 1 and 2

Day 8
· Commence new sheet, do not transcribe admission data. Keep forms together for easy reference

Discharge Plan
· Commence on admission
· Continue progressively

**APPROVED PAIS TECHNICAL ACTIVITIES**

· Pre-operative preparation

· Nebulised medications / peak flow
· Oxygen therapy
· Cardiac monitoring

· Tracheostomy care
· Management of naso-gastric tube
· Management of under-water sealed drains
· Insertion of urinary catheter
· Stomal care
· Enema / bowel washout

· Venepuncture
· Finger-prick blood sugar levels

· Traction
· Team lifting (more than 2 persons)
· Peritoneal dialysis procedures
· Central line change
· Applying Thrombo-embolic Deterrent Stockings

· Assisting a clinical procedure
· Specialised nursing procedures

ADMISSION DATE ............ SHEET NO ............

PROVISIONAL DIAGNOSIS ............

OPERATION(S) ............

**PATIENTS PERSONAL PROFILE**

RELIGION (OPTIONAL) ............ WISH TO SEE A MINISTER? YES ☐ NO ☐

PERSON FOR NOTIFICATION ............ PHONE NO ............

LIVING ARRANGEMENTS - TYPE ............ WITH WHOM ............

FIRST LANGUAGE ............ NEED AN INTERPRETER? YES ☐ ARRANGED ☐

ANY PARTICULAR WORRIES ABOUT BEING IN HOSPITAL? ............

**ALLERGIES**
DRUGS ............ FOOD ............ OTHERS ............

**MEDICATIONS BROUGHT TO HOSPITAL** ............

**ORIENTATION TO WARD**
INTRODUCTION TO OTHER PATIENTS ☐ NURSE UNIFORM EXPLANATION ☐ BUZZER ☐ TELEPHONE ☐

VISITING HOURS ☐ TOILET / BATHROOM ☐ SITTING ROOM ☐ NO SMOKING ☐ MEAL TIMES ☐

**VALUABLES**
SENT HOME ☐ HOSPITAL SAFE ☐ OTHER ☐

**SPECIAL INSTRUCTIONS**

NURSING DATA BASE AND ACTION PLAN

| PAIS INDICATORS | DAY Date: | DAY Date: | DAY Date: | DAY Date: | DAY Date: | DAY Date: | DAY Date: |
|---|---|---|---|---|---|---|---|
| HYGIENE | | | | | | | |
| MOBILITY | | | | | | | |
| OBSERV-ATIONS | | | | | | | |
| NUTRITION | | | | | | | |
| INVESTIGA-TIONS PROCEDURES OPERATIONS | | | | | | | |

DISCHARGE PLANNING SHOULD BE COMMENCED ON ADMISSION - SEE BACK PAGE FOR PLAN

PREDICTED DATE OF DISCHARGE ............ DISCHARGE PLAN COMMENCED ............ Date ............

FIGURE 26.1. The Nursing Data Base and Action Plan (front and back pages)

AFFIX
PATIENT'S
I.D LABEL
HERE

PATIENT'S SURNAME, CHRISTIAN OR GIVEN NAMES, TITLE     WARD | | | | | HOSPITAL NUMBER

PATIENT'S ADDRESS

| | | | | DATE OF BIRTH | |    SEX

MEDICAL OFFICER

| PAIS INDICATOR ASSESSMENT | INITIAL PLAN OF CARE ADMISSION DAY...... DATE | DAY...... EVALUATION & REVISED PLAN DATE | DAY...... EVALUATION & REVISED PLAN DATE | DAY...... EVALUATION & REVISED PLAN DATE | DAY...... EVALUATION & REVISED PLAN DATE | DAY...... EVALUATION & REVISED PLAN DATE | DAY...... EVALUATION & REVISED PLAN DATE |
|---|---|---|---|---|---|---|---|
| **MENTAL HEALTH** Confusion : Present ☐ Absent ☐ Level of consciousness Fully conscious ☐ Impaired ☐ Emotional status assessed ☐ | | | | | | | |
| **SENSORY DEFICITS** Present ☐ Absent ☐ Type: | | | | | | | |
| **ISOLATION** Risks identified: Protective strategies Body substances management | | | | | | | |
| **ELIMINATION** Incontinence Yes ☐ No ☐ Type: Usual elimination pattern: Urine: Faeces: Indwelling catheter Yes ☐ No ☐ | | | | | | | |
| **URINALYSIS** Abnormalities on admission Present ☐ Absent ☐ TESTING FAECES Indicated ☐ Not indicated ☐ | | | | | | | |
| **FLUID BALANCE** Level of hydration assessed ☐ Fluid balance chart Indicated ☐ Not indicated ☐ | | | | | | | |
| **PRESSURE AREA CARE** Norton Scale score: | | | | | | | |
| **I.V. LINE** Present ☐ Absent ☐ Type(s): Site(s): Date inserted: Line change M ☐ T ☐ W ☐ Th ☐ F ☐ S ☐ Su ☐ | | | | | | | |
| **WOUND CARE** Wound site(s): | | | | | | | |
| **TECHNICAL ACTIVITIES** Types: | | | | | | | |
| **SPECIFIC PATIENT EDUCATION** N/A ☐ Topic required: | | | | | | | |
| **SPECIFIC PATIENT PROBLEMS** | | | | | | | |
| **NURSE'S NAME** (PRINT), SIGNATURE, DESIGNATION | | | | | | | |

**FIGURE 2.6.2:** The Nursing Data Base and Action Plan (middle page)

FIGURE 2.6.3: An example of the Standards Evaluation tool (courtesy of St Vincent's General Hospital, Darlinghurst)

---

STANDARD 2. SEPARATION OF PATIENT

A plan is commenced and continued throughout the length of stay, to prepare the patient for separation to another environment.

Criteria

Documentation indicates:

★ plan for discharge/transfer, commenced at the time of admission;
★ involvement of nursing and allied health resources in development of the separation plan where appropriate;
★ personal belongings have been returned to the patient (including receipt for valuables);
★ follow-up appointments have been made;
★ discharge summary has been completed prior to departure from the ward;
★ time of departure from the ward and who accompanied the patient.

NURSING DIVISION POLICY

Discharge of Patient
Discharge Planning
Discharge Medications

STANDARDS EVALUATION                                 WARD NAME .............................................
                                                      PATIENT NAME .........................................

STANDARD 2. SEPARATION OF PATIENT

INSTRUCTIONS FOR USE

A. Photocopy this page.
B. Examine the patient's documentation.
C. Tick the relevant box — Y (YES), N (NO), N/A (NOT APPLICABLE) for each criterion.
D. For each "Y" or "N/A" answer, add 16.67; if all criteria have been met, score = 100.
E. Enter score here .................... ☐

| Documentation indicates: | Y | N | N/A |
|---|---|---|---|
| ★ plan for discharge/transfer, commenced at the time of admission; | ☐ | ☐ | ☐ |
| ★ involvement of nursing and allied health resources in development of the separation plan where appropriate; | ☐ | ☐ | ☐ |
| ★ personal belongings have been returned to the patient (including receipt for valuables); | ☐ | ☐ | ☐ |
| ★ follow-up appointments have been made; | ☐ | ☐ | ☐ |
| ★ discharge summary has been completed prior to departure from the ward; | ☐ | ☐ | ☐ |
| ★ time of departure from the ward and who accompanied the patient. | ☐ | ☐ | ☐ |

Comment ..................................................................................................................................
................................................................................................................................................
................................................................................................................................................
................................................................................................................................................

Evaluated by: ....................................................................    Date: ......................

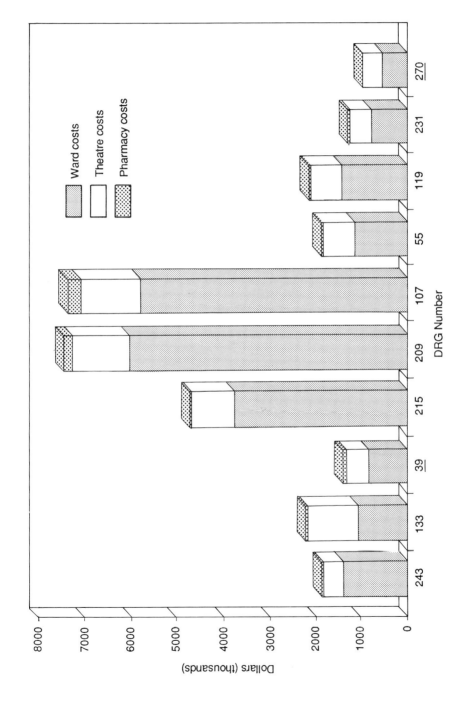

**FIGURE 2.6.4:** Comparison average total cost/patient top 10 DRGs

# APPENDIX

Selected standards from the Nursing Quality Assurance Committee of St Vincent's Hospital, Sydney.

## STANDARD 2: SEPARATION OF PATIENT

There is a planned systematic approach to the continuity of patient care to facilitate separation to another setting.

### Interpretation

Discharge planning is a process that begins on the patient's admission to the unit/ward and is addressed in their initial action plan.

The action plan will identify and indicate that the issues of the patient's self-reliance during and after separation and the need for community resources have been addressed.

### Criteria

The patients' records indicate that:

☐ the plan for their discharge/transfer was commenced at time of their admission;

☐ nursing and allied health resources have been utilised in development of the plan;

☐ property (including receipt for valuables) accompanied patient;

☐ discharge summary was completed prior to their departure.

## STANDARD 7: THE PATIENT'S NUTRITIONAL REQUIREMENTS (excluding total parenteral nutrition and intravenous supplementation)

There is a planned systematic approach to ascertain the patient's nutritional requirements. The nurse uses knowledge of biophysical and psychological sciences to determine the appropriate intake absorption and assimilation of nutrients. The patient's records indicate that the patient's diet during hospitalisation has been evaluated.

### Sub-Standard 7.1: Oral Feeding

Nutrition is the sum of the processes involved in the taking in of nutrients, their assimilation and utilisation for proper body functioning and maintenance of health. The patient's disease process will determine the type of diet. The patient's social, cultural and religious beliefs and preferences as well as their appetite at any given time will affect their choice of food and are considered in the organisation and supervision of their diet. The environment and the method of feeding are to be conducive to their enjoyment of their food.

## Criteria

The patient's records indicate that:

☐ the patient's nutritional status has been assessed;

☐ their diagnosis and treatment have been considered in the selection of their diet;

☐ their specific nutritional requirements have been discussed with the dietitian;

☐ their personal beliefs, preferences and appetite have been considered;

☐ they have received appropriate instruction about nutritional requirements and diet;

☐ an appraisal has been made in consultation with them of their capacity to organise their own meals and feed themselves;

☐ their response to their diet has been evaluated.

# SUMMARY

Case mix and clinical costing information systems are proving to be extremely useful tools for the nurse manager. However information systems are only useful to the extent that the data provided is reliable and valid. Nursing dependency systems which are part of an overall nursing information system which includes a nursing data base and action plan supported by nursing standards can assist in ensuring the best possible patient outcomes are achieved.

# BANGALOW CASE STUDY

Juli Donaghy was appointed Executive Director of the Bangalow Health Services Nursing Division 10 months ago. Bangalow is located in a metropolitan area and has 602 approved beds. The Bangalow Health Services, which are directed from the hospital, includes four community health centres established in the surrounding districts, nursing homes, a rehabilitation centre and a home nursing service. Bangalow Hospital and Health Service is the major teaching hospital for the nearby Bangalow University.

The Bangalow Health Service has applied for accreditation and a date has been scheduled in nine months' time. However there are a number of issues which are of concern to Juli and the other members of the executive staff. The introduction of Medicare saw many people opt out of private insurance and this has resulted in increased pressure on beds in the public hospital system. This, combined with the shortage of nurses, has meant the closure of 45 beds, extremely high occupancy rates and a decreased length of stay for acute patients. The pressure on beds has also meant that the number of inappropriately placed patients has increased to 50–60 at any one time. This combination of factors, plus the high demand for beds by emergency patients, has led to a reduction in the number of beds available for elective surgery.

Meanwhile the two private hospitals in the region, the Drakea Hospital and Mulla Mulla Hospital have been finding it difficult to maintain their daily occupancy rates at 60 per cent.

There has also been an acute shortage of nursing staff in the region. Bangalow is currently running a refresher course which commenced as one strategy to attract nurses back to the workforce. Attempts have also been made to recruit nurses from overseas. Both groups of nurses are due to commence in the wards in four weeks' time. A number of the overseas nurses use English as a second language. Doubts have been expressed by members of both the nursing and medical staff of the capabilities of these nurses and of their successful integration into the nursing workforce.

The nursing division was recently reorganised to implement the new career structure for nurses. Hospital services are structured on divisional lines with a professor from the university as divisional head. The hospital and community health divisions represented are surgical, medical, obstetric, accident and emergency, operating theatres, intensive care, diagnostic, geriatric and rehabilitation, psychiatry, mental health, palliative and terminal care, family and child health, adolescent, developmental disability, drug and alcohol, dental, health promotion, domiciliary and community health. Each division has an Assistant Director of Nursing, or Nursing Unit Manager in the case of the smaller divisions, in charge of nursing services for the division. They are responsible for the overall management of the division's nursing services. Each division also has either a nursing clinical consultant or clinical nurse specialist attached. The various wards in each unit are under the control of the nursing unit manager who is also responsible for the ward budget.

In the Bangalow Health Service there are 230 acute medical and surgical beds comprised of seven x 30 bed wards and a 20 bed neurosurgical ward; five operating theatres and one theatre for caesarians; 10 intensive care beds; 10 accident and emergency beds; eight day only beds; 14 convalescent care beds; 26 geriatric assessment beds; 60 bed hospice; 60 bed hostel; 60 bed nursing home; 50 bed obstetric ward; 25 bed paediatric ward; six intensive care bassinets; 20 bed adolescent ward and a 23 bed acute psychiatric ward. Currently there are 390 FTEs employed in the nursing services with 43 FTEs in the community services still classified as public servants. They will be reclassified to the Bangalow Health

Service in November. Nursing accounts for 35 per cent of overall staffing numbers with paramedical accounting for 24 per cent, support services 20 per cent, administration 14 per cent and medical seven per cent.

During rounds Juli and Jo van Witt, the Director of Medical Services, have been concerned about the state of patients' records. Although the standard of reporting has improved in recent years, nursing services are still keeping separate records which are not read by the medical staff. This has recently led to a number of cases where patients have suffered as a consequence. One patient is now sueing the hospital for negligence. The patient claims that a bedsore resulted from inadequate nursing care and lack of medical treatment. The

Quality Assurance Co-ordinator reported that other problems have also resulted from inadequate documentation and the use of separate records. Several cases of drug reactions were not followed up as rapidly as they should have been and there are instances of pathology results not being notified to the attending doctor.

At a meeting of the nursing executive recently the problem of an improved nursing information system was discussed. A number of the ADONs expressed the view that the hospital should be using a nursing dependency system for allocation of nursing staff. The Deputy Director of Nursing, Lindsay Rutkowski, suggested that if a nursing dependency system was to be introduced that this would be an opportune time to revise the care plans and look at nursing care standards.

1.  As the Accreditation Co-ordinator you have been asked to look at options for dealing with each of the issues which are of concern to Juli and Jo and the executive staff and propose a plan for implementation of the selected options prior to the accreditation survey.

# REFERENCES

Abernethy, M. A., Magnus, A. and Stoelwinder, J. U. (1990), *Costing nursing services,* Monash Medical Centre, Clayton, Victoria.
Broadhead, P. (1991), 'Approaches to public funding of Australia's health care', *Australian Health Review,* 14, 3, 223–234.
Cuthbert, M. (1983), 'Patient classification for nurse staffing', No. 52, *Australian studies in health service administration,* School of Health Administration, University of New South Wales.
Cuthbert, M. (1990), 'DRGs, length of stay and nursing resource use', *Proceedings of the Australian Nursing Federation and the Department of Community Services and Health, The Nursing and Casemix Conference,* 20th and 21st of May, 1990.
Cuthbert, M., Hawkins, A. and Goodwin, M. (1989), 'PAIS nursing dependency system validation study, 1988–1989', St Vincent's Hospital, Sydney.
Fetter, R. B., Thompson, J. D., Ryan., Diers, D., et al (1987), *Diagnosis related groups (DRGs) and nursing resources,* Health Systems Management Group, Yale University, New Haven.

Fletcher, A. (1990), 'Labour force issues: DRGs and their possible effects on nurse supply and demand', *Proceedings of the Australian Nursing Federation and the Department of Community Services and Health,* The Nursing and Casemix Conference, 20th and 21st of May, 1990

Grant, C. and Lapsley, H. (1991), 'The Australian health care system', 1990. No. 71, Australian studies in health service administration, School of Health Administration, University of New South Wales.

Hovenga, E. (1985), *Patients assessment information system* (PAIS), Health Department Victoria, Melbourne.

Jackson, T. (1990), 'Ambulatory casemix in Australia: APGs or AVGs?', *Australian Health Review,* 14, 3, 335–345.

Meehan, T. (1991), Interim report on the patient dependency system at the Rozelle Hospital project, Rozelle Hospital, Rozelle, Sydney.

Palmer, G., Aisbett, C., Fetter, R., et al (1991), 'Estimates of costs by DRG in Sydney teaching hospitals: an application of the Yale cost model', *Australian Health Review,* 14, 3, 314–334.

Phelan, P. D., Baxter, K., Bishop, J. et al (1991), 'The problem of neonatal diagnosis related groups', *Australian Health Review,* 14, 3, 346–353.

Reid, B., Palmer, G. and Aisbett, C. (1991), 'Choosing a DRG grouper for Australia: issues and options', *Australian Health Review,* 14, 3, 285–300.

# GLOSSARY

**ADO** Accrued day off. Occurs every 20th working day because of the difference between the award of 38 hours and the 40 hours worked weekly. The ADO may be taken on the 20th day or at a mutually convenient time.

**Art of nursing** This is performed by any nurse be they practitioner, educator, manager or researcher. It is the sum total of innate capacity, education, practical experience and initiative; the skills by which a nurse performs nursing.

**Assertive communication** This includes active listening, separation of ideas from feelings and saying what you want to happen. Demonstrating assertive communication empowers staff to assume accountability for their own rights.

**Break-even analysis** The analysis of the relationship of costs to volume and profit of a product or service to facilitate management decisions.

**Bureaucracy** The most common form of organisational structure particularly in large complex organisations, originally defined by Max Weber in 1921. There are two main features of his model.

**Case-management** This model is common in multi-disciplinary community health settings. Care delivery is co-ordinated by either the person with the greatest expertise in the case area or by the person who was the patient's first point of contact with the system.

**Casemix** The mix of patients or clients treated in a specific health care area, such as a ward, unit or service, over a specific time period. There are a number of ways of classifying the case mix including diagnosis related groups (DRGs), ambulatory visit groups (AVGs), refined DRGs (RDRGs) and patient management categories (PMCs).

**Casemix development programme** A five year Commonwealth Department of Community Services and Health funded programme of research to develop casemix information systems and examine options for allocation of funds to acute care health services.

**Chain of command** This is displayed in the organisational chart and identifies to whom each staff member reports. The chart displays the heirarchy of authority and the line of management. In all except the matrix structure it is usual for each person to report to only one superior.

**Clinical costing** A method of allocating all costs, direct, indirect and fixed, incurred in patient care to specific cost centres so the costs incurred within each DRG can be averaged and an average cost obtained for each DRG. Costs can also be allocated to individual cases using software designed for this purpose, ie the MDIS Clinical Costing Module.

**Common law** This consists of decisions made by judges which are based on the doctrine of precedent. Judges look to past cases to determine the principle of law to be applied to the facts in the case before them. Important cases are reported in law reports relevant to particular courts. Most of the law relating to clinical nursing practice is found within the common law, for example law relating to assault, false imprisonment, negligence and negligent advice.

**Consent** To be valid consent must be voluntarily given, cover the treatment to be carried out, be informed to some degree, and be given by a person legally competent to do so.

**Continuing education** This is carried out externally to the health care service. It includes workshops, seminars, specialty courses and post-graduate courses to provide specific development to those people already working in a field related to the content of the programme.

**Continuing professional education** Includes both inservice education and staff development. Other terms such as adult education, life-long education and on-the-job training are also included under continuing professional education. It is part of an individual's broader education which continues over their life-span.

**Coronial law** Each state has its own Coroner's Court which is set up under legislation to provide the means whereby certain types of death, such as violent, unnatural or suspicious deaths, and fires can be investigated. In some states the coroner must hold an inquest into deaths under anaesthetics and deaths in mental hospitals irrespective of the cause. Coroner's courts are conducted by magistrates and usually as courts of inquiry rather than adversarial courts.

**Cost per unit of service** Unit costs relate to patient days and include the costs incurred by departments or units on a daily basis, for example surgery minutes and anaesthesia minutes for the operating room or meals for the dietary department.

**Criminal law** Criminal law operates to protect interests which are important to society. Criminal law offences relevant to health care include criminal assault, negligence and child abuse.

**Delegation** A managerial tool for allocation of work, authority and responsibility to employees. If there is a small span of control the work delegated can be more easily supervised than is possible with a wide span of control. A wide span of control requires more autonomous employees. Delegation places a greater responsibility on employees for communication.

**Diagnosis related groups (DRGs)** Short-term acute care patients are classified into 477 DRGs according to 23 major diagnostic categories (MDCs) based mostly on body systems. Prior to classification patient records are coded using the International Classification of Diseases 9th clinical modification (ICD-9-CM) method. The next step is to use special computer software to group patients according to their principal diagnosis and sometimes their age and sex, into the appropriate MDC. Whether patients have had a surgical procedure determines their grouping into a medical or surgical DRG and the presence of other diseases (comorbidity) and complications also helps stratify cases.

**Differentiation** This refers to the degree of difference between sub-systems of an organisation. In an unstable environment there is a greater need for differentiation and a greater need for co-ordination of the activities which occur within. When differentiation occurs there is more likely to be decentralised decision making, greater use made of informal communication and a more rapid response to customer demands and needs.

**Direct costs** Costs that are directly connected to the delivery of patient services such as nursing services and medical supplies.

**'Emic' science** This form of science relies on the powers of observers to describe their experience which for the purpose of investigation is within a circumscribed time period. The method seeks through descriptive language to increase knowledge of the context in which human interaction occurs. This method is often referred to as 'qualitative' research.

**Ethics committee** In major hospitals this committee or the research and ethics committee is responsible for vetting all research proposals. In smaller institutions this role may be undertaken by the Patient Care Review committee. Most institutions have a formal written policy about how proposals are to be judged and approved, and how research is to be conducted. This policy is usually based on the National Health and Medical Research Committee's recommendations.

**'Etic' research** This is the kind of research performed by most modern western scientists. In this form the investigator seeks to find explanations for causal relations or to discover interventions which will alter an undesirable effect. The most rigorous approach to science in this form is the controlled experimental trial. This method uses a 'quantitative' approach.

**Fixed costs** Those costs incurred by the health care service irrespective of the volume of patients such as salaries of permanent staff, insurance, capital financing.

**Formal leaders** These leaders hold an appointed managerial position in the heirarchy of the organisation, their role being to lead a specified group towards the attainment of the organisation's goals.

**Functional or task nursing** Tasks are delegated to individual team members who subsequently document completion of the tasks. It is an economical way of delivering care but it can lead to promotion of task rituals and to depersonalisation of the patient.

**Goals** A goal is a general statement of a desired or expected outcome. Goals are usually written for an expected time-frame which may be short term, as in goals for this quarter, or medium term as in goals for this year, or long term as in a five-year or more strategic plan.

**Historical funding** Health care funding based on past funding requirements with an added allowance for inflation.

**Horizontal communication** This follows workflow patterns. It occurs between members of a work group and between members of different work groups. In health care organisations clients are included as part of the work group in this context. It also occurs between different departments and between those employed in a line capacity and those in an advisory or resource capacity.

**Hours per patient day (HPPD)** This refers to the number of nursing staff hours required to provide the nursing care needed by a patient over a 24 hour period. The number of hours may be averaged over a group of patients with similar medical diagnosis, similar diagnosis related groups, nursing needs or dependencies.

**Human resource management** Assists in the achievement of the organisation's goals by planning for, attracting, selecting, developing and compensating people who are willing and capable of contributing to these goals.

**Human resource planning** Involves forecasting short and long term human resource requirements.

**Indirect costs** Costs that are not specifically directed to patient care such as engineering costs or administration costs.

**Informal communication** Informal communication networks known also as the 'grapevine'. Serves social and work-related informal communication functions and is often much faster in operation than formal communication.

**Informal leaders** An informal leader is appointed by the work group itself, usually as the result of some outstanding characteristic such as personality, job knowledge or experience. This individual tends to be the spokesperson for the group, the person to whom others go for advice or assistance. Their objectives may or may not be congruent with those of the organisation. If the objectives are congruent they may be a potential ally for the manager; if incongruent then the nurse manager has a potential problem.

**Inservice education** This education is provided within the institution in order to maintain infrequently used skills, to update staff skills, or to ensure acquisition of new skills and knowledge.

**Job analysis** The process where data is gathered which provides information on the duties of a job and the required qualifications or characteristics an employee must possess to perform it. The information is converted into job descriptions and job specifications.

**Job description** This is a simple concise statement describing the duties, responsibilities and tasks of a particular job which is to be performed. Out of this a job specification is developed.

**Job specification** States the knowledge, skills and abilities required of a person to adequately perform a particular job.

**Law of bailment** This is a form of contract and applies when one person delivers goods to another (the bailee) so that they may be used or stored until they are delivered back to the bailor. When patient's goods are handed to the hospital for safekeeping the law of bailment governs the relationship. Bailment may be for reward or gratuitous. In the case of patient's property which has been handed to the hospital, the hospital is considered to be a 'bailee for reward'.

**Law of contract** This law governs agreements made between parties which give rise to the rights of and obligations to those parties. The law is concerned with the rights of individuals with regard to, inter alia, health care and personal property. Patients who enter hospitals and other health care centres enter into a contract with the institution. Nurses and other employees enter into a contract of employment (refer also to contract of service). The rights and obligations of the parties are referred to as the terms and conditions of the contract. A contract may be written or implied.

**Leadership** The process of influencing and directing others to achieve the organisation's goals. A strong leader will bring forth a willing and eager co-operation releasing energy in others to achieve goals beyond what is prescribed or expected.

**Legislation** Legislation is law made by parliamentarians through the parliamentary process. In Australia legislation is promulgated by each state and federal parliaments. The federal parliament's law making powers are restricted by the Australian constitution. In some cases it has exclusive powers, in other cases there is concurrent powers with state governments. Where there is an inconsistency between federal and state law on the same matter, then federal law prevails. In all other matters the states retain the right to make laws. Legislation affecting all employees includes occupational health and safety and work care acts and regulations.

**Line management** These positions are directly associated with the achievement of the organisation's goals. Line managers are directly responsible for delivering the service that the organisation offers.

**Maintenance education** This is the education required to maintain little used skills at a reasonably high level, for example annual revision of cardio-pulmonary resucitation skills; or when new equipment is introduced to the work situation, for example a new vital signs monitoring unit requires demonstrations in its use.

**Management** Management is a goal oriented activity accomplished through other people. It is a process involving the application of principles and techniques — a practice methodology — which takes place within an organisation.

**Management by objectives** The setting of objectives based on organisational aims and goals. The objectives may be determined by management, or the employee or the supervisor and employee conjointly. Employees' performance can be measured against the predetermined objectives.

**Mandatory continuing education** Compulsory education for nurses in order to retain or renew their nurses' registration. It ensures that registered nurses maintain a minimum level of competence. Mandatory education is contrary to principles of adult learning and if enforced may lead to professionals resenting the continuing education experience.

**Matrix organisation** This is a multiple command system which is organised according to two different dimensions. These two dimensions are often according to function and programme. Consequently there are two heirarchies involved in decision making, one responsible for a programme and one responsible for a specific function. Programmes are frequently service oriented while functions are professionally oriented.

**Mechanistic organisation** The mechanistic structure is highly bureaucratic with centralised decision making, rules, procedures, a precise division of labour, narrow spans of control and formal methods of co-ordination. This structure is more suited to a stable environment.

**Modular nursing** Modular nursing breaks down patient care into small groups of team members. The modules are often dictated by the geographical layout of the patient care unit.

**Motivation** The internal or external factors which impel the employee or the manager to perform a job. These factors also affect the level at which the job is performed and the level of job satisfaction attained.

**Negligence** The tort of negligence is applicable where a person suffers harm because of a breach of a duty of care owed by another. Negligence is conduct that falls below the standard regarded as normal or desirable in a given community. Criminal negligence, in contrast to the tort of negligence, occurs when an act causing death goes beyond a mere matter of civil compensation to show a reckless disregard for the life and safety of another.

**Negligent advice** The tort of negligent advice is a form of negligence action which can be brought for damage caused by the giving of advice, or information, as distinct from advice, where the defendant has sufficient interest to see that the information is correct.

**Networks-Professional** Process in which managers use contacts for information, advice and moral support for the development of their careers. Important factors in successful networking are trust among participants; communication feedback; movement towards set goals; and genuine interdependence in the system.

**Noise** Any factor that disturbs, confuses or otherwise interferes with or distorts communication.

**Nurse-managed care** Nurses involved in provision of this mode of care delivery are self-directed professionals who are willing to work flexible hours as required to provide care when needed and when acceptable for 'their' patients.

**Nurses' registration** The registration of nurses is a matter of state law. All states and territories in Australia have enacted legislation creating Registration Boards (known in Victoria as a Council) which are required to establish and maintain acceptable standards of nursing care. The Boards are required to maintain rolls and registers of nurses. Nurses must be registered in order to practice. Registration is granted upon proof that a nurse has completed a recognised course, has reached a prescribed age, is of good character and is proficient in the English language.

**Nursing dependency system** These are a means of classifying patients according to the intensity of their nursing needs. They were developed as a means of assessing the staffing levels required and distributing available staff to wards according to patient needs. The most commonly used system in Australia is the Patient Assessment Information System (PAIS).

**Objectives** An objective describes the expected outcome of a specific activity. In order to be useful it must be stated in terms of the results to be achieved so that it can be used for evaluation of the level of achievement.

**Occupier's liability** Refers to the duty of care owed by occupiers of premises to persons entering therein. The duties are exclusively linked to occupation since responsibility is based on control, not ownership, as a corollary of the power to admit and exclude. The duty of the occupier is to exercise reasonable care to avoid harm to invitees which may be caused by unusual dangers of which the occupier is aware or ought to be aware.

**One-way communication** The sender is neither expecting nor responding to feedback from the receiver. Usually a more orderly and faster way of communicating.

**On-the-job training** This is directly related to the development of expertise required for a specific job or task. This utilises teaching skills such as task analysis, and the demonstration method and is usually conducted on a one-to-one basis or in small groups. Preceptors may be used for the purpose of on-the-job training.

**Orientation** The process of inducting a new employee into the organisation, or an established employee into a new position. It provides the introductory education and socialisation required to adjust the new situation. It is also provided to patients on entry to the health service organisation.

**Organic organisation** This type of organisation is decentralised, has fewer rules, regulations and procedures, a less precise division of labour, wider spans of control and less formal methods of co-ordination than the mechanistic organisation. This structure is more suited to an unpredictable environment where greater flexibility is required.

**Organisation** An organisation is formed by a group of people who have joined together in a systematic structure for a specific purpose.

**Organisational culture** This is determined to a large extent by the philosophy and mission of the organisation and the extent to which these are accepted by its members. Each organisation develops its own set of norms which become part of the prevailing culture. These are behaviours judged by the organisations members to be acceptable or not according to their own particular standards.

**Output-based payment** This method of funding is a fee-for-service payment and is used for Medicare reimbursement to doctors who bulk-bill and for reimbursing pharmacists. It is also a method of funding hospitals based on the number of patient days in a given period. When used for this purpose this method does not account for the intensity or complexity of care provided and does little to promote efficiency.

**Participative management** The inclusion of staff in the decision-making process. The decision made by management may or may not reflect staff input. (Refer also to management by objectives)

**Patient assignment or total patient care** During each tour of duty the nurse is fully responsible for the total care of a group of patients. The number of patients assigned to each nurse depends on the nurse's abilities and the dependency level of the patients.

**Patient classification systems** Methods by which patients can be classified into groups according to the resources used in their care. The resources included may be only the direct costs incurred such as the costs of nursing services and consumables, or may include also the indirect costs such as cleaning and administration.

**Performance appraisal** A management initiated system designed to provide feedback and motivation to nursing staff regarding their performance. Appraisal tools are usually based on professional standards. Results are used to reward performance or correct deficiencies.

**Philosophy** An organisation's philosophy identifies its beliefs and values and formally prescribes the ways in which goals and objectives should be achieved. A philosophy is a written statement, which is widely communicated to staff and clients; is recognised in the practice of members; is a reflection of current values and a direction for future planning and is updated periodically to reflect changes in attitudes and influences. The philosophy of the nursing division, and the other divisions and departments within the organisation, should be determined by the overall organisational philosophy.

**Planning** This is a part of every phase of management. It is the basic process of defining objectives and determining how to achieve them. The plan assigns responsibilities and communicates them to those involved in its implementation. Plans require regular evaluation and revision and should be sufficiently flexible to change when necessary.

**Planned change** This relates to internal changes within the organisation. It implies forethought on the part of the manager as to what the problem is, an analysis of the ways in which it can best be resolved, a selection of the best strategy to effect change and an evaluation of the effectiveness of this strategy.

**Population-based funding** This method of funding is based on a formula which takes into consideration geographic location and population characteristics. It attempts to ensure geographical funding equity but the system falls down because their is no check on how the resources are used within each location.

**Preceptors** Very experienced nurses who have participated in a teaching skills training programme and are prepared to work alongside new graduates or new nurses to help them adjust to the workplace.

**Primary nursing** The primary nurse is responsible for individual patient assessment, care planning, care delivery and evaluation of care during the entire stay of the patient. The primary care nurse is assisted by associate nurses who implement the planned care in the primary nurse's absence. Associate nurses will also be primary care nurses for other patients.

**Recruitment** Involves attracting the right people, in the right numbers, with the required knowledge, skills, abilities and attitudes to fill identified vacancies.

**Reliability** Refers to the ability of the researcher or researchers to use the survey tool or instrument in the same way on repeated occasions. In order to do this the instrument must be clearly worded and unambiguous and the researchers and subjects should be unaffected by weather, moods, fatigue or other factors.

**Remedial education** Remedial education is the education required to remedy gaps in professional knowledge or skills. It may be provided internally or externally. It also includes the learning of new skills when a nurse moves into a new position or returns to nursing after a period of absence.

**Science of nursing** This is a description of the what, how and why of nursing. It is a set of methods fundamentally based on the concept of falsifiability; if a proposition is true then it will only hold to be true if it cannot be demonstrated to be false. Conversely, if a proposition is not true then it can be demonstrated to be false. There are three essential features: first it is an investigative process; second it is systematic; and third, it is open to public scrutiny.

**Scientific method** A planned systematic method of investigating a question or assumption in order to draw a rational conclusion based on the evidence obtained from the data collected. It includes a set of conventions or accepted set of practices developed from a set of cognitive values and normative assumptions shared by adherents to the perspective.

**Selection** The process of shortlisting and/or interviewing candidates for a position. Candidates' knowledge, skills, abilities and attitudes are compared to the criteria specified for the position.

**Span of control** The number of staff members who report to each superior. The wider the span of control the fewer the levels of hierarchy which appear in the organisation's structure.

**Specialised or specialty nursing** Provision of nursing care is related to each nurse's area of expertise. It is associated with 'progressive patient care' as patients 'progress' through the health care system as their needs change, for example a cardiac patient may progress through the cardiac ward to the operating room, to intensive care, to the post-surgical cardiac unit, or to the cardiac rehabilitation unit and on discharge come under the care of the community nurse.

**Staff development** This is concerned with developing the potential of the individual for the benefit of the organisation or the individual at some future date, for example nurse managers displaying leadership or executive potential are encouraged to serve on committees, relieve in higher positions, or attend advanced management courses in order to develop the skills and confidence required to apply for senior positions.

**Staffing plan** A document which identifies the numbers and types of staff members required for patient care. It is flexible enough to guide current human resources practices within the organisation, as well as to enable adaptation as changes occur as a result of influences from the internal and external environment. The plan's components should help substantiate requests for resources, and account for the manner in which the abilities and qualities of staff members will help achieve the organisation's goals.

**Staff management** These managers provide a service or specialist advice to those in line positions and only indirectly contribute to the achievement of the organisation's goals. Staff managers usually work in such positions as accounting, financial control, personnel, research, office management, cleaning and other support services.

**Standing committee** A committee which is a formal part of the organisation's heirarchy with written terms of reference to guide it.

**Team nursing** Nursing unit staff are assigned to teams each of which is responsible for care for a group of patients. The care provided may be either task or patient oriented. However, which system is used depends to a large extent on the abilities of the team leader and staff members. It is thought that as fewer nurses interact with each patient this system encourages caring for the patient as an individual.

**Tort** Civil wrongs. The law of torts serves to protect an individual's right to autonomy, self-determination and bodily integrity. Examples of torts are assault and battery, false imprisonment, negligence and negligent advice.

**Total quality management (TQM)** The general philosophy of TQM is that workers are the people best able to identify and deal with production problems. Participative management is the keystone. The aim of TQM is continuous improvement in the quality of nursing care through improved management and communication processes and continual improvement in nursing knowledge and skills.

**Two-way communication** The receiver provides acknowledged feedback to the sender. Usually more accurate as interpretation by receiver can be checked with the sender.

**Validity** If an instrument is valid it is actually measuring what it is designed to measure. It is possible for an instrument to be valid in one setting but not in another and without reliability there is no validity. An internally valid design is one that endeavours to hold constant extraneous factors and thus prevent the likelihood of an alternative explanation for results obtained. External validity is generally concerned with generalisability of results to other settings.

**Values of nursing** These cover the question of what 'ought a nurse to do' in the myriad contexts in which they practise. Values are often very personal, linked to culture and are metaphysically based. For example, the caring demeanour adopted by a 'good' nurse is based on the altruistic value and a belief that no matter what the condition, care is warranted and should be delivered in a kindly and respectful manner.

**Variable costs** Those costs which vary with the volume of patients such as medical supplies, food and linen.

**Variance analysis** Analyses changes in expected and actual services provided. It includes both volume variance, for example changes in actual volume from budgeted volume of patient days or patient classification intensities; and efficiency variance, for example changes in efficiency levels and changes in rates of wages and salaries.

**Vertical communication** May be either downward or upward. Downward communication flows from top management through the hierarchy of line-management to line workers and non-supervisory personnel. Upward communication flows in the reverse order. Problems occur through filtering, altering, condensing or stopping the communication. Thus communications are often partially inaccurate or incomplete.

**Vicarious liability** Under the law of vicarious liability an employer can be held responsible for the acts of employees carried out in the course of their employment.

**Workers' compensation** This is essentially a form of insurance. Employers pay premiums on a compulsory policy which insures them against the costs associated with a worker suffering injury or disease associated with their employment, which results in death, incapacity for work, permanent loss or impairment of a part of the body or faculty, or the incurring of medical or hospital expenses.

# INDEX

2 3 4 5 6 7 8 9 0 1
B C D E F G H I J

**(Tape shut)**

- - - - - - - - - - - - - - - - - - - - - - - - - - - - - - - - - - - - - - - - - -

**BUSINESS REPLY POST**
Permit No. 7323 - SYDNEY
Postage and fee will be paid on delivery to

Managing Editor, College Division
**Harcourt Brace Jovanovich, Australia**
Locked Bag 16
MARRICKVILLE NSW 2204

# TO THE OWNER OF THIS BOOK

We are interested in your reaction to the *Management in nursing* by Marjorie Cuthbert, Christine Duffield and Joanne Hope.

1. What was your reason for using this book.

    _____ university course _____ continuing education course
    _____ college course _____ personal interest
    _____ other (specify)

2. In which school are you enrolled? _____

3. Approximately how much of the book did you use?
    _____ 1/4 _____ 1/2 _____ 3/4 _____ all

4. What is the best aspect of the book?

5. Have you any suggestions for improvement?

6. Would more diagrams help?

7. Is there any topic that should be added?

**Fold here**